D1573004

...........................
**Immunology of Intracellular Parasitism**

# Chemical Immunology

## Vol. 70

Series Editors      *Luciano Adorini*, Milan
                         *Ken-ichi Arai*, Tokyo
                         *Claudia Berek*, Berlin
                         *J. Donald Capra*, Oklahoma City, Okla.
                         *Anne-Marie Schmitt-Verhulst*, Marseille
                         *Byron H. Waksman*, New York, N.Y.

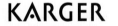

**KARGER**    Basel · Freiburg · Paris · London · New York ·
                     New Delhi · Bangkok · Singapore · Tokyo · Sydney

......................

# Immunology of
# Intracellular Parasitism

Volume Editors  *Foo Yew Liew*, Glasgow
*Frank E.G. Cox*, London

17 figures and 6 tables, 1998

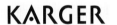

**KARGER**  Basel · Freiburg · Paris · London · New York ·
New Delhi · Bangkok · Singapore · Tokyo · Sydney

# Chemical Immunology

Formerly published as 'Progress in Allergy'
Founded 1939 by Paul Kallòs

........................

## Foo Yew Liew

Department of Immunology
University of Glasgow
Western Infirmary
UK-Glasgow G11 6NT
(United Kingdom)

## Frank E.G. Cox

Department of Infectious & Tropical Diseases
London School of Hygiene & Tropical Medicine
Keppel Street
UK-London WC1E 7HT (United Kingdom)

Bibliographic Indices. This publication is listed in bibliographic services, including Current Contents® and Index Medicus.

Drug Dosage. The authors and the publisher have exerted every effort to ensure that drug selection and dosage set forth in this text are in accord with current recommendations and practice at the time of publication. However, in view of ongoing research, changes in government regulations, and the constant flow of information relating to drug therapy and drug reactions, the reader is urged to check the package insert for each drug for any change in indications and dosage and for added warnings and precautions. This is particularly important when the recommended agent is a new and/or infrequently employed drug.

# Contents

....................
# Preface

The intracellular habitat provides a secure environment for many micro-organisms but those that parasitize the cells of the immune system, particularly macrophages and lymphocytes, live on a knife edge between survival and triggering a potentially destructive immune response. All intracellular organisms have, therefore, evolved ways of evading the immune response with the consequence that the infections they cause tend to be long and chronic and accompanied by immune responses that are not necessarily protective and may actually be counter-protective. For many years it was accepted dogma that immunity to such organisms was largely cell-mediated and characterized by the development of delayed-type hypersensitivity (DTH) reactions. A fuller understanding of the actual mechanisms of both survival in the immune host and the protective immune responses evoked was not possible until a decade ago when Tim Mosmann, Robert Coffman and their colleagues showed that cell-mediated responses resulted from the activities of cytokines produced by Th1 CD4+ T lymphocytes and that humoral immune responses were under the control of Th2 CD4+ cells. This provided a framework within which the various components of the immune response, particularly to infectious organisms, could be analysed. Over the past decade, there have been a number of additions and modifications to this overall pattern, including the findings that CD8+ T cells have similar properties to CD4+ cells. However, the basic dichotomy still holds and it is now generally held that clear-cut Th1-type and Th2-type responses represent polar positions and that, in most infections, it is the actual balance between Th1 and Th2 cytokines that determines the overall pattern and outcome of any particular immune response.

Central to our understanding of the immune response to intracellular parasites is the role of IFN-$\gamma$ in macrophage activation culminating in the release of toxic reactive oxygen radicals (ROI), nitric oxide (NO) and tumor necrosis factor (TNF) that separately or together are responsible for the destruction of many intracellular parasites. IFN-γ is also a product of natural killer (NK) cells under the influence of IL-12. The overall immune response in any particular infection is, therefore, the result of the activities of a number of cytokines some of which drive protective antiparasitic immune responses and some of which are counter-protective and are induced by the parasite itself in order to manipulate the immune response in such a way as to ensure its own survival. This overall pattern is common to all infections caused by intracellular parasites and this volume explores both these common features and also the special features whereby particular parasites evade immune attack and how they are destroyed. An understanding of the roles of lymphocytes, macrophages, NK cells and cytokines in the immune response is essential for the development of vaccines, for strategies for ameliorating immunopatholog-ical responses and for explaining why some infections are important concomi-tants in AIDS while others are not.

The organisms discussed in this volume include prokaryotes and eukary-otic protozoa and these will be used to illustrate and expand on the principles outlined above. Listeriosis has long been regarded as the prototype of DTH (Th1) responses but this situation is no longer as clear cut as it was once thought to be and there is now evidence that CD8+ lymphocytes, macro-phages, neutrophils and NK cells are also involved, the last three in the absence of T lymphocytes. In mycobacterial infections the essential role of Th1 CD4+ cells is not in doubt but there is increasing evidence that CD8+ cells and IL-12 are also involved. Turning to the protozoa, cutaneous leishmaniasis is usually regarded as a paradigm of the Th1/Th2 dichotomy with CD4+ Th1 products having a protective role and Th2 products being counter-protective. This remains the case but, in addition, IL-12 and CD8+ cells are now known to be involved in protection and the outcome of the infection is determined by the balance between the Th1 and Th2 cytokines. In toxoplasmosis, more than any other protozoan infection, the Th1/Th2 balance is crucial in determin-ing whether the outcome is chronic or acute and during the infection there is a swing from the production of protective cytokines to the production of regulatory cytokines that prevent the development of pathology.

Cryptosporidiosis is an emerging infection particularly in AIDS patients and here, as in most other intracellular infections, CD4+ Th1 cells predomi-nate in the immune response particularly during the early phases of the infec-tion but NK cells and IL-12 also play minor but significant roles. In Chagas disease, caused by *Trypanosoma cruzi*, the immune response is complicated by the fact that there is immunodepression early in the infection but later there is an autoimmune component and, although IFN-γ-activated macrophages are involved in parasite killing, this is inhibited by other cytokines. Malaria is the most complicated of all the infections discussed here as the infection comprises a number of antigenically distinct phases, some intracellular and some extracellular, each evoking a specific immune response. In the erythrocytic stages of the infection antibodies play a major role in protection but the role of macrophages is ambiguous as there is evidence that macrophage products such as NO and TNF are both protective and involved in the disease process. In theileriosis, the only wholly veterinary infection discussed here, the parasites live in lymphocytes and this is the only protozoal infection in which immunity is mainly effected by CD8 + CTL cells and is class I restricted. Finally, African trypanosomiasis is different from the other parasites described here in that the infection is extracellular and immunity is largely antibody-mediated. It is included here for comparison because the overall picture is one in which evasion of the immune response results from antigenic variation but there is also evidence that Th1 cytokines are manipulated by parasite factor(s) to permit parasite survival. In addition, macrophages are instrumental in immunosuppression, NO is infection-enhancing and IFN-γ stimulates parasite growth.

The purpose of this volume is to explore the immune responses to a selection of important intracellular parasites in order to stimulate interest in a comparative approach from which lessons concerning the development of vaccines, ameliorating deleterious immune responses and preventing the complications of concurrent infections with HIV can be learned.

*Foo Yew Liew*, Glasgow
*Frank E.G. Cox*, London

Liew FY, Cox FEG (eds): Immunology of Intracellular Parasitism.
Chem Immunol. Basel, Karger, 1998, vol 70, pp 1–20

...........................

# Immunity to *Listeria monocytogenes*

*Robert J. North, J. Wayne Conlan*

The Trudeau Institute, Saranac Lake, N.Y., USA

## Listeria and Listeriosis

*Listeria monocytogenes* is a gram-positive, non-spore-forming bacterium
that is ubiquitous in nature. It is a facultative intracellular pathogen capable
of causing disease in domestic and wild animals and in humans [1]. Because
it is enteroinvasive, it infects naturally via the oral route from which it can give
rise to a spectrum of diseases ranging from localized enteritis to disseminated
infection that can involve any or all major organs including the brain [1, 2]. It
is an opportunistic pathogen of immunosuppressed patients such as transplant
recipients on immunosuppressive drugs and patients undergoing chemotherapy for malignant disease. Neonates can be particularly susceptible to listeriosis. Even so, the incidence of the disease is very low, being of the order
of 0.7 cases per 100,000 population. Therefore, *Listeria* is not virulent for the
majority of humans. Neither is listeriosis a common secondary infection of
AIDS patients, in spite of the fact that the organism is widespread in the
environment.

On the other hand, recent investigations have revealed that *Listeria* is well
equipped for intracellular parasitism [3, 4]. Although once thought to be
exclusively a pathogen of permissive macrophages (the professional phagocytes
that clear it from the circulation), it is now known that *Listeria* is endowed
with 'virulence' factors that enable it to gain entry to and multiply in the
cytoplasm of a variety of mammalian cells, and that it has the potential to
parasitize the parenchymal cells of major organs. This knowledge is important
from the point of view of understanding host immune defense, because the
requirements for expression of successful immunity against a pathogen residing
exclusively in macrophages are likely to be different from those needed to
combat the same pathogen living inside parenchymal cells. Indeed, the surpris-

ing revelation several years ago [5, 6] that specific immunity is not mediated by CD4 T cells, as originally believed, but by CD8 T cells, is in keeping with the knowledge that *Listeria* parasitizes nonphagocytic cells. It also serves to explain why AIDS patients are not commonly infected with *Listeria*. Most humans either have preexisting innate defense mechanisms which can prevent *Listeria* from establishing infection, or they can quickly acquire defense mechanisms capable of inactivating *Listeria* after infection is established. Regardless, *Listeria* is potentially pathogenic because of its possession of mechanisms which enable it to induce nonphagocytic host cells to ingest it, and which enable it to multiply to large numbers intracytoplasmically and thence directly infect neighboring host cells. By these means it can give rise to cell-to-cell spread of infection without entering the extracellular environment where it would be exposed to host defenses.

The molecular mechanisms possessed by *Listeria* which enable it to establish intracellular infection are the subject of some recent excellent reviews [3, 4, 7]. First, *Listeria* expresses surface proteins (internalins) that on contact with the host cell induce it to perform phagocytosis and carry the pathogen into its cytoplasm in a membrane-bound phagocytic vacuole or phagosome. After being ingested, *Listeria* secretes molecules that enable it to escape from the phagocytic vacuole and avoid being subjected to the microbicidal factors that are discharged into this compartment. The most important factor that *Listeria* secretes to escape from the phagosome is the pore-forming protein, listeriolysin, which acts to cause dissolution of the phagosome membrane. Once free in the cytoplasm, *Listeria* uses a protein (Act A) expressed at one of its poles to initiate polymerization of host cell actin. In this way the pathogen takes advantage of the cytoskeleton machinery of the host cell to move through the cytoplasm. Movement results from the continuous polymerization of actin in close proximity to the Act A-expressing pole of the bacterium coupled with continuous depolymerization of actin at a distance from the opposite pole. This process enables *Listeria* to reach the periphery of the host cell where it induces the formation of cytoplasmic protrusions or filopodia in which it becomes localized. The *Listeria*-containing filopodia are ingested on contact by neighboring host cells. The organism then proceeds to escape from the phagosomes of these cells and to multiply in the cytoplasm and to infect other host cells in turn by way of the same sequence of events. Given that these virulence factors enable *Listeria* to infect large numbers of nonphagocytic cells by direct cell-to-cell infection, successful defense against listeriosis requires that the host possess the means to detect the presence of *Listeria* in these cells and kill it. In this way the pathogen is released into the extracellular environment where it can be dealt with by professional phagocytic cells with the ability to ingest and kill it. In other words, successful host defense requires that cell-to-cell spread of infection be aborted. The way in which the antimicrobial defenses of the mouse achieve this and bring infection to an end will be dealt with under the headings that follow.

## Murine Listeriosis as a Model of Cellular Immunity to Infection

The mouse model of listeriosis was first used more than 35 years ago [8] to analyze mechanisms of acquired antibacterial immunity of the type that does not depend on the production of humoral antibodies, but on the generation of a state of delayed-type hypersensitivity (DTH) to bacterial antigens. Immunity associated with a state of DTH was referred to as cellular immunity, and it was believed that this type of immunity constituted the major defense against infections caused by intracellular, as opposed to extracellular, bacterial pathogens. Because DTH was known to be generated in response to listeriosis in mice, it was reasoned that mouse listeriosis could serve as a model with which to analyze immunity to infection with intracellular bacterial pathogens in general, for example, to analyze immunity to salmonellosis, brucellosis and tuberculosis. It was known that acquired immunity to these infections is also associated with the acquisition of a state of DTH that enables a host to express a delayed (24-hour) inflammatory response at a site of injection of bacterial antigen in the skin. This type of sensitivity is in contrast to a state of immediate hypersensitivity which is mediated by serum antibodies and which enables a host to mount an immediate (1- to 3-hour) inflammatory reaction in response to injected bacterial antigens. It was also known that DTH can be transferred from sensitized donor animals to naive recipients with lymphoid cells, but not with serum, whereas immediate sensitivity is transferrable with serum.

Mackaness discovered that, like species of *Salmonella, Brucella* and *Mycobacterium, Listeria* is capable of surviving and multiplying in mouse peritoneal macrophages. He made the important additional observation that peritoneal macrophages from mice in the process of resolving a primary *Listeria* infection display a heightened capacity to restrict the growth of *Listeria* in vitro, as assessed by the superior ability of monolayers of these macrophages, compared to monolayers of control macrophages, to inhibit *Listeria*-induced plaques of cell destruction during a 24-hour incubation period. Because macrophages with increased anti-*Listeria* activity were acquired in concert with a state of systemic DTH to *Listeria* antigens, Mackaness [8] proposed that acquired anti-*Listeria* immunity is expressed by activated macrophages, but is mediated by a mechanism of specific immunity associated with DTH. Histological evidence showing that resolution of infection occurred when macrophages replaced neutrophils at infectious foci in the liver and spleen was an additional reason for proposing a central role for macrophages in the expression of immunity. However, all of this early evidence that anti-*Listeria* immunity is cellular in nature was correlative, rather than cause-and-effect.

It was not until 1969 that cause-and-effect evidence that lymphocytes mediate anti-*Listeria* immunity was published in the form of results showing [9] that a high level of resistance to a lethal *Listeria* challenge infection can be conferred on naive recipient mice by infusing them with splenic lymphoid cells from donor mice in the process of resolving a primary infection. Because it was also demonstrated that the spleen cells that transferred immunity were destroyed by treatment with heterologous antithymocyte serum and complement it was concluded that the cells responsible were lymphocytes. On the other hand, attempts to transfer immunity with serum antibodies completely failed. It was shown several years later [10, 11] that the transfer of anti-*Listeria* immunity can be prevented by treating the donor spleen cells with anti-Thy-1.2 antibody. This implied that *Listeria*-protective spleen cells are thymus-derived T lymphocytes, rather than B lymphocytes. These adoptive immunization results were taken to mean, in addition, that transferred donor T cells function to up-regulate the listeriacidal activity of the recipients' macrophages. In vitro evidence consistent with this interpretation was supplied by a publication [12] showing that spleen cells from *Listeria*-immunized guinea pigs, on incubation with *Listeria* antigens, secreted soluble products capable of causing macrophages to acquire enhanced listericidal activity.

According to the results of adoptive immunization studies [13] that measured the capacity of one organ equivalent of donor spleen cells harvested at progressive stages of infection to protect normal recipients against a standard lethal challenge infection, protective T cells are first produced on day 2 of infection, reach peak numbers on day 6, and decline in number thereafter. These kinetics of protective T-cell production support the interpretation that T cells are responsible for the progressive resolution of primary infection which occurs from day 2 onwards. According to adoptive immunity results, then, immunity to listeriosis is a model of T-cell-mediated macrophage-expressed immunity. However, to gauge the relevance of results obtained with the adoptive immunization assay, it is necessary to understand its limitations. These will be discussed under the next heading.

**Limitations of the Adoptive Immunization Assay**

Adoptive immunization experiments provided the first cause-and-effect evidence that anti-*Listeria* immunity is T-cell-mediated. As an analytical tool, adoptive immunization is still considered one of the most acceptable ways to demonstrate that a given population of antigen-specific T cells generated in vitro or in vivo is involved in immune defense against a microbial pathogen or tumor in vivo. In the case of adoptive immunization against listeriosis, the immunity conferred on the recipient animal by immune T cells can apparently be very powerful. For example, when measured on day 2 of a challenge infection and expressed as the $\log_{10}$ difference between bacterial numbers in the spleens of adoptively immunized mice and the spleens of control mice, 3 logs of protection are routinely obtained [13–15]. However, on close examination, this degree of protection proves to be more apparent than real, because it is to a large extent a reflection of uninterrupted log linear growth of *Listeria* in the lethally challenged control mice, and to a lesser extent a reflection of the destruction of *Listeria* in adoptively immunized mice, as mediated by donor T cells. An appreciation of the meaning of results obtained with the adoptive immunity assay requires a consideration of the bacterial growth curves in the spleens of mice inoculated with a lethal versus a sublethal number of *Listeria*. In the former case, *Listeria* grows exponentially without interruption until the animals die with 8 or more logs of bacteria in their spleen on days 4 and 5 of infection. In the case of a sublethal infection, in contrast, *Listeria* grows progressively for only 24 h, after which infection is controlled, and, beginning at 48 h, is progressively resolved. Thus if the number of *Listeria* present in internal organs is below a given threshold at 24 h, infection is sublethal, and host defenses are capable of resolving it. Typically, an infusion of *Listeria*-immune spleen cells provides recipient mice with a capacity to significantly reduce the rate of growth of *Listeria* to the point of converting an otherwise lethal number of bacteria to a sublethal number by the end of the first day. Therefore, the course of a challenge infection in adoptively immunized mice can be explained by the ability of the recipient's own defense mechanisms to inactivate a now sublethal number of bacteria. During the same time, the lethal *Listeria* challenge in control mice grows unabatedly. The longer the duration of the assay, the larger the number of *Listeria* in internal organs of the control mice and the greater the levels of adoptive immunity measured according to $\log_{10}$ protection. However, because protection afforded by adoptive immunization is almost certainly finished at 24 h of the challenge infection, the longer the duration of the assay after this time, the more misleading the results are likely to be. For example, a population of T cells with a weak ability to adoptively immunize as measured at 24 h can be made to show a strong protective ability if $\log_{10}$ protection is calculated at 72 or 96 h, as is sometimes done. It is also worth keeping in mind that a population of T cells that provides a recipient with 3 logs of protection is not greatly more protective than a population that provides 1 log protection. In the first case the reduction in bacterial number is 99.9%, whereas in the second case it is 90%.

Another limitation of the adoptive immunity assay is that transferred *Listeria*-specific T cells cannot protect recipient mice against an already established infection [15]. A typical adoptive immunization experiment involves infusing immunocompetent recipient mice with donor T cells within an hour of inoculating *Listeria* intravenously. This results in the expression of adoptive immunity as evidenced by a reduction in bacterial numbers at 24 h. However, adoptive immunity is not expressed against a *Listeria* challenge infection if the time between inoculating *Listeria* and infusing donor T cells is delayed for 12 h or more [15]. This has important implications, because it means that immune T cells can mediate anti-*Listeria* function if they are given when *Listeria* is still predominantly located in fixed macrophages of the liver and spleen, but are not capable of mediating anti-*Listeria* function when *Listeria* has induced the formation of microabscesses. This suggests that *Listeria*-specific T cells may have a limited role in the control and resolution of a sublethal primary infection, because they are not generated until the primary infection has progressed for at least 2 days, by which time *Listeria* is well known to be exclusively confined to microabscesses. This suggestion might seem difficult to accept, given that it generally has been believed without question that immunity to murine listeriosis is a model of T-cell-mediated immunity. However, when one considers publications showing the important roles played by neutrophils [16–19] and NK cells [20], on the one hand, and a limited role for T cells on the other [21–23], it is apparent that the original hypothesis formulated to explain the resolution of primary *Listeria* infection is no longer tenable. The cellular events that are important in the resolution of primary listeriosis will be dealt with under headings that follow.

## Resolution of Primary Infection

### *Role of Tissue Macrophages in Initial Defense*
Most of an intravenous inoculum of *Listeria* is removed from the blood by the liver, with most of the remainder going to the spleen [8]. Blood clearance is rapid and is complete in less than an hour. Of the bacteria removed by the liver, 60–80% are inactivated during the first 8–12 h of infection [16]. It is the surviving bacteria in the liver, with those in the spleen, that multiply to give rise to a lethal or sublethal infection, depending on the size of bacterial inoculum. In the spleen, there is little killing of *Listeria* during the first 24 h of infection [18, 22]. Consequently, the organism grows progressively without interruption during the first day in this organ. For this reason, the spleen contains more bacteria than the liver at 24 h of infection, even though the initial bacterial load in the liver is 10 times greater.

An extensive histological examination of the livers of *Listeria*-infected mice has revealed [24] that during the first several hours of infection *Listeria* is located exclusively in the cytoplasm of elongated, mononuclear phagocytic cells in the sinusoids. These by definition are resident liver macrophages (Kupffer cells) and the exclusive location of *Listeria* in these macrophages, even following the inoculation of lethal numbers of the organism, makes it unlikely that other cells of the liver are initially infected. In the spleen, *Listeria* is first seen in the phagocytic cells that line the marginal zone sinuses that border the lymphoid follicles [25]. It is well known that the mononuclear phagocytic cells of the marginal zone sinuses are responsible for removing particulate material that enters the spleen. Failure of these phagocytic cells to significantly reduce the number of *Listeria* during the first hours [18–27] of infection suggests that, in contrast to Kupffer cells, they are permissive of *Listeria* growth. As will be described below, *Listeria* infection in the liver moves from Kupffer cells to parenchymal cells that are highly permissive of *Listeria* growth. In the spleen, on the other hand, infection moves from the marginal zone into the white pulp where *Listeria* parasitizes phagocytic and as yet to be identified other cells [18, 25], some of which have the morphology of dendritic cells.

*The Essential Early Role of Neutrophils*

Because of early studies [8] showing that resolution of primary listeriosis does not begin until macrophages replace neutrophils at infectious foci, it was believed that neutrophils play little or no protective role in anti-*Listeria* defense. This view was in keeping with the belief that DTH was of central importance in acquired immunity to infection with *Listeria* and other intracellular pathogens. DTH reactions in the skin were known to be dominated by macrophages and other mononuclear cells to the near exclusion of neutrophils, and it was generally believed that the cellular events that characterize a DTH reaction at a site of injection of bacterial antigen in the skin are similar to those that occur in response to the same antigen at sites of bacterial infection. Neutrophil accumulation, on the other hand, is a feature of immediate sensitivity reactions as mediated by serum antibodies that appeared to play no role in resistance to infection with intracellular pathogens.

It has become clear over the past few years, however, that neutrophils play an essential role in resistance to listeriosis. This was first indicated by the results of experiments designed to determine whether listeriosis is exacerbated by treating mice with a monoclonal antibody (mAb; 5C6) directed against the CD11b chain of the $\beta_2$ integrin, Mac-1, a leukocyte adherence receptor involved in the extravasation of myelomonocytic cells to sites of inflammation [26]. The results of this study demonstrated [16] that treating mice with mAb 5C6, or a similar mAb [27], resulted in severe exacerbation of listeriosis, in that a sublethal infection was rapidly converted to a lethal one that gave rise to log linear *Listeria* growth in the liver and spleen. In the liver, 5C6 treatment caused *Listeria* to multiply much more rapidly over the first 24 h, and this was associated with the almost complete absence of inflammatory cells at foci of infection. Under these conditions it was strikingly clear that the target cells of *Listeria* in the liver are hepatocytes, in that each infectious focus in this organ consisted of a group of heavily infected hepatocytes that apparently had become infected with *Listeria* by cell-to-cell spread. Most of these infected hepatocytes were morphologically intact, in spite of their heavy burdens of *Listeria*. Recent published evidence indicates that these hepatocytes eventually die from infection-induced apoptosis [28].

In control mice, the slower growth of *Listeria* in the liver during the first 24 h was associated with the accumulation of large numbers of neutrophils at infectious foci, and with the presence of fewer *Listeria* at these sites [16, 18, 24, 27]. It was obvious, moreover, that neutrophils that accumulated at infectious foci occupied space that was once occupied by hepatocytes, meaning that the hepatocytes had been destroyed. This destruction was not caused directly by *Listeria*, as even heavily-infected hepatocytes in 5C6-treated mice remained intact. On the contrary, it was obvious at the periphery of infectious foci that infected hepatocytes were undergoing dissolution where they were in close contact with neutrophils. In fact, neutrophils were frequently seen within the cytoplasm of these disintegrating hepatocytes. This striking morphological evidence for the close association of neutrophils with infected hepatocytes undergoing dissolution, together with an extensive literature attesting to the tissue-destructive powers of neutrophils [29] and the part played by these cells in the pathology of a number of human inflammatory diseases [30–33], justified the interpretation [16, 24] that neutrophils function to lyse *Listeria*-infected hepatocytes and thereby to abort cell-to-cell spread of infection in the liver. It was suggested that destruction of infected hepatocytes serves also to ensure the exposure of *Listeria* to the extracellular compartment for attack by neutrophils themselves or macrophages. It has been shown [34, 35], in this regard, that neutrophils as well as macrophages can phagocytose and kill *Listeria* in vitro. Thus although in neutropenic mice *Listeria* can eventually kill the hepatocytes it infects by inducing them to undergo apoptosis [28], in normal mice neutrophils are mobilized to directly destroy these hepatocytes as quickly as possible in order to keep cell-to-cell spread of infection to a minimum.

Published evidence that other cells with lytic function are not responsible for early lysis of *Listeria*-infected hepatocytes is of two types. First, it was demonstrated [36] that lysis of hepatocytes at infectious foci, as well as the growth kinetics of *Listeria* at these sites, are not affected by depleting mice of NK cells, CD4 T cells, or CD8 T cells by treatment with appropriate mAbs. Second, lysis of hepatocytes failed to occur and extensive cell-to-cell spread of infection occurred in mice selectively depleted of neutrophils by treatment with a neutrophil-specific mAb [18]. However, it is the evidence as a whole, rather than that obtained with the antineutrophil mAb that allows a strong case to be made for an essential role for the lytic function of neutrophils in early defense against listeriosis. There is also evidence [19, 37] that neutrophils contribute to defense at later stages of infection. It needs to be realized, however, that whereas the evidence for a cytolytic role for neutrophils in resistance to listeriosis in the liver seems unequivocal, the way that neutrophils contribute to anti-*Listeria* resistance in the spleen has yet to be determined [18, 25]. A nonphagocytic target cell of *Listeria* in this organ has yet to be identified.

### The Role of NK Cells

NK cells, like neutrophils, are considered components of host innate defense [38, 39], as opposed to specific, acquired defense that is mediated by clonally-expanded, antigen-specific T cells or B cells. The NK cells are mobile cells that are continuously produced in bone marrow and released into blood from which they can be directed to extravasate into sites of inflammation and microbial colonization. There is now convincing evidence that NK cells play an important early role in anti-*Listeria* defense and that they play this role by virtue of their ability to produced IFN-γ [20]. Earlier published evidence for a role for NK cells in resistance to listeriosis is to a large extent correlative in nature. It resulted from an investigation [40] of the basis for the anomalously high level of anti-*Listeria* resistance expressed by severe combined immunodeficient (SCID) mice that are essentially devoid of T cells and B cells. This investigation revealed that the macrophages of SCID mice up-regulate their MHC class II expression in response to *Listeria* infection and that this is associated with the ability of the mice to control *Listeria* growth in internal organs and to cause infection to plateau. It was shown, in addition, that IFN-γ was needed for the up-regulation of macrophage class II expression, and that this lymphokine is produced by SCID mouse spleen cells in response to incubation with heat-killed *Listeria*. Because the only cells other than T cells with the capacity to produce IFN-γ are NK cells, it was reasonable to propose that NK cells are the cells that produce IFN-γ in SCID mice in response to listeriosis. Indeed, treating SCID mice with anti-NK cell reagents eliminated the ability of their spleen cells to make IFN-γ [39]. This evidence plus that which shows that treating conventional mice with an anti-IFN-γ mAb causes exacerbation of *Listeria* infection [20, 41] supported the interpretation that the high levels of anti-*Listeria* resistance expressed by SCID mice is mediated by NK cells via the secretions of IFN-γ. It has since been shown [42] that activation of NK cells to secrete IFN-γ in response to heat-killed *Listeria* requires the presence of IL-12 and TNF-α that presumably are secreted by macrophages.

Athymic nude mice which are essentially devoid of T cells also can express high levels of resistance against a *Listeria* infection, in that they can cause infection to plateau and become chronic [43, 44]. Moreover, chronically-infected nude mice display an acquired stable capacity to rapidly inactive a lethal intravenous *Listeria* challenge infection [45]. The finding [45] that this acquired resistance to secondary infection and the capacity to stabilize the underlying primary infection can be essentially ablated by treating nude mice with anti-Thy-1.2 mAb suggest that acquired resistance is based on the function of Thy-1.2⁺ NK cells. Presumably these are the same cells that can control and then slowly resolve infection in conventional mice depleted of CD4 and CD8 T cells by treatment with mAbs [21–23]. Obviously, then, nude mice acquire a T-cell-independent mechanism which, although capable of quickly destroying *Listeria* introduced into the blood, is not capable of completely eliminating primary *Listeria* infection confined to the microabscesses that populate the livers and spleens of these mice. It should be kept in mind that the SCID and nude mice that have been used to study anti-*Listeria* resistance were of the susceptible BALBc strain. The possibility that SCID and nude mice of resistant strains can resolve infection needs investigating.

Convincing cause-and-effect evidence that NK cells participation is necessary for successful defense against a primary *Listeria* infection in immunocompetent mice was supplied by a detailed investigation of the generation and function for IFN-γ-producing cells in the lymph node draining a subcutaneous site of *Listeria* infection [20]. This investigation showed that subcutaneous infection resulted in the generation of a large number of IFN-γ-producing cells in the draining lymph node. Enumeration of these cells by a spot ELISA assay showed that they were produced in peak numbers at 24 h of infection, i.e., at the time that the rate of growth of *Listeria* at the site of infection and in the draining node was reduced. Most of the IFN-γ-producing cells proved to be large granular lymphocytes that were NK-1.1⁺. Eliminating these cells from mice with anti-NK-1.1 mAb or anti-asialo-GM1 antibody resulted in severe exacerbation of infection. In contrast, depleting mice of CD4 and CD8 T cells had no effect on the production of IFN-γ-producing cells or the level of infection at 24 h.

Presumably the protective function of NK cells is expressed at sites of *Listeria* infection in lymphoid and nonlymphoid tissue, because it is at these discrete sites that *Listeria* needs to be ingested and destroyed by macrophages after they are activated microbicidally by IFN-γ. Moreover, it is at these sites that *Listeria*-infected macrophages would be expected to secrete IL-12 and TNF-α that serve to activate NK cells to secrete IFN-γ. There is in vitro evidence [46], in this connection, that macrophages secrete these and other cytokines following ingestion of live, but not dead *Listeria*. Needless to say, it is at infectious foci that *Listeria*-specific T cells would also be expected to mediate their protective function. However, given the results of T-cell-depletion studies there is now some doubt about the absolute requirements for T cells for the resolution of primary infection. It may well be asked what *Listeria*-specific T cells do at sites of infection that cannot be done by NK cells.

*The Role of T Cells*

The most convincing evidence that resolution of *Listeria* infection is mediated by T cells comes from adoptive immunization studies of the type originally performed by Mackaness and Hill [9] in 1969. These studies and many performed since leave no doubt that mice in the process of resolving a sublethal *Listeria* infection can acquire T cells capable of transferring high levels of protective immunity to immunocompetent, syngeneic recipient mice. It seemed logical to conclude that these T cells must also be responsible for the inactivation of *Listeria* in donor mice which are the subjects of analysis. The protective T cells were shown not only to be present in the spleens of donor mice, but also in their blood, as evidenced by the ability of the cells to extravasate into the peritoneal cavity in response to an inflammatory stimulus [47]. Therefore, *Listeria*-protective T cells are equipped to extravasate into sites of infection where immunity needs to be expressed.

Because of the prevailing conventional wisdom that immunity to listeriosis, like immunity to infections with intracellular microbial pathogens in general, is dependent on DTH, the first surprising recent revelation regarding anti-*Listeria* immunity is that, according to the results of T-cell-depletion experiments immunity is mediated by CD8 T cells [5]. In other words, depleting mice of CD8 T cells completely reduced their capacity to express immunity, whereas depleting them of CD4 T cells was without significant effect. In fact, on the basis of adoptive immunization results [14], anti-*Listeria* immunity can be dissociated from DTH on the grounds that CD8 T cells transfer immunity without DTH, whereas CD4 T cells transfer DTH without immunity. Whether this holds true under all experimental circumstances in all strains of mice needs to be examined. In the meantime, there is no doubt that CD8 T cells are greatly more important than CD4 T cells in the mediation of adoptive anti-*Listeria* immunity. This is the case in spite of the fact that high levels of DTH are generated in response to infection.

Evidence in keeping with the importance of CD8 T cells in anti-*Listeria* immunity *is* the knowledge that *Listeria* is capable of parasitizing nonphagocytic cells in vitro and of causing infection of liver parenchymal cells in vivo. Because *Listeria*-infected nonphagocytic cells would be expected to present *Listeria* antigens in the context of Class I MHC, these cells could only be specifically recognized as harboring *Listeria* by T cells of the CD8 subset. Indeed, the elegant studies of Pamer et al. [48] and Sijts et al. [49] leave no doubt that *Listeria* antigens are processed and presented by nonphagocytic cells in the context of Class I MHC. According to these studies, *Listeria*-specific CD8 T cells are directed against Class I-associated immunodominant peptides of listerolysin and P60, both proteins secreted by *Listeria* inside host cells. Other *Listeria* proteins presumably can be immunogenic [50] and induce *Listeria*-specific CD8 T-cell production. Target cells expressing the dominant epitope of listeriolysin are susceptible to lysis by *Listeria*-specific CD8 T cells generated in vivo in response to infection [48]. Conversely, T-cell clones expanded in vitro in response to exposure to *Listeria*-infected target cells are capable, on intravenous infusion, of protecting mice against a *Listeria* challenge infection [51]. However, the immunity provided by T-cell clones was measured with a 72-hour adoptive immunity assay which can overestimate the immunity transferred, as discussed above.

Needless to say, the foregoing evidence has been interpreted as showing that the protective function of *Listeria*-specific CD8 T cells is based on their ability to lyse *Listeria*-infected target cells in vivo. It is envisaged that cytolysis would serve to release *Listeria* from permissive phagocytic or parenchymal cells, thereby making the pathogen accessible to attack by phagocytes with up-regulated listeriacidal capacity. The alternative, or additional way that CD8 T cells could mediate protection is by secreting IFN-γ to up-regulate the listeriacidal ability of macrophages at sites of infection. It is known, in this connection, that *Listeria*-specific CD8 T cells are both lytic and capable of secreting IFN-γ [52]. The claim that the CD8 cells mediated their function in an IFN-γ-independent manner is based on the published results claiming to show [53] that the expression of adoptive immunity transferred by CD8 T cells can take place in recipient mice treated with an anti-IFN-γ mAb to neutralize endogenously produced IFN-γ. It is known that treatment with the same mAb can exacerbate primary listeriosis [41] under certain conditions. A problem with these adoptive immunization experiments, however, is that they did not include a positive control to show that the mAb had the capacity to exacerbate infection. If the mAb did have this capacity one might have expected it to reduce the expression of adoptive immunity to a degree corresponding to the recipients' own contribution to immunity measured by the assay. There is evidence [54], in this regard, that an anti-IFN-γ mAb capable of exacerbating a *Listeria* infection initiated via an extravascular route is not capable of exacerbating infection initiated intravenously. Even so, it has yet to be shown unequivocally that IFN-γ produced by any subset of T cells plays a role in the resolution of *Listeria* infection. If T-cell-produced IFN-γ were important, one would expect *Listeria*-specific CD4 T cells to be capable of transferring high levels of anti-*Listeria* immunity. However, in spite of the fact that relatively large numbers of *Listeria*-specific CD4 T cells are generated during sublethal infection, and the knowledge that these T cells by virtue of their ability to transfer DTH are TH-1 cells, they are not capable of transferring a significant level of immunity [14]. Presumably, therefore, *Listeria* antigens are not presented in the context of Class II MHC at sites of infection, in spite of the fact that these antigens when injected subcutaneously give rise to a vigorous CD4 T-cell-mediated DTH reaction that depends on the antigens being recognized in the context of Class II.

There is also no formal evidence that lysis of target cells by CD8 T cells is essential for resolution of listeriosis in vitro. *Listeria*-specific CD8 T cells are not produced until 48 h of a primary *Listeria* infection, by which time most of the lysis of infected target cells, as seen by histology, has already taken place. Moreover, at 48 h, resolution of infection is well under way. Evidence against a role for CD8 T-cell-mediated lysis in resolution of infection is that resolution of primary listeriosis has been shown to proceed in a normal fashion in gene knockout mice incapable of producing perforin [55] or granzyme [56], the proteins believed to provide CD8 T cells with the ability to lyse target cells, as measured by the short-term $^{51}$Cr-release assay. Taken as a whole, therefore, the published evidence that CD8 T cells mediated resolution of listeriosis by virtue of their lytic function is not compelling. In fact, there is evidence that their role in resolution of primary infection is not essential.

*Evidence against a Role for T Cells*

The results of adoptive immunization have provided most of the evidence that supports a central role for T cells in immunity to listeriosis. It needs to be brought to mind, moreover, that this procedure has been employed to analyze the immunological basis of resolution of infection in the donor mouse from which *Listeria*-specific T cells are harvested at about their time of peak production on day 6. However, the acquisition of T cells capable of transferring an increased capacity to resolve infection to recipient mice does not prove that the T cells were resolving infection in the donor mice. In fact, there is reason to believe that the same T cells play only a minimal role in resolution of primary listeriosis.

Evidence against an essential role for conventional αβ T cells in anti-*Listeria* immunity consists of the demonstration [21–23] that mice essentially devoid of αβ T cells remain capable of resolving infection, although at a slower than normal rate. For example, the results of experiments that employed anti-

CD4 and anti-CD8 mAb to deplete thymectomized CB6F1 mice of CD4 or CD8 T cells respectively, showed [22] that in the absence of either, or both, T-cell subsets, resolution of a primary sublethal *Listeria* infection proceeded to completion. It was only in mice depleted of CD8 T cells that the time of resolution of infection was significantly extended. This same study also demonstrated that if T-cell-depleted mice were treated with anti-Thy-1.2 mAb to deplete them of Thy-1.2$^+$ cells, resolution of infection failed to occur. On the contrary, infection was greatly exacerbated and the mice died in several days. It was concluded on the basis of these results that the control and resolution of primary infection is not dependent on either CD4 or CD8 T cells, but is dependent, instead, on a population of Thy-1.2$^+$ CD4 CD8$^-$ cells. On the basis of evidence discussed under a preceding heading, at least some of these cells are likely to be NK cells [20]. They presumably are the same cells that enable athymic nude mice to control listeriosis [45]. This evidence against a role for CD4 and CD8 T cells is supported by the results of more recent experiments showing [57, 58] that gene knockout mice that are essentially incapable of generating CD8 T cells or CD4 T cells are capable of completely resolving a primary *Listeria* infection, although at a somewhat slower rate than normal mice. Therefore, while these studies show on the one hand that CD8 T cells enable infection to be resolved somewhat more efficiently, they show on the other that CD8 T cells are not essential. Similarly, gene knockout mice that are incapable of generating γδ T cells are capable of resolving primary infection [59].

In view of the foregoing evidence against an absolute requirement for CD8 or CD4 T cells for resolution of primary listeriosis, it remains to be explained why infection in nude mice and SCID mice is not resolved, but remains chronic [39, 43, 44]. One possible explanation is that the need for T cells for complete resolution of infection may depend on the native resistance of the mouse strain being studied. It is apparent that the nude and SCID mice that have been employed to study anti-*Listeria* resistance were of the *Listeria*-susceptible BALB/c strain. It is possible that susceptibility and resistance to listeriosis is determined by NK cell function.

## Immunity to Reinfection

Resolution of primary infection leaves the murine host with a long-lived state of heightened resistance to reinfection. It has been assumed that this immunity to reinfection is based on the function of a population of *Listeria*-specific memory T cells of the subset believed to be responsible for resolution of primary infection, namely, the CD8 subset. It has been shown [60–62] that long-lived memory immunity to reinfection can be distinguished from the state of active immunity associated with resolution of primary infection on the grounds that the latter state, but not the former, is associated with high levels of nonspecific resistance to infection with heterologous bacteria. This has been taken to mean that resolution of primary infection is associated with a highly activated macrophage system that decays after the primary infection resolves. Obviously, therefore, memory-based resistance to reinfection should not be measured until nonspecific resistance has decayed. This occurs after about 3 weeks. Unfortunately, very little analysis of memory immunity to listeriosis has been performed. It has been the experience in this laboratory that it is difficult to transfer high immunity from immunized donor mice to normal mice, unless 2 spleen equivalents of donor cells are used. Attempts to show that *Listeria*-immune mice have an increased capacity to generate high levels of transferable T-cell-mediated active immunity in response to secondary infection were successful [60]. They revealed that T cells capable of transferring active immunity were produced earlier than in unimmunized mice, but that they were lost more quickly, in keeping with the faster resolution of secondary infection.

As for whether conventional αβ T cells are really responsible for resolving a secondary challenge infection in the immunized donor mice themselves, some published evidence suggests that they are not. According to the results of a study that employed thymectomized mice depleted of T-cell subsets with mAbs [22], the absence of CD4, CD8, or both subsets of T cells does not prevent resolution of primary infection or the ability to acquire heightened resistance to a lethal challenge infection given well after primary infection has resolved. Interestingly, acquired immunity to reinfection could be ablated by treating mice depleted of CD4 and CD8 T cells with anti-Thy-1.2 mAb, thereby showing that, as is the case with immunity to primary infection [22], immunity to secondary infection is dependent on Thy-1.2$^+$ CD4$^-$CD8$^-$ cells. Some of these cells are probably T cells, as evidenced by the finding [58] that secondary infection is exacerbated in mice treated with a mAb directed against the γδ T-cell receptor. Supporting evidence that the cells are neither CD4 on CD8 T cells is in publications showing that gene knockout mice devoid of CD8 [57, 58] or CD4 [57] T cells are surprisingly capable of acquiring heightened resistance to secondary infection. Lastly, immunity to reinfection is not dependent on specific antibodies or B cells, because knockout mice incapable of generating mature B cells display a normal ability to resolve primary infection and acquire high levels of immunity to secondary infection [J.W. Conlan, manuscript submitted]. All in all, then, published evidence is mostly against an essential role for conventional αβ T cells in acquired immunity to secondary listeriosis.

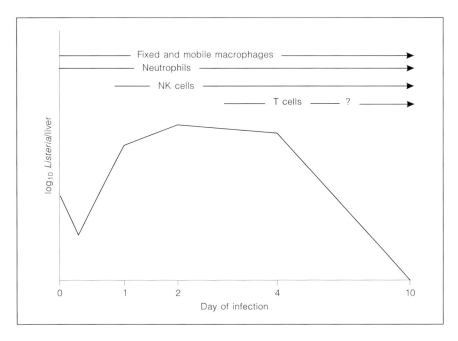

*Fig. 1.* Interpretation of the time of action and relative importance of different types of host cells involved in the resolution of primary listeriosis. Macrophages, neutrophils and NK cells are essential for defense, whereas T cells, although participants, need not be essential.

## Conclusion

Immunity to murine listeriosis has been considered a prototype model of T-cell-mediated immunity to microbial infection. It was believed that information revealed about mechanisms responsible for resolution of listeriosis would help to explain resistance to infection with other microbial pathogens that also can survive and multiply inside cells. As a model, murine listeriosis has generated a great deal of useful information from a large number of laboratories. It has served to draw attention to the antimicrobial function of macrophages, neutrophils, NK cells and T lymphocytes, and the way in which the functions of these different cell types are activated and coordinated by cytokines. The purpose of this article is to draw attention to some of the discrepancies and contradiction in the literature dealing with this subject. On close examination the literature as a whole shows that immunity to listeriosis can no longer be considered a clear-cut, convincing model of T-cell-mediated immunity. The facts are that depleting mice of most of their T-cell function need not result in lethal exacerbation of listeriosis, whereas depleting them of neutrophils or NK cells does. A simple interpretation of the relative importance of these different types of host cells in resolution of primary infection is shown in figure 1. There is no doubt, however, that resolution of listeriosis is associated with the generation of *Listeria*-specific CD4 T cells capable of mediating DTH, and of *Listeria*-specific CD8 T cells capable of transferring high levels of adoptive immunity to naive recipients. In our opinion, the results of adoptive immunization experiments showing that protective CD8 T cells are produced during resolution of infection need not contradict T-cell-depletion studies showing that these T cells are not essential for resolution. *L. monocytogenes,* although equipped for intracellular parasitism, is an opportunistic pathogen of low virulence that can be inactivated by the microbicidal functions of macrophages, neutrophils and NK cells in the absence of CD8 and CD4 T cells. Nevertheless, infection with *Listeria* is of long enough duration to induce the generation of CD8 T cells and CD4 T cells that are specific for epitopes of *Listeria*-secreted proteins. The evidence that these T cells are of minimal importance in the resolution of infection does not mean that they would not function protectively against a strain of *L. monocytogenes* of sufficient virulence to resist destruction by non-T-cell defenses. Therefore, murine listeriosis remains a legitimate model with which to analyze the properties and functions of T cells generated against intracellular bacterial pathogens, provided its limitations are realized.

### References

1   Gray ML, Killinger AH: *Listeria monocytogenes* and listeric infections. Bacteriol Rev 1966;30: 309–382.
2   Lorber B: Clinical listeriosis – implications for pathogenesis; in Miller AJ, Smith JL, Somkuti GA (eds): Food-Borne Listeriosis. Amsterdam, Elsevier Science, 1990, pp 41–50.
3   Cossart P, Mengaud J: *Listeria monocytogenes.* A model system for the molecular study of intracellular parasitism. Mol Biol Med 1989;6:463–474.
4   Portnoy DA, Chakraborty T, Goebel W, Cossart P: Molecular determinants of *Listeria monocytogenes* pathogenesis. Infect Immun 1992;60:1263–1267.
5   Mielke ME, Ehlers S, Hahn H: T-cell subsets in delayed-type hypersensitivity, protection, and granuloma formation in primary and secondary *Listeria* infection in mice: Superior role of Lyt-2$^+$ cells in acquired immunity. Infect Immun 1988;56:1920–1925.
6   Berche P, Decrueusefond C, Therodorou I, Stiffel C: Impact of genetically regulated T cell proliferation on acquired resistance to *Listeria monocytogenes.* J Immunol 1989;142:932–939.
7   Southwick FS, Purich DL: Intracellular pathogenesis of listeriosis. N Engl J Med 1996;334:770–776.
8   Mackaness GB: Cellular resistance to infection. J Exp Med 1962;116:381–406.
9   Mackaness GB, Hill WC: The effect of anti-lymphocyte globulin on cell-mediated resistance to infection. J Exp Med 1969;129:993–1012.
10  Blanden RV, Langman RE: Cell-mediated immunity to bacterial infection in the mouse. Thymus-derived cells as effectors of acquired resistance to *Listeria monocytogenes.* Scand J Immunol 1972; 1:379–391.
11  North RJ: Importance of thymus-derived lymphocytes in cell-mediated immunity to infection. Cell Immunol 1973;7:166–176.

12 Simon HB, Sheagren JN: Cellular immunity in vitro. I. Immunologically mediated enhancement of macrophage bactericidal capacity. J Exp Med 1971;133:1377–1389.

13 North RJ: Cellular mediators of anti-*Listeria* immunity as an enlarged population of short-lived replicating T cells. J Exp Med 1973;138:342–355.

14 Baldridge JR, Barry RA, Hinrichs DJ: Expression of systemic protection and delayed-type hypersensitivity to *Listeria monocytogenes* is mediated by different T-cell subsets. Infect Immun 1990;58:654–658.

15 Dunn PL, North RJ: Limitations of the adoptive immunity assay for analyzing anti-*Listeria* immunity. J Infect Dis 1991;164:878–882.

16 Conlan JW, North RJ: Neutrophil-mediated dissolution of infected host cells as a defense strategy against a facultative intracellular bacterium. J Exp Med 1991;174:741–744.

17 Rogers HW, Unanue ER: Neutrophils are involved in acute, nonspecific resistance to *Listeria monocytogenes* in mice. Infect Immun 1993;61:5090–5096.

18 Conlan JW, North RJ: Neutrophils are essential for early anti-*Listeria* defense in the liver, but not in the spleen or peritoneal cavity, as revealed by a granulocyte-depleting monoclonal antibody. J Exp Med 1994;179:259–268.

19 Czuprynski CJ, Brown JF, Maroushek N, Wagner RD, Steinberg H: Administration of anti-granulocyte mAb RB6-8C5 impairs the resistance of mice to *Listeria monocytogenes* infection. J Immunol 1994;152:1836–1846.

20 Dunn PL, North RJ: Early gamma interferon production by natural killer cells is important in defense against murine listeriosis. Infect Immun 1991;59:2892–2900.

21 Sasaki T, Mieno M, Udono H, Yamaguchi K, Usui T, Hara K, Shiku H, Nakayama E: Roles of $CD4^+$ and $CD8^+$ cells, and the effect of administration of recombinant murine interferon-$\gamma$ in listerial infection. J Exp Med 1990;171:1141–1154.

22 Dunn PL, North RJ: Resolution of primary murine listeriosis and acquired resistance to lethal secondary infection can be mediated predominantly by $Thy-1^+$ CD4 CD8$^-$ cells. J Infect Dis 1991;164:869–877.

23 Czuprynski CJ, Brown JF: Effects of purified anti-Lyt-2 mAb treatment on murine listeriosis: Comparative roles of Lyt-2$^+$ and L3T4$^+$ cells in resistance to primary and secondary infection, delayed-type hypersensitivity and adoptive transfer of resistance. Immunology 1990;71:107–112.

24 Conlan JW, North RJ: Roles of *Listeria monocytogenes* virulence factors in survival: Virulence factors distinct from listeriolysin are needed for the organism to survive an early neutrophil-mediated host defense mechanism. Infect Immun 1992;60:951–957.

25 Conlan JW: Early pathogenesis of *Listeria monocytogenes* infection in the mouse spleen. J Med Microbiol 1996;44:295–302.

26 Rosen H, Gordon S: Monoclonal antibody to the murine type 3 complement receptor inhibits adhesion of myelomonocytic cells in vitro and inflammatory cell recruitment in vivo. J Exp Med 1987;166:1685–1701.

27 Conlan JW, North RJ: Monoclonal antibody NIMP-R10 directed against the CD11b chain of the type 3 complement receptor can substitute for monoclonal antibody 5C6 to exacerbate listeriosis by preventing the focusing of myelomonocytic cells at infectious foci in the liver. J Leukoc Biol 1992;52:130–132.

28 Rogers HW, Callery MP, Deck B, Unanue ER: *Listeria monocytogenes* induces apoptosis of infected hepatocytes. J Immunol 1996;156:679–684.

29 Weiss SJ: Tissue destruction by neutrophils. N Engl J Med 1989;320:365–376.

30 Jaeschke H, Farhood A, Smith CW: Neutrophil-induced liver cell injury in endotoxin shock is a CD11b/CD18-dependent mechanism. Am J Physiol 1991;261:1051–1056.

31 Mulligan MS, Polley MJ, Bayer RJ, Nunn MF, Paulson JC, Ward PA: Neutrophil-dependent acute lung injury. Requirement for P-selectin. J Clin Invest 1992;90:1600–1607.

32 Repine JE, Beehler CJ: Neutrophils and adult respiratory distress syndrome: Two interlocking perspectives in 1991. Am Rev Respir Dis 1991;144:251–252.

33 Birdsall HH: Induction of ICAM-1 on human neural cells and mechanisms of neutrophil-mediated injury. Am J Pathol 1991;139:1341–1350.

34 Stecha PF, Heynen PA, Roll JT, Brown JF, Czuprynski CJ: Effects of growth temperature on the ingestion and killing of clinical isolates of *Listeria monocytogenes* by neutrophils. J Clin Microbiol 1989;27:1572–1576.

35  Czuprynski CJ, Canono BP, Henson PM, Campbell PA: Genetically-determined resistance to listeriosis is associated with increased accumulation of inflammatory neutrophils and macrophages which have enhanced listericidal activity. Immunology 1985;55:511–518.

36  Conlan JW, Dunn PL, North RJ: Leukocyte-mediated lysis of infected hepatocytes during listeriosis occurs in mice depleted of NK cells or CD4$^+$ CD8$^+$ Thy-1.2$^+$ T cells. Infect Immun 1993;61: 2703–2707.

37  Rakhmilevich AL: Neutrophils are essential for resolution of primary and secondary infection with *Listeria monocytogenes.* J Leukoc Biol 1995;57:827–831.

38  Trinchieri G: Biology of natural killer cells. Adv Immunol 1989;47:187–386.

39  Bancroft GJ: The role of natural killer cells in innate resistance to infection. Curr Opin Immunol 1993;5:503–510.

40  Bancroft GJ, Schreiber RD, Bosma GC, Bosma MJ, Unanue ER: A T-cell-independent mechanism of macrophage activation by interferon-γ. J Immunol 1987;139:1104–1107.

41  Buchmeier NA, Schreiber RD: Requirement of endogenous interferon-γ production for resolution of *Listeria monocytogenes* infection. Proc Natl Acad Sci USA 1985;82:7404–7408.

42  Tripp CS, Wolf SF, Unanue ER: Interleukin-12 and tumor necrosis factor alpha are costimulators of interferon gamma production by natural killer cells in severe combined immunodeficiency mice with listeriosis, and interleukin-10 is a physiologic antagonist. Proc Natl Acad Sci USA 1993;90:3725–3729.

43  Emmerling P, Finger H, Bockemühl J: *Listeria monocytogenes* infection in nude mice. Infect Immun 1975;12:437–439.

44  Newborg MF, North RJ: On the mechanism of T-cell-independent anti-*Listeria* resistance in nude mice. J Immunol 1980;124:571–576.

45  Dunn PL, North RJ: Stabilization of *L. monocytogenes* infection by athymic nude mice is dependent on the presence of Th-1$^+$ CD4 CD8$^-$ cells and is associated with acquired systemic resistance to blood-borne bacteria. Immun Infect Dis 1994;4:3–11.

46  Zhan Y, Cheers C: Differential induction of macrophage-derived cytokines by live and dead intracellular bacteria in vitro. Infect Immun 1995;63:720–723.

47  North RJ, Spitalny G: Inflammatory lymphocytes in cell-mediated antibacterial immunity: Factors governing the accumulation of mediator T cells in peritoneal exudates. Infect Immun 1974;10: 489–498.

48  Pamer EG, Harty JT, Bevan MJ: Precise prediction of a dominant class I MHC-restricted epitope of *Listeria monocytogenes.* Nature 1991;353:852–855.

49  Sijts AJ, Villanueva MS, Pamer EG: CTL epitope generation is tightly linked to cellular proteolysis of a *Listeria monocytogenes* antigen. J Immunol 1996;156:1497–1503.

50  Daugelat S, Ladel CH, Schoel B, Kaufmann SHE: Antigen-specific T-cell responses during primary and secondary *Listeria monocytogenes* infection. Infect Immun 1994;62:1881–1888.

51  Harty JT, Bevan MJ: CD8$^+$ T cells specific for a single nonamer epitope of *Listeria monocytogenes* are protective in vivo. J Exp Med 1992;175:1531–1538.

52  Harty JT, Lenz LL, Bevan MJ: Primary and secondary immune responses to *Listeria monocytogenes.* Curr Opin Immunol 1996;8:526–530.

53  Harty JT, Schreiber RD, Bevan MJ: CD8 T cells can protect against an intracellular bacterium in an interferon γ-independent fashion. Proc Natl Acad Sci USA 1992;89:11612–11616.

54  Dunn PL, North RJ: The importance of route of infection in determining the extent of exacerbation of listeriosis by anti-interferon-γ monoclonal antibody. J Interferon Res 1991;11:291–295.

55  Kägi D, Lederman B, Bürki K, Hengartner H, Zinkernagel RM: CD8$^+$ T cell-mediated protection against an intracellular bacterium by perforin-dependent cytotoxicity. Eur J Immunol 1994;24: 3068–3072.

56  Ebnet K, Hausmann M, Lehmann-Grube F, Mullbacher A, Kopf M, Lamers M, Simon MM: Granzyme A deficient mice retain potent cell-mediated cytotoxicity. EMBO J 1995;14:4230–4239.

57  Ladel CH, Inge EA, Arnoldi J, Kaufmann SHE: Studies with MHC-deficient knockout mice reveal impact of both MHC-I and MHC-II dependent T cell responses on *Listeria monocytogenes* infection. J Immunol 1994;153:3116–3122.

58  Fu Y-X, Roark CE, Kelly K, Drevets D, Campbell P, O'Brien R, Born W: Immune protection and control of inflammatory tissue necrosis by γδ T cells. J Immunol 1994;153:3101–3115.

59  Mombaerts P, Arnoldi J, Russ F, Tonegawa S, Kaufmann SHE: Different roles of αβ and γδ T cells in immunity against an intracellular bacterial pathogen. Nature 1993;365:53–56.

60  Mackaness GB: The immunological basis of acquired cellular resistance. J Exp Med 1964;120: 105–120.

61  North RJ: Nature of 'memory' in T cell-mediated antibacterial immunity: Anamnestic production of mediator T cells. Infect Immun 1975;12:754–760.

62  North RJ, Diessler JF: Nature of 'memory' in T cell-mediated immunity: Cellular parameters that distinguish between the active immune response and a state of 'memory'. Infect Immun 1975;12: 761–767.

Robert J. North, PhD, DSc, The Trudeau Institute, PO Box 59, Saranac Lake, NY 12983 (USA)
Tel. +1 518 891 3080, fax +1 518 891 5126

Liew FY, Cox FEG (eds): Immunology of Intracellular Parasitism.
Chem Immunol. Basel, Karger, 1998, vol 70, pp 21–59

........................

# Immunity to Mycobacteria with Emphasis on Tuberculosis: Implications for Rational Design of an Effective Tuberculosis Vaccine

*Stefan H.E. Kaufmann*[a,b]*, Peter Andersen*[c]

[a] Department of Immunology, University of Ulm and [b] Max-Planck-Institute for Infection Biology, Berlin, and [c] The TB Research Unit, Statens Seruminstitut, Copenhagen, Denmark

Of the more than 50 different species of the genus *Mycobacterium* only a minority is pathogenic for humans [1]. Yet, mycobacteria impose a major health threat to humans globally, primarily because a single member of this group, the tubercle bacillus, *Mycobacterium tuberculosis*, alone is responsible for approximately 3 million deaths annually and hence kills more individuals than any other infectious agent [2, 3]. Although *Mycobacterium bovis* and *Mycobacterium africanum* also cause human tuberculosis, their share is relatively small as compared to that of *M. tuberculosis* [4]. The second important mycobacterial disease is leprosy which is caused by *Mycobacterium leprae* [5]. The so-called atypical mycobacteria encompass all other mycobacteria, some of which cause disease, particularly in immunocompromised patients [6]. Growth of many mycobacteria, in particular the pathogenic ones, is slow with a generation time of 12 h for tubercle bacilli and more than 10 days for the leprosy bacterium. Mycobacteria are acid-fast, i.e., stained microbes cannot be destained even by harsh methods such as acid treatment. This acid fastness is caused by the robust lipoid-rich cell wall [7]. This is not only of interest for the microbiologist. More recently, it has also caught the attention of immunologists because several of the mycobacterial lipoglycans have been found to modulate the macrophage and to serve as specific ligands for T lymphocytes [8].

## Mycobacterial Diseases

The major, if not exclusive, biotope of pathogenic mycobacteria is the mononuclear phagocyte. Their specific survival strategy allows mycobacterial replication or persistence in resting macrophages. The tubercle bacilli are typically inhaled and, therefore, arrive in lung alveoli where they are engulfed by alveolar macrophages. Other pathogenic mycobacteria, including *M. leprae*, typically enter the host through mucosal surfaces. In any case, mycobacteria persist within macrophages at the site of entry or are transported inside mononuclear phagocytes to draining lymph nodes. There, T lymphocytes are activated which induce granuloma formation at the site of mycobacterial implantation. Within granulomas, the intricate interplay between T cells, cytokines and mononuclear phagocytes succeeds in containing pathogenic mycobacteria, but fails to fully eradicate them. This labile balance may persist for years without development of clinical disease. Therefore, mycobacteria principally cause chronic diseases. Several atypical mycobacteria, such as members of the *Mycobacterium avium* complex are efficiently combated by the competent immune system and, therefore, generally only cause disease in immunocompromised patients. The tubercle and leprosy bacilli and some atypical mycobacteria, such as *Mycobacterium ulcerans*, resist attack by a proficient immune response and, therefore, ultimately cause disease in immunocompetent individuals. Yet, even these pathogens frequently establish stable infection without clinical disease. For example, it has been estimated that less than 10% of the 2 billion individuals infected with *M. tuberculosis* will eventually develop disease [2]. The pathogens persist in the rest of these individuals and are controlled as long as specific immunity prevails. At later time points – in most cases through reactivation of dormant foci – disease may develop as a consequence of a weakened immune response.

Tuberculosis is typically a disease of the lung, that is, the lung is the major port of entry, the site of microbial persistence, and the location of disease outbreak and manifestation. Granulomas at the site of bacterial persistence serve to contain the pathogen [9]. Once these lesions lose their structured organization and liquefy, the *M. tuberculosis* organisms can grow unrestrictedly and spread to other tissue sites. Moreover, if open cavernous lesions are formed, bacteria can be disseminated via the aerogenic route thus infecting other individuals. Maintenance of a proficient granuloma is the outcome of complex interactions between different T-cell populations and macrophages with the help of various cytokines. Elucidation of the immune mechanisms which are essential, auxiliary, or harmful is a major goal of research into the immune response against mycobacteria.

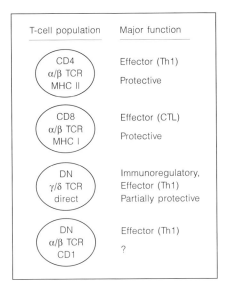

| T-cell population | Major function |
|---|---|
| CD4<br>α/β TCR<br>MHC II | Effector (Th1)<br>Protective |
| CD8<br>α/β TCR<br>MHC I | Effector (CTL)<br>Protective |
| DN<br>γ/δ TCR<br>direct | Immunoregulatory,<br>Effector (Th1)<br>Partially protective |
| DN<br>α/β TCR<br>CD1 | Effector (Th1)<br>? |

*Fig. 1.* Major T cells and their main functions in tuberculosis.

Leprosy is a polar chronic disease typically afflicting skin and peripheral nerves [10, 11]. At the tuberculoid pole a strong immune response develops capable of containing bacteria in granulomatous lesions similar to those in tuberculosis. At the more malign lepromatous pole, the cell-mediated immune response is markedly impaired and, as a consequence, lesions fail to control microbial growth resulting in dissemination of the leprosy bacillus. At these polar as well as at intermediate forms, encounters between the immune response and the leprosy bacillus occur in skin lesions which are accessible to immunologic research. Therefore, much has been learned from this disease about the immune mechanisms underlying protection, pathology or suppression.

## T Cells as Central Mediators of Protection

The essential role of T lymphocytes in protection against mycobacteria is without doubt. Although it is generally agreed that different T-cell populations must be activated for an optimum response, the precise role of these T-cell subsets in protection requires further investigation. The following four phenotypically distinct T-cell populations are currently considered as participants in the immune response to mycobacteria (fig. 1).

The CD4 T cells, without doubt, are essential players in the field as most impressively illustrated by increased incidences of tuberculosis in AIDS patients [12, 13]. Although studies in the murine system have brought forward convincing evidence that CD8 T cells are important, the situation in the human system is less clear [14–18]. Accumulation of γδ T cells in certain mycobacterial lesions and vigorous responses of human γδ T cells to mycobacterial components in vitro suggest a role of this T-cell subset in immunity against mycobacteria [19–21]. Consistent with this, γδ T-cell-deficient mutant mice succumb to tuberculosis [22]. Finally, double-negative (DN) αβ T cells have been identified recently which respond to mycobacterial glycolipids and thus may be implicated in antimycobacterial immunity [23, 24].

### Mycobacterial Localization and Antigen Presentation

Activation of CD4 or CD8 T cells requires appropriate processing and presentation of mycobacterial antigens by gene products of the major histocompatibility complex (MHC) [25]. Following phagocytosis, mycobacteria like other particulate matters, end up in the phagosome [9]. Because of their remarkable resistance to intracellular killing, mycobacteria, in contrast to many other bacteria, persist in phagosomes of macrophages for long periods. The phagosomal compartment is the starting point for MHC class II processing and hence for CD4 T-cell activation. In contrast, protein antigens which are present in the cytosol are processed through the MHC class I pathway, giving rise to CD8 T lymphocytes [25]. The intracellular bacterium, *Listeria monocytogenes*, is able to egress from the endosome into the cytosol and stimulates CD8 T cells in addition to CD4 T cells. In fact, CD8 T cells are the major mediators of acquired resistance against listeriosis [26; see also chapter 1 in this volume]. General agreement exists that the antituberculosis vaccine strain, *M. bovis* BCG, resides in the phagosome [27]. Although some evidence has been presented that *M. tuberculosis* and *M. leprae* leave the phagosome and enter the cytosol, the vast body of evidence suggests that these pathogens remain entrapped in the phagosome [27–29]. The intracellular localization of mycobacteria in the phagosomal compartment would predict processing through the MHC class II and exclusion from the MHC class I pathway. Consistent with this, mycobacteria are potent stimulators of CD4 T cells both in the human and in the murine system [9, 12]. Yet, mycobacteria-reactive CD8 T cells have been isolated and their contribution to protection has been demonstrated in the mouse [14–16, 30]. More recent findings in several systems have provided compelling evidence for an alternative pathway of MHC class I processing of antigens originating from the endosomal compartment [31, 32]. Although incompletely understood, it appears that peptides from particulate antigens are translocated from the endosome to the cytosol and thus processed through MHC class I. Because mycobacteria persist in macrophages, it is conceivable that mycobacterial peptides can be presented by MHC class I molecules.

## CD4 T Lymphocytes

The key role of CD4 T cells in acquired resistance against mycobacterial infections is without doubt [9, 12]. Because the role of CD4 T cells in mycobacterial infections has been reviewed extensively, we will not reiterate these data. This brevity should not be misunderstood as argument against the importance of CD4 T lymphocytes in all mycobacterial infections. The in vitro response against mycobacterial antigens of T cells from BCG-vaccinated individuals, as well as tuberculosis and leprosy patients, primarily resides in the CD4 T-cell set [33, 34]. Selected CD4 T cells from *M. bovis* BCG-vaccinated or *M. tuberculosis*-infected donor mice confer protection against experimental tuberculosis, and reciprocally, depletion of CD4 T cells from *M. bovis* BCG or *M. tuberculosis*-infected mice exacerbates disease [14, 15, 35–37]. Consistent with this, MHC class II-deficient gene deletion mutant mice lacking conventional CD4 effector T cells severely suffer from experimental BCGiosis and tuberculosis [30, C.H. Ladel and S.H.E. Kaufmann, unpubl. data]. Altogether, these data indicate that CD4 cells are probably the single, most important, subset in the immune response to tuberculosis.

## CD8 T Cells

Contribution of CD8 T cells to protection against tuberculosis was indicated by adoptive transfer experiments and antibody depletion studies in the mouse model [14, 15]. More recently, tuberculosis and also *M. bovis* BCG infection were found to be exacerbated in mutant mice with a disrupted $\beta_2$-microglobulin ($\beta_2$m) gene [16, 30]. Because stable surface expression of MHC class I is $\beta_2$m-dependent, conventional CD8 T cells do not develop in such mice [38]. However, $\beta_2$m also fulfils other functions which may influence mycobacterial growth. For example, CD1 surface expression is $\beta_2$m-contingent and CD1-dependent T cells may contribute to antimycobacterial immunity (see below) [39]. Moreover, the iron load in different organs, including lung and liver, is regulated in a $\beta_2$m-dependent way [40]. Iron is an essential factor both for mycobacterial growth and host defense [41]. Therefore, $\beta_2$m deficiency may influence mycobacterial infections independent from CD8 T lymphocytes. Yet, evidence from experimental mouse models emphasizing a role of CD8 T cells in resistance against tuberculosis is compelling. Only few studies have demonstrated mycobacteria-reactive CD8 T cells in humans [17, 18]. In contrast to viable bacteria and particulate antigens, soluble proteins are generally prevented from entering the MHC class I pathway [31]. Therefore, the failure to identify CD8 T cells after in vitro stimulation with soluble proteins – notably purified protein derivates (PPD) – must be interpreted carefully. Indeed, recent experiments reveal dependency on viability of *M. bovis* for successful in vitro restimulation of human mycobacteria-specific CD8 T cells [17].

## γδ T Cells

The CD4 and CD8 T lymphocytes constitute more than 90% of all peripheral T cells in human and mouse. They use the same type of T-cell receptor (TCR) for antigen recognition which is composed of an α- and a β-chain. A second T-cell population exists which utilizes an alternate TCR of a γ- and a δ-chain [21]. These γδ T cells are generally DN, i.e., they lack CD4 and CD8 markers. Although the biological role of these γδ T cells remains elusive, strong evidence both from the human and the murine system exists to suggest some role in protection against mycobacteria. Gene deletion mutant mice lacking γδ T cells are only slightly more susceptible to *M. bovis* BCG infection [22] and antibody-based depletion of this subset has been reported not to change the outcome of infection [42]. In contrast, tuberculosis is markedly exacerbated in γδ T-cell-deficient mutants [43]. After infection with relatively high doses of *M. tuberculosis*, they die more rapidly than heterozygous controls and even earlier than αβ T-cell-deficient mutants. These findings suggest an early role of γδ T cells in protection against experimental tuberculosis. Accumulation of γδ T cells has been described in lesions of leprosy patients caused by reversal reaction or lepromin skin test [20]. However, in tuberculoid and lepromatous lesions of leprosy patients, no such increase was found [20] and accumulation of γδ T cells in tuberculous lymphadenitis lesions remains controversial [44, 45]. Importantly, γδ T lymphocytes respond vigorously to non-proteinaceous low molecular weight fractions of mycobacteria in vitro [46]. More recent studies have revealed that phosphate is an essential component of these ligands [47–49]. Although isopentenyl pyrophosphate is the first chemically defined ligand, other phospholigands, containing carbohydrates or oligonucleotides, may exist, in addition [50]. Recognition of these phospholigands apparently requires anchoring in the host cell membrane, but appears independent from additional accessory molecules [51]. Recognition of purified isopentenyl pyrophosphate does not require intracellular processing [51]. Yet, macrophages infected with viable mycobacteria are potent γδ T-cell stimulators and recent evidence suggests intracellular transport of phospholigands from the phagosome to the cell surface in mycobacteria-infected macrophages [B. Schoel and S.H.E. Kaufmann, unpubl. data].

Although stimulation by phospholigands is TCR-dependent, the receptor-ligand interaction markedly differs from conventional peptide/MHC recognition by the αβ TCR. Available evidence suggests binding of the ligands to a conserved region of the γδ TCR [21]. Consistent with this, the phospholigands stimulate all γδ T cells expressing the Vγ9Vδ2 combination independent from their fine specificity. Although γδ T-cell-stimulating ligands are not exclusive for mycobacteria and have been identified in various pathogenic and nonpathogenic bacteria, the available data strongly support a role of γδ T cells in mycobacterial infections [21]. Oligoclonal stimulation of γδ T cells by phospholigands, of course, does not exclude γδ T-cell stimulation by bacterial proteins which may result in clonal T-cell expansion [52, 53]. In contrast to their human counterparts, murine γδ T cells apparently do not recognize phospholigands and preferential responsiveness to mycobacterial heat-shock protein (hsp) peptides has been described [21, 54]. Interestingly, these hsp peptides are oligoclonal stimulators of Vγ1-expressing cells with junctional diversity. Hence, binding to a conserved site in Vγ1, independent from fine antigen specificity, appears likely.

## DN αβ T Cells

Recently, a minor population of DN TCRαβ lymphocytes has been isolated from the peripheral blood of humans which recognize mycobacterial glycolipids in the context of CD1 molecules [23, 24]. The CD1 molecules are nonpolymorphic gene products which are encoded outside the MHC [39]. Similar to MHC class I molecules, CD1 surface expression is $\beta_2$m-dependent. The murine CD1 complex encompasses four isotypes, CD1a–d, whereas mice only possess CD1d cognates [39]. Thus, the CD1b and CD1c molecules which are responsible for presentation of mycobacterial glycolipids to DN αβ T cells do not exist in mice [23, 24, 55]. Two major cell wall components have been identified as ligands for DN αβ T cells, namely the mycolic acids and lipoarabinomannans (LAM) [23, 24]. The LAM contain a variety of sugars notably arabinose and mannose as well as fatty acid residues linked to phosphatidylinositol [7]. The mycolic acids are large (up to C90) β-hydroxy, α-alkyl fatty acids which characteristically form esters with arabinogalactan. Presentation of glycolipids by CD1 processing involves the phagosomal compartment. Consistent with this, CD1 localization to phagosomes has been described recently [56].

## Cytokines

T cells, though being essential for acquired resistance against mycobacteria, are not protective by themselves, but rather through their cooperation with macrophages [57]. In fact, the concept of macrophage activation is inseparable from investigations of immunity to mycobacteria. Macrophages are both activators and targets of T-cell responses to mycobacteria. Although antigen-specific T-cell activation is cell-cell dependent, cytokines are the crucial signal transmitters between macrophages and T cells. Macrophages infected with mycobacteria produce various cytokines which modulate the host response in a positive or negative way. Thus, cytokines are not only important mediators of protection, but also of pathology and susceptibility. Whilst macrophage activation by cytokines is the central mechanism underlying defense against mycobacteria, it would be an oversimplification to consider it sufficient. In vivo, the attraction of professional phagocytes to the site of mycobacterial growth, as well as the formation and sustaining of granulomas, are crucial parts of the protective host response which elude direct in vitro analysis to great extent. Therefore, the cytokines responsible for these effector functions are less well understood than those mediating macrophage activation. More recently, application of mutant mice with disrupted cytokine genes has provided adequate tools for analyzing these issues more directly. These studies have been performed with *M. bovis* BCG and *M. tuberculosis*. Because *M. leprae* is not a mouse pathogen, direct information about the immune response against leprosy is missing. However, relatively easy access to leprosy lesions has made possible cytokine analysis in situ, thus providing important and often complementary information about the role of cytokines in protection and susceptibility in leprosy and probably other mycobacterial infections.

The protective T-cell response against mycobacteria is characteristically of Th1 type [58]. Accordingly, interferon-$\gamma$ (IFN-$\gamma$) is the major mediator of macrophage activation by T cells and interleukin (IL)-12 is the major inducer of protective T cells [59–64]. Consistent with this, IFN-$\gamma$ or IFN-$\gamma$ receptor gene deletion mice are highly susceptible to *M. tuberculosis* or *M. bovis* BCG infection [62–64]. Conversely, IL-4 production is only weakly induced in tuberculosis [65, 66]. Studies from other models have provided compelling evidence that prompt production of IL-12 and IL-4 by cells of the innate immune system determines the degree of Th1/Th2 cell polarization. Evidence has been presented that IL-4 dominates over IL-12, i.e., in the presence of both cytokines the system is biased towards Th2 cell differentiation [67]. At later stages, Th1 and Th2 cells control each other via their major cytokines, IFN-$\gamma$ or IL-4, respectively [58]. Despite its oversimplification, the concept of Th segregation according to cytokine patterns has been extremely helpful. It is beyond question that Th1 cells are the central mediators of protection against intracellular pathogens, including mycobacteria, whereas Th2 cells are involved in defense against helminths. Evidence has been presented that human Th1 and Th2 cells can be distinguished by differential surface expression of CD30 with Th1 cells being CD30$^+$ and Th2 cells being CD30$^-$ [68]. However, it was found that CD4 T cells secreting IFN-$\gamma$ in response to stimulation with *M. tuberculosis* antigens express high CD30 levels [69]. These findings indicate that *M. tuberculosis* is a CD30 inducer in Th1 cells and argue against an exclusive link between CD30 expression and Th2 cell responses. The seminal studies in experimental leishmaniasis of mice have revealed a harmful effect of Th2 cells once they are produced [70]. Although a recent study has provided indirect evidence for a disease-exacerbating role of Th2 cytokines induced by experimental tuberculosis subunit vaccines in animal models, Th2 activation appears minimal during human tuberculosis [71]. Rather, exaggerated Th1 responses and Th2-independent immune deficiency appear likely elements of pathology in tuberculosis. The development towards the tuberculoid or lepromatous leprosy pole at present is best explained within the framework of the Th1/Th2 concept [11]. Towards the lepromatous pole, Th2 cytokines preponderate, whereas Th1 cytokines are abundant at the more benign tuberculoid pole [11]. In contrast to other Th1/Th2 systems, however, CD8 rather than CD4 T cells appear to be a predominant source of the Th2 cytokines, IL-4 and IL-5. Thus, it appears that IFN-$\gamma$-producing CD4 T cells are counteracted by IL-4-secreting CD8 T cells in leprosy.

*Proinflammatory cytokines*, notably IL-1, IL-6, and TNF, are produced by various cell types with macrophages infected with bacteria being the major source [72–74]. Increased secretion of IL-1, IL-6 and TNF by bronchoalveolar lavage cells from pulmonary tuberculosis patients has been described [75]. In tuberculosis, TNF represents the most important member of the group of proinflammatory cytokines [74]. Because of its central role in granuloma formation and maintenance, it is considered both protective and pathologic [76, 77]. Although TNF is not essential for induction of tuberculostatic macrophage functions, it is an important costimulator of IFN-$\gamma$ [78]. Accordingly, macrophage activation is delayed in mutant mice with a deficient TNF receptor 1 (TNFR1) gene and these mice suffer severely from exacerbated tuberculosis [76]. Although granulomas develop, they apparently fail to contain tubercle bacilli. The lesions in TNFR1-deficient mutants show extensive necrosis, arguing against an exclusive role of this cytokine in the formation of necrotic lesions. Exacerbated tissue destruction in the absence of TNF suggests an important role of cytokines other than TNF. In situations where TNF production is exaggerated, TNF down-modulation may be desirable. For example, TNF has been implicated in reversal reactions in leprosy as well as in extensive tissue necrosis and in cachexia in tuberculosis. Treatment with thalidomide which is known to inhibit TNF production was found to ameliorate reversal reactions in leprosy patients and to increase body weight in tuberculosis patients [79–81].

Information about the role in antimycobacterial immunity of the other major proinflammatory cytokines, IL-1 and IL-6, is scarce. However, IL-6 has been shown to activate mycobacterial growth inhibition in murine macrophages [82] and circumstantial evidence has been presented that protective immunity against *M. avium* is affected by IL-6 neutralization in vivo [83]. More recently, IL-6 gene-deficient mice have been infected with *M. tuberculosis* [83a]. Tuberculosis was dramatically exacerbated and resulted in death of the mutant mice at inocula which were still tolerated by controls. Consistent with this, high IL-6 production has been found in *M. tuberculosis*-infected mice [65]. It is likely that detrimental consequences of IL-6 deficiency are related to two effects: first, reduced proinflammatory response and second, impaired Th cell development. It was found that *M. tu- berculosis*-infected IL-6-deficient mutant mice have higher IL-4 and reduced IFN-γ titers and increased antibody responses. This finding could be explained best by immune deviation towards the Th2 pole.

*Chemokines* are a distinct group of proinflammatory cytokines [84, 85]. Various chemokines are produced by mycobacteria-infected host cells, suggesting that they play a role in early control of mycobacterial infections. Recently, evidence for rapid mRNA induction for various chemokines in response to *M. tuberculosis* infection has been reported [86, 87]. However, much more work needs to be done before exact information about the precise role of chemokines in tuberculosis becomes available. One recent study analyzed *M. tuberculosis* infection in transgenic mice which overexpress MCP-1 [88]. These mice were found to be more susceptible to tuberculosis. However, this should not be interpreted to mean negative effects of MCP-1 on resistance against tubercle bacilli. Rather, it appears from this study that constant high level expression of MCP-1 led to desensitization of macrophages. Hence, these data only point to a role of MCP-1 in host resistance against *M. tuberculosis* and it remains to be established whether MCP-1 supports protective or pathogenic reactions.

*IL-12* is an important regulatory cytokine produced by macrophages infected with mycobacteria [60]. Its major function is the activation of NK cells and the promotion of Th1 cell development. IL-12 administration increases resistance of mice against tuberculosis and, reciprocally, IL-12 neutralization delays clearance of tubercle bacilli [89, 90]. However, reduction is modest, arguing against exclusive IL-12 dependency of acquired host resistance against tuberculosis. Probably IL-12 increases host protection indirectly via stimulation of increased IFN-γ secretion. A recent study has described disseminated *M. avium* complex infections in familial patients suffering from an intrinsic IL-12 defect [91]. Similarly, protection against *M. avium* is also impaired by IL-12 neutralization in a mouse model [92]. IL-12 secretion is affected in BCG-immunized IFN-γR gene deletion mutant mice, suggesting that IL-12 secretion by BCG-infected macrophages depends on costimulation by IFN-γ [93]. Although such a dramatic effect on IL-12 secretion is not observed with *M. tuberculosis* [93a], agonistic effects of IFN-γ and tubercle bacilli appear likely.

*IFN-γ*: Whilst the essential role of IFN-γ in defense against tuberculosis is without doubt in the murine system, its role in tuberculosis of humans remains controversial. In vitro stimulation with IFN-γ induces potent tuberculostasis in murine, but not in human, macrophages [94, 95]. Only a cocktail of additional cytokines together with 1,25-dihydroxyvitamin $D_3$ has been found to cause some macrophage activation [96, 97]. Yet, local administration of IFN-γ to patients led to improved resistance against mycobacterial infections [59]. Moreover, hereditary IFN-γ deficiencies are associated with increased incidences of mycobacterial infection [98, 99]. In these studies IFN-γR deficiency was associated with idiopathic *M. bovis* BCG infection and elevated susceptibility to infections with atypical mycobacteria [98, 99]. This high susceptibility was accompanied by impaired formation of granulomas which resembled those in lepromatous leprosy patients. Similarly, mouse mutants with a disrupted IFN-γ gene succumb to *M. tuberculosis* and *M. bovis* BCG infection [62, 63]. In these gene deletion mutants, tuberculosis becomes disseminated and causes exaggerated tissue destruction and necrosis. Yet, the mutants develop granulomas, arguing against a central role of IFN-γ in granuloma formation.

*IL-4*: Although *M. tuberculosis* infection seems to strongly counteract Th2 cell development, IL-4 secretion has been observed at later stages of disease [65]. Consistent with this, human T cells produce IL-4 subsequent to IFN-γ during in vitro culture with *M. bovis* BCG [100]. Moreover, high IL-4 mRNA was observed in peripheral blood leukocytes from patients suffering from pulmonary tuberculosis and increased numbers of IL-4-producing cells have been detected amongst peripheral blood lymphocytes from tuberculosis patients as compared to healthy control donors [66]. On the contrary, IL-4 mRNA levels were low in lymph nodes of patients suffering from tuberculous lymphadenitis [101]. In vitro studies suggest that secretion of Th1 or Th2 cytokines by mycobacteria-activated human T cells is influenced by the type of accessory cells responsible for antigen presentation and T-cell stimulation [102]. Mononuclear phagocytes favor Th1 responses, whereas the presence of B cells promotes a shift towards the Th2 pole. It, therefore, appears that a modest Th2 response develops in tuberculosis. The late appearance of such Th2 cells does not necessarily imply a pathologic role, but may suggest that they participate in down-regulation of the protective Th1 response to avoid exaggerated pathologic consequences [58]. Yet, it is conceivable that disturbances in the balance encompassing strong Th1 and modest Th2 responses which lead to elevated IL-4 production, promote disease exacerbation [71]. It, therefore, appears important to strictly control Th2 cell development at any stage of tuberculosis.

Although mycobacteria are potent IL-12 inducers, stringent down-regulation of early IL-4 production may occur in adjunct. Recent studies in the mouse have identified an unconventional T cell population, coexpressing CD4 and TCRαβ as T-cell markers and NK1 as an NK marker [103]. These cells are early IL-4 producers and thus probably involved in Th2 cell promotion [104, 105]. Infection with intracellular bacteria, including *M. bovis* BCG, causes down-regulation of these early IL-4 producers [106]. It is, therefore, possible that mycobacteria promote Th1 cell development not only by potent IL-12 induction, but also by curtailment of IL-4 secretion.

*Transforming growth factor β* (TGF-β), in addition to IL-4, seems to participate in down-regulation of Th1 responses [107]. TGF-β is primarily produced by mononuclear phagocytes. Increased levels of TGF-β in granulomatous lesions and heightened TGF-β secretion by blood monocytes from tuberculosis patients are consistent with an inhibitory, and perhaps disease-exacerbating, role of TGF-β in tuberculosis [108, 109]. TGF-β acts on macrophages and hence may directly interfere with its anti-mycobacterial capacities. Because TGF-β also down-regulates secretion of macrophage cytokines, it may impair Th1 cell development, in addition.

## Cytolytic T Lymphocyte Responses

In most experimental systems both in humans and mouse, cytolytic T-cell functions are preferentially associated with the CD8 phenotype [26] and cytolytic CD8 T cells have been isolated from mycobacteria-immune mice [110]. In humans, cytolytic activities may be preferentially associated with CD4 T cells, although more recently, CD8 T cells capable of lysing mycobacteria-infected target cells have been identified [17, 18, 111, 112]. Despite the ease with which target cell lysis is demonstrated in vitro, little evidence exists for its in vivo relevance. Yet, it is tempting to speculate that lysis of host cells infected by tubercle bacilli may contribute to protection through microbial release from incapacitated host cells, thus allowing their uptake by more proficient phagocytes [9]. Although macrophages are considered a major habitat of tubercle bacilli, evidence to suggest infection of other host cells, in particular lung parenchyma cells, has been presented [113]. Moreover, mycobacteria deactivate macrophages in which they persist [114]. Thus, both professional and nonprofessional phagocytes exist which are insufficiently equipped for killing of the tubercle bacilli. In contrast, blood phagocytes with high bactericidal capacities are better suited to combat *M. tuberculosis*. Hence, bacterial transition from a less hostile to a more aggressive host cell may contribute to protection. At the same time, lysis of host cells could result in tissue destruction and promote mycobacterial dissemination. Therefore, stringent control of cytolytic T-cell activities represents an important parameter within this scenario. Recently listeriosis has been found to be exacerbated in perforin gene deletion mutant mice which suffer from impaired cytolytic T-cell functions [115]. In contrast, support for a measurable influence of perforin deficiency on early control of tuberculosis is lacking [116]. It remains to be established whether cytolytic mechanisms are involved in protection against late or secondary tuberculosis.

### T Cells Mediating Immunological Memory

Immunological memory is expressed as a more potent and accelerated response in hosts that have already encountered a pathogen or a foreign antigen previously. The accelerated kinetics of secondary responses in general, occurs as a consequence of an increased precursor frequency of antigen specific T cells generated after the first encounter with the antigen [117], and due to a potentiated and accelerated initiation of effector functions in already primed and differentiated T cells [118–120]. Classical studies by Lefford and McGregor [121] demonstrated that long-lived memory immunity to tuberculosis does not depend upon the presence of viable bacteria. In this study, live bacteria were cleared from the animals by chemotherapy without abolishing the generation of immunological memory. This initial observation has formed the basis for most of the experimental attempts to address memory immunity to tuberculosis in animal models. Orme [35] used mice cured from a primary infection by chemotherapy and the technique of adoptive transfer to demonstrate that the cells responsible for immunological memory are long-lived, nondividing T cells insensitive to antimitotic drugs, in agreement with observations made in animal models of infection with *L. monocytogenes* previously [122]. By separating T cells into subsets, it was further found that long-lived resistance to tuberculosis in the mouse model was mediated by CD4 T cells with only a minor contribution by the CD8 T-cell subset [35]. The cytokines secreted by CD4 T cells during the recall of immunological memory are typically of Th1 type characterized by high levels of IFN-γ and IL-2 accumulating in the infected target organs as soon as 24 h after infection [123].

Evidence from studies of recall responses to various antigens have suggested that naive and memory T cells can be distinguished phenotypically on the basis of a number of alterations of cell surface marker expression. In particular, down-regulation of high molecular mass isoforms of the surface exposed tyrosine phosphatase CD45 and up-regulation of several adhesion molecules have been associated with differentiation of naive cells into memory cells [119, 124] In murine tuberculosis it was recently demonstrated that the cells which accumulate in the spleen and lymph nodes during recall of memory immunity are of the phenotype CD4$^+$ CD45RB$^{low}$ CD44$^{high}$ [123, 125]. By direct magnetic cell separation, additional evidence was provided by the finding that mycobacteria-reactive memory effector cells are predominantly found in the CD4$^+$ CD45RB$^{low}$ CD44$^{high}$ LFA$^{high}$ L-selectin$^{low}$ population [123]. It is presently debated whether this phenotype represents true memory cells or simply activated T cells which can revert to the naive phenotype during rest [126, 127]. Basic studies of lifespans of different lymphocyte subpopulations in vivo have shown that cells with the memory phenotype have a higher turnover than naive cells [128], but that over time a low proportion of the activated pool of cells may revert to a resting state with a very slow turnover and this subset may represent true resting memory cells [129]. In the mouse model of memory immunity to tuberculosis, recent evidence suggests that resting memory T cells are nonresident, contained in the recirculating pool of lymphocytes and recruited to the site of infection in a highly accelerated manner leading to a 500- to 1,000-fold increase in the frequency of mycobacteria-reactive T cells within the first few days of infection [130].

The memory T-cell repertoire primed in mice rendered memory immune by a primary infection and a subsequent antibiotic cure is broad, directed at both somatic and extracellular antigens [131]. This is not surprising because such animals have probably seen all classes of mycobacterial antigens at this time point. Interestingly, the first phase of the recall of memory immunity in this model involves almost exclusively IFN-γ producing T cell, reactive with culture filtrate antigens, a finding in agreement with the idea that T cells directed to extracellular antigens will recognize macrophages harboring multiplying mycobacteria early after infection [131]. Only very few target molecules dominate the response at this early time point and as many as 25–30% of the total mycobacteria-reactive T-cell repertoire recognizes the low mass secreted antigen ESAT-6 and antigen 85 during recall immunity [130].

The highly efficient immune surveillance manifested by the immune system controls infection but without sterilizing immunity. A few bacilli, possibly about 1–5% of the total inoculum, typically escape and will lead to a chronic or recrudescent form of disease [36]. These surviving bacteria may be buried deep in the center of granulomas controlled by the immune system and probably the low oxygen tension in the necrotic center. The factors which subsequently lead to reactivation of disease are presently totally unknown. Eventually immune suppression either as a consequence of advancing age, or other infectious diseases may tilt the balance in favor of the pathogen and result in reactivation of clinical disease.

## Mycobacterial Antigens

*M. tuberculosis* comprises thousands of proteins. The complexity of the mycobacterial antigen repertoire was initially illustrated by the crossed immune electrophoresis reference system introduced for *M. bovis* BCG [132]. Although only a limited number of the proteins had been characterized when the reference system was introduced, it underlined the need for a systematic approach to the dissection of the mycobacterial antigen repertoire. Within the last few years this field of research has witnessed considerable progress. From a few defined mycobacterial antigens, more than 15 have been characterized in detail today and have either well-described functions in mycobacterial physiology or immunological relevance (table 1) [for recent reviews, see 133, 134]. Mycobacterial antigens can be divided into somatic proteins bound to the bacteria and extracellular proteins which can be obtained in culture filtrates at early time points of bacterial culture. This division is possibly over-simplified as many proteins, in particular molecules from the outer cell wall, will be present both in bacteria-derived antigen preparations (such as sonicates) and in culture filtrates [135]. Recent attempts to characterize components in culture filtrates by two-dimensional gels have emphasized the complexity of this mixture, possibly containing as many as 100 different spots [136; K. Weldingh and P. Andersen, unpubl. data].

Initial attempts to purify single mycobacterial T-cell antigens were mostly random and led to the biochemical purification of molecules selected either as a consequence of their abundance in various mycobacterial preparations, or due to the availability of monoclonal antibodies (mAb) defining the molecule [137–139]. The establishment of expression libraries of *M. tuberculosis* greatly promoted the definition of mycobacterial antigens and provided the tools for a detailed characterization [140]. Most of the genes initially isolated were identified in expression libraries with mAb, but recently the screening of libraries with degenerate oligonucleotide primers based on N-terminal sequence data has allowed a very direct approach to the isolation of new genes. Expression gene libraries have also been used for the identification of T-cell antigens

*Table 1.* Defined protein antigens of *M. tuberculosis*

| Name | kD[1] | Localization | Protective efficacy | Functions/activity | References |
|---|---|---|---|---|---|
| DnaK | 70 | Somatic/extracellular | | Heat shock protein | 212–214 |
| GroEL | 65 | Somatic | + | Heat shock protein | 212, 215, 216 |
| Urease | 62 | Somatic | | Involved in nitrogen metabolism | 217 |
| Glutamine synthase | 58 | Somatic/extracellular | | Involved in cell wall synthesis(?) | 218 |
| Proline-rich complex | 45–47 | Extracellular | | Target for DTH and antibody responses after immunization with live bacteria; glycosylated | 219–221 |
| L-Alanine dehydrogenase | 40 | Outer cell wall | | Involved in cell wall synthesis(?) | 222 |
| Phosphate-binding protein | 38 | Outer cell wall | | Anchored in cell membrane by lipid moiety; involved in phosphate metabolism | 223, 224 |
| Ag 85 complex | 30–32 | Extracellular | + | Fibronectin binding; antigen 85b holds mycolyl transferase activity; prominent T-cell target. | 180, 225–227 |
| HBHA (heparin binding hemagglutinin) | 28 | Outer cell wall | | Adherence to cell surfaces | 228 |
| MPT51 | 27 | Extracellular | | Homology to antigen 85 | 229 |
| MPT64 | 26 | Extracellular | | Deleted in some strains of BCG; potent inducer of DTH | 154, 191 |
| Superoxide dismutase | 23 | Somatic/extracellular | | Cleaves toxic superoxide radicals | 135, 230 |
| 19-kD lipo-protein | 19 | Outer cell wall | | Anchored in outer cell wall by lipid moiety; glycosylated | 224, 231 |
| α-Crystallin | 16 | Somatic/extracellular | | Heat shock protein; forms oligomeric structures with nine monomers | 232, 233 |
| GroES | 10 | Somatic/extracellular | | Heat shock protein; forms heptameric configuration | 212, 234, 235 |
| ESAT-6 | 6 | Extracellular | + | Key target for long-lived memory cells; deleted in all strains of BCG | 123, 130, 155, 170; Andersen, unpubl. data |

[1] As determined by separation in SDS-PAGE.

by direct screening with T-cell clones derived from human tuberculosis patients [141]. The intrinsic problem with lipopolysaccharide and *Eschericia coli* proteins in such preparations requires the use of cloned T cells which limits use of this approach in the search for new mycobacterial T-cell antigens.

Recombinant technology enables the production of large amounts of defined material and circumvents exhausting attempts to purify native proteins present in low concentrations in mycobacterial preparations. Some recent reports have, however, only found limited T-cell responses to a number of the major mycobacterial antigens available as recombinant preparations [142, 143]. In a model of experimental encephalomyelitis, Ben-Nun et al. [144] found a marked proliferative response to native GroES purified from PPD whereas a preparation of recombinant GroES was found to be almost totally inactive. Likewise, in a recent study of recombinant MPT64 expressed in *Mycobacterium smegmatis*, this preparation was found to be superior to an analogous preparation produced in *E. coli*, in eliciting DTH reactions in sensitized guinea pigs [145]. One possible explanation of such differences would be a lack of critical posttranslational modifications in products expressed in *E. coli*. In this regard, a recent study has demonstrated that mutagenesis of residues required for the glycosylation of the 19-kD antigen led to a changed pattern of proteolytic cleavage of the molecule, something which may influence processing and result in the presentation of different T-cell epitopes [146]. In a recent comparative study of T-cell recognition of native and recombinant GroES from *M. tuberculosis*, the two preparations were found to differ markedly. Whereas the native protein induced high levels of INF-$\gamma$ in cell cultures, the recombinant preparation was totally inactive [Rosenkrands et al, unpubl. data]. This study addressed the potential differences of the two preparations, but found no apparent differences with a range of sensitive biochemical analyses including mass spectrometry analysis. Hence, the background for these differences is unclear but the potential difference in the recognition of recombinant and native versions of the same protein should be taken into consideration when evaluating T-cell responses to defined antigens.

### Mycobacterial Antigens Recognized by T Cells

As the number of mycobacterial proteins identified and characterized is still relatively small compared to the total number of molecules in lysates or culture filtrates, various attempts have been made to screen T-cell recognition of complex protein mixtures. The need for a rapid direct screening of T-cell recognition was initially met by the T-cell Western blot method introduced by Young and Lamb [147]. Protein antigens which had been separated by gel electrophoresis and transferred to nitrocellulose paper were used to stimulate T cells in vitro. The method was employed in a number of studies to map T-cell recognition in human tuberculosis patients and animal models [148, 149]. Today the method is used less frequently probably due to the potential influence of the nitrocellulose particles on the cellular assay and the fact that proteins used to stimulate T cells cannot be quantified. The investigation of T-cell responses to complex mixtures has more recently been addressed by methods based on soluble protein fractions eluted from SDS-PAGE gels [131, 150]. Because SDS is highly toxic in cell cultures it is generally removed from the protein fractions by high-pressure dialysis or detergent binding affinity columns. Recently, two improved methods based on direct electroelution of proteins separated in either one- or two-dimensional gels were described [151, 152]. In these methods the SDS problem is circumvented either by running nondenaturing gels [151], or by an efficient removal of SDS during the electroelution process [152]. The latter technique, called the multielution method, was demonstrated to yield nontoxic products with unchanged stimulatory abilities in vitro compared to native proteins [152]. The methods have been used extensively since to study T-cell antigen recognition in human tuberculosis patients and in experimental animals infected with tuberculosis [123, 136, 153, 154]. Hasløv et al. [154] screened a panel of antigen fractions using delayed-type hypersensitivity (DTH) and cellular proliferation as read out in the guinea pig model. This study pointed to low mass antigens as the major targets for proliferative responses and the 26-kD secreted molecule MPT64 as a potent inducer of DTH responses in guinea pigs infected with *M. tuberculosis*. The methods have been used to produce antigen fractions in a highly reproducible manner which have enabled the comparison of antigen recognition patterns in independent experiments. Antigen recognition at various stages of infection has been the subject of a number of studies in the mouse model of tuberculosis. Culture filtrate antigens within the molecular mass range 4–11 and 26–35 kD were found to constitute the major targets for T cells at the peak of a primary infection [150]. Memory immune animals in which the primary infection had been cured by chemotherapy recognized the same culture filtrate antigens, but exhibited a broader T-cell recognition directed at somatic antigens as well [131]. Interestingly, evidence was provided in this study that secondary infection predominantly boosted T-cell responses targeted to culture filtrate antigens below 10 kD. A subsequent detailed study of the antigen recognition during the recall of protective immunity led to the identification of the low mass secreted antigen ESAT-6 and the 31–32 kD antigen AG85B as key target molecules for IFN-$\gamma$ producing memory effector T cells [123]. The preferential recognition of the low mass region and ESAT-6 was shared in 5/6 genetically different strains of mice [130]. Further evidence for conserved antigen recognition pattern focused on low mass culture filtrate antigens in the first phase of infection was recently provided by a study in cattle experimentally infected with *M. bovis* [154a, 154b]. In this study IFN-γ responses to culture filtrate antigens were found from week 2 of infection and these early responses were clearly focused on low mass culture filtrate antigens and in particular ESAT-6. That this striking antigen recognition pattern is characteristic for the first phase of infection was strongly supported by the finding that cattle at later stages of infection recognized a range of culture filtrate antigens of various masses.

It has been a consistent finding that tuberculosis patients recognize multiple targets found both in the somatic and secreted pool and that a considerable heterogeneity exists within donor groups [136, 142, 149]. Using the high resolution of the two-dimensional separation method, Daugelat et al. [136] reported a complex antigen recognition pattern in human patients characterized by a cluster of highly stimulatory secreted antigens located in the region from 30 to 100 kD and with a pI of 4–5. In a study by Boesen et al. [142], tuberculosis patients were classified based on a clinical investigation and X-ray, and patients with minimal tuberculosis had much higher levels of Th1 reactivity to culture filtrate antigens. Of importance, 6/8 patients with minimal tuberculosis shared the preferential recognition of the low mass culture filtrate fraction highly enriched for ESAT-6.

Although protein antigens and in particular extracellular antigens constitute important T-cell antigens, recent years' research have provided evidence for the recognition of nonproteinaceous antigens recognized by rare T-cell subsets such as DN αβ as well as γδ T cells. The γδ cells recognize small phosphorylated ligands with an estimated molecular mass of 500–600 daltons [46–50], whereas the DN TCRαβ-positive T cells recognize lipoglycans presented by the non-MHC encoded CD1 molecule [23, 24]. Although no ample evidence for a role of these subsets in protective immunity to tuberculosis exists, the potential importance of these nonproteinaceous target molecules should be borne in mind when designing future subunit vaccines.

## Extracellular versus Somatic Antigens – Early versus Late Antigens

A number of studies have provided evidence to suggest that mycobacterial antigens become available for the immune system in a sequential manner (reviewed by Andersen [134]). Culture filtrate antigens are important target molecules in the first phase of infection, whereas later during the course of infection the emergence of host immunity leads to killing of the bacterial pathogen and the release of somatic antigens. As reviewed above, the conserved

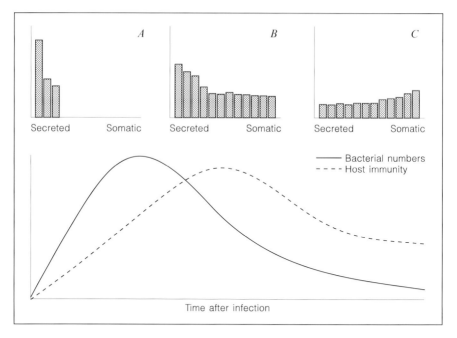

*Fig. 2.* Schematic overview of antigenic targets recognized by T cells during the course of tuberculosis infection. The first phase of infection (*A*) is characterized by unrestrained bacterial multiplication and an emerging host response restricted to relatively few antigenic targets in the secreted part of the  protein repertoire. (Up-regulated by the pathogen in response to the phagolysosomal environment?) Later time points (*B*) are characterized by gradual bacterial clearance, the release of antigens from degraded bacteria and a fully developed host response directed to antigens of all classes. At late time points (*C*) host immunity will have controlled the infection and only low numbers of bacteria reside and will give rise to either a chronic manifestation or a reactivation disease at late time points. This phase is characterized by a host response directed to all classes of antigens with a marked contribution from somatic antigens.

recognition of particular culture filtrate antigens such as ESAT-6 in the first phase of infection in several species, supports the idea that initially only a limited repertoire of antigens is available for host recognition (fig. 2). The paradox that ESAT-6 is such a prominent target in vivo but is present only in trace amounts in culture filtrates [155], raises the possibility that proteins like ESAT-6 may be part of a distinct protein repertoire which is up-regulated in response to the hostile environment inside the macrophage. Host recognition of such key target molecules would be expected to result in the early detection of infected macrophages. Results from several laboratories have provided evidence that high levels of protective immunity can be obtained with vaccines based on culture filtrate proteins (see later in this chapter). Because the composition of proteins expressed by mycobacteria is markedly influenced by growth conditions [156, 157], the future challenge will be to identify molecules up-regulated by stress or intracellular growth and to enrich culture filtrates with these relevant antigens.

Vaccines based on culture filtrate antigens would be expected to prime T cells of particular importance for immune surveillance in the first phase of tuberculosis, whereas immunological control at later and more chronic stages of infection may require involvement of other antigen specificities. At later time points the molecules available for T-cell recognition may predominantly be somatic antigens released from killed bacteria. The recent finding of protective immunity to tuberculosis induced by a DNA vaccine encoding the somatic 65-kD hsp [158] favors this notion suggesting that an efficient future vaccine should include both early and late antigens.

Recent evidence has provided a new conceptional angle on the intepretation of the immunological relevance of secreted antigens. A study by Hess et al. [159] suggests that antigens secreted from live bacteria may have a built-in advantage as they are more efficiently presented to the immune system. By introducing the naturally secreted antigens listeriolysin or the p60 antigen of *L. monocytogenes* into *Salmonella typhimurium* either in secreted or somatic form, it was shown that the secretion of these antigens induced protective immune responses, whereas somatic display gave low and insignificant levels of immunity. Even the naturally somatic antigen, superoxide dismutase, when displayed in secreted form, induced protective immunity [159a].

### The Design of Novel Vaccines against Tuberculosis

*M. bovis* BCG is presently the only vaccine against tuberculosis. Besides being the most widely used vaccine in the world, BCG is the most controversial vaccine in use today. Although BCG generally induces high levels of protective immunity in experimental animals [160], a pronounced variation has been found in human field trials with efficacies as high as 80% in some trials whereas other trials have failed to show protection [161]. The BCG vaccine was developed using traditional principles of attenuation, tested in animal models, followed by human trials and was taken into clinical practice with no knowledge of the mechanisms underlying its efficacy. Still today, the immunology underlying the efficacy of BCG is largely unknown and the huge variation found in vaccine efficacy from one trial to another is a totally unresolved problem. A generally accepted hypothesis is that exposure and sensitization to environmental mycobacterial strains will influence the outcome of BCG vaccination [162]. The absence of prior sensitization seems a prerequisite for high efficacy and studies using the most stringent criteria for exclusion of sensitized individuals have generally found high vaccination efficacy [163, 164]. There is, furthermore, an unbroken record of success with BCG campaigns in newborn children [165, 166]. The frequency and variety of environmental exposures is known to differ greatly between geographic regions and is particularly pronounced in tropical regions of the world. There is disagreement about the mechanism of these interactions, whether they involve adverse effects through the induction of antagonistic immune reactions [167, 168], or masking of BCG's protection through exposure to environmental mycobacteria which themselves induce similar levels of protection [169]. With the information which has become available in recent years it seems clear now that there are two potential immunologic pitfalls with the BCG vaccine in its present form: (1) BCG lacks important antigens expressed in virulent mycobacteria such as ESAT-6 [170] and (2) BCG may be an insufficient stimulator of CD8 responses relevant for protection against tuberculosis [9].

There are only few reports on human immune responses induced by BCG. In a recent study of cell-mediated immune responses induced by intradermal BCG vaccination, a group of nonsensitized donors (based on both PPD-negative skin tests and lack of in vitro responsiveness to PPD) were followed over a period of 1 year postvaccination [171]. In these individuals, potentially protective effector functions such as antigen-specific IFN-$\gamma$ responses and cytotoxicity were observed to peak between 56 days and 1 year postvaccination. Distinct differences in the emergence of T cells recognizing different classes of mycobacterial antigens were found. Of importance, some donors with high levels of prevaccination sensitization exhibited only a limited increase in mycobacterial responsiveness postvaccination.

Although the reasons for the lack of BCG vaccine efficacy is still unresolved, the urgent need for efficient means to control tuberculosis worldwide has stimulated a major international effort to develop new and improved vaccines. This work is currently conducted along parallel lines.


### Subunit Vaccines

Early attempts to construct tuberculosis subunit vaccines were focused on different cell-wall-derived mycobacterial subfractions. When given in oil-based vehicles, these subfractions, in a number of studies, induced detectable levels of protection measured both as increased survival and reduced number of bacteria recovered from target organs in guinea pigs and mice [for a review, see 160]. Some of the most successful attempts along this line were made by Ribi's group [172, 173] using different combinations of cell wall and mineral oil in murine tuberculosis. Today most of these results should be interpreted cautiously because mycobacterial cell walls contain considerable amounts of highly stimulatory components mediating inflammatory reactions. In this regard, both trehalose dimycolate and muramyl dipeptide have been shown to stimulate nonspecific resistance in animal models [174, 175].

Based on classical observations of high efficacy of live vaccines in contrast to killed vaccine preparations [176, 177], recent research has focused on the use of extracellular proteins from *M. tuberculosis* as a source of protective antigens [135, 178]. These efforts have so far resulted in a number of successful studies from several laboratories [179–183]. In the mouse model of tuberculosis, a vaccine based on a defined short-term culture filtrate (ST-CF) mixed with the mild adjuvant dimethyl deoctadecyl ammonium bromide (DDA) induced a potent MHC class II restricted CD4 T-cell response [179]. The optimal dose was 100 mg inducing a Th1 response whilst higher doses were found to induce Th2 responses. In its optimal concentration, this vaccine induced acquired resistance at the same level as BCG. In two other studies late culture filtrates from *M. tuberculosis* have been given in incomplete Freund's adjuvant (IFA). Both studies reported significant protection to an aerosol challenge with virulent *M. tuberculosis*, monitored as reduced numbers of bacteria in the target organs [181, 182]. In the study by Roberts et al. [181], a waning of the immune response induced by the subunit vaccine was observed 5 months after immunization, whereas BCG induced high and consistent vaccine efficacy. This finding differs from the high levels of memory immunity, as late as 22 weeks after vaccination, with the ST-CF DDA vaccine [179]. Subunit vaccines based on extracellular proteins have also been tested in the aerosol guinea pig model. This model, which more closely resembles the advanced stage of human tuberculosis, was used to demonstrate low but significant levels of protection by a vaccine based on a culture filtrate fraction in IFA [183]. The study used both bacterial numbers in the target organs and weight loss as a read-out of protection. Later, a number of single mycobacterial culture filtrate antigens in the Syntex adjuvant [180] was investigated. In this study only antigen 85B induced low but detectable levels of protective immunity and reduced immunopathology.

It is known that different adjuvants prime markedly different immune responses with some adjuvants inducing preferentially cell-mediated immunity and others skewing towards humoral immune responses [184, 185]. The mouse model of tuberculosis infection has recently been used to evaluate a range of different adjuvants for tuberculosis subunit vaccines [71]. This study demonstrated markedly different immune responses by the adjuvants and a clear relationship between the Th1/Th2 character of the mRNA signal for cytokines in the regional lymph node, the isotype of the resulting antibody response and the subsequent resistance to a virulent *M. tuberculosis* challenge. The study pointed to a few potent Th1 inducing adjuvants in particular DDA, whereas alum, being the only adjuvant approved for human use today, was found to give a nonprotective Th2 response.

The adjuvants tested for tuberculosis subunit vaccines so far, have predominantly been chosen to stimulate the generation of a CD4 T-cell response. In the light of the potential importance of CD8 T cells in protective immunity to tuberculosis, future studies will have to address the use of adjuvants reported to promote the development of MHC class I restricted antigen presentation such as ISCOMS [186].

Although the results obtained with subunit vaccines so far are promising, the studies indicate that both antigen, dosage and the adjuvant need to be carefully evaluated in various animal models including primate models before a successful vaccine for human testing can be constructed.

### Recombinant Carriers

*BCG*

So far no experimental vaccine has proven to be more efficient than BCG. One obvious approach to the development of an improved tuberculosis vaccine could therefore be in the form of recombinant (r) BCG overexpressing key antigens from virulent mycobacteria. Recent research on vectors for the introduction of genes into mycobacteria has provided the necessary technological basis for this approach [187, 188]. A number of nonmycobacterial antigens have been tested in this system and have paved the road for the development of a new multivalent live vaccine based on BCG [189, 190]. No mycobacterial antigens have been tested in this system probably due to the extensive antigenic identity between the virulent strains and the vaccine which would complicate the interpretation of results. Recent progress in the definition of antigens expressed in *M. tuberculosis* but absent in BCG has emphasized the potential of such an approach. MPT64 has been found to be expressed in virulent mycobacteria but is absent in some BCG strains [191], whereas the important T-cell antigen ESAT-6 is absent in all strains of BCG [170]. A recent analysis of the genetic differences between virulent *M. bovis* and avirulent BCG confirmed these differences as part of larger deletions from the genome of the vaccine strains [192]. Reintroduction of genes within these regions, such as *esat6* and *mpt64*, without reversion to virulence may lead to an efficient vaccine enriched with critical epitopes from the virulent strain.

An alternative approach to improvement of BCG may be to modulate the immune responses induced by the vaccine, e.g. by the integration of genes encoding critical cytokines. A recent study demonstrated that r-strains of BCG-secreting murine cytokines potentiated the immune response in immunized mice [193]. The expression of both IL-2, IFN-γ and GM-CSF in the vaccine enhanced the response.

### Other Carriers

Recombinant *Salmonella* aroA and vaccinia virus have been widely used as vaccine carriers for the delivery of heterologous antigens from various pathogens to the immune system. Vectors for the transformation of *Salmonella* have been constructed to allow genetic fusions to carrier proteins such as tetanus toxoid either as full-size proteins or as repeats of single epitopes [194, 195]. Recently, a r-*Salmonella* strain was described which is capable of secreting virtually any heterologous antigens by means of the *E. coli* hemolysin export apparatus [159]. This construct represents a promising carrier for tuberculosis antigens. Vaccinia virus has been used for the expression of *M. tuberculosis* as well as *M. leprae* proteins [196, 197].

### Attenuated Mycobacterial Strains

Live attenuated bacteria generally provide high levels of protection. Experiments with other bacterial pathogens have revealed that by rational attenuation it is possible to limit replication of the bacteria in vivo, while stimulating immunity to the parental strain [198]. Conventional approaches to the generation of mutants, such as chemical and physical mutagenesis, are inadequate for mycobacteria which grow in clumps and where the generation of clones based on single cells is virtually impossible. Recent progress towards the attenuation of mycobacteria has been conducted along two lines which both employ selectable marker genes (such as antibiotic resistance genes) which allow an easy selection of mutants.

*Allelic exchange*: Successful reports of allelic exchange have recently been reported in slow-growing mycobacteria [199–201]. The methodology employs disrupted versions of a gene in a suicide vector to replace a target gene by homologous recombination. In a number of recent reports the methodology has been used to construct mutants of *M. tuberculosis* or *M. bovis* in which different biosynthetic pathways were destroyed leading to auxotrophic [200] or urease-negative strains [201]. None of these strains have been tested as vaccines so far, but the potential disruption of any desired gene makes the general strategy very promising.

*Transposon mutagenesis*: This methodology has been used in several studies as an efficient means of generating auxotrophic mutants in mycobacteria. Recently, this research led to the development of leucine and methionine *auxotrophic* mutants of *M. bovis* BCG [202]. These strains had a markedly reduced virulence and did not replicate in SCID mice in contrast to BCG which causes death of these highly susceptible mice within 8 weeks. Surprisingly, replication of the vaccine strain was not necessary for protection, as is the case for BCG, and the auxotrophic strain gave rise to comparable levels of protection to a virulent challenge with *M. tuberculosis* [203]. In the light of the spreading of the HIV epidemic such low virulent strains may have a potential for prophylaxis of tuberculosis in populations at risk for HIV.

## DNA Vaccines

The most recent achievement in experimental vaccines is the efficient induction of immune responses by direct delivery of DNA encoding the protein antigens of interest. By using a strong promoter such as the cytomegalovirus promoter, injection of plasmid DNA leads to the expression of foreign proteins in vivo and the generation of humoral and cell-mediated immune responses [204, 205]. The methodology has now been applied successfully in a number of animal models of infectious diseases; influenza, HIV, herpes, malaria and leishmaniasis [206]. Two recent reports indicate that this method may have a major potential for the development of tuberculosis vaccines. Tascon et al. [158] injected the gene encoding the 65-kD hsp as well as a 36-kD proline-rich antigen from *M. leprae* and found significant levels of protection against tuberculosis with both constructs. The best protection (equivalent to that obtained by BCG), was provided by the plasmid encoding the hsp and a correlation with high levels of cytotoxicity as well as IFN-$\gamma$ release was found. The second study by Huygen et al. [207] focused on Ag85A and evaluated constructs which encoded cytoplasmic and secreted forms of the antigen. The immunizations gave rise to a predominant Th1 response with high levels of IFN-$\gamma$ and detectable levels of protective immunity, although at a somewhat lower level than after BCG vaccination.

DNA vaccines will by their nature primarily give rise to endogenously processed peptides and MHC class I restricted responses. Hence, the technology has an obvious potential for the development of vaccines against viral diseases. However, in the study by Huygen et al. [207] the DNA vaccine was found to induce a predominant Th1 response and some CD8 cytotoxicity.

The pathway leading to MHC class II presentation after DNA vaccination is not precisely defined, but may occur through macrophage uptake of antigen from lysed transfected muscle cells. The MHC class II restricted pathway can be further improved by constructing DNA vaccines which allow the antigen in question to be secreted, pinocytosed by professional antigen presenting cells and processed through the MHC class II pathway.

Unanswered safety issues such as the risk of genomic integration and inadvertent generation of autoimmune diseases prevents the present use of DNA vaccines in humans, but in animal models the technology may permit rapid identification of protective antigens for future vaccines. A recent study in another infection model (*Mycoplasma*) has provided interesting results which indicate that direct immunization with expression libraries divided into sublibraries may be one feasible way toward the identification of genes encoding protective antigens from different pathogens [208].

## Testing of Experimental Vaccines in Animal Models

The evaluation of new tuberculosis vaccines should ideally be conducted in animal models that closely resemble human disease. Such a model could be a primate model, but there is a need for a rational screening procedure of new candidate vaccines which will allow a larger number of candidates to be tested in less expensive models. The choice of animal model has a profound influence on the conclusions reached and a calculation of all the variables in a protection experiment has revealed that more than 20,000 combinations exist [160] with the obvious risk that a model can be tailored to give the desired results [for extensive reviews of animal models, see 160 and 209].

The mouse model is generally regarded as a useful, cost-effective first choice for screening new vaccine candidates. Mice are easy to handle and a large range of immunological reagents is available for the investigator. Mice are relatively resistant to tuberculosis and succumb only to high doses of the more virulent strains such as the Erdman strain [109]. The protective window (the difference in mycobacterial numbers in vaccinated and naive mice) is not as large as in more susceptible species and will in most strains be a 20–40 times decrease in bacterial numbers in BCG-vaccinated mice [160, 179]. As a consequence of this, a fine ranking of vaccines with similar overall level of efficacy is impossible in the mouse model. However, as a first screening of candidate vaccines for further testing the model is fully appropriate. Moreover, it is the best model for precise definition of underlying immune responses.

The guinea pig is the classical experimental animal for tuberculosis research and clearly a superior model to the mouse in terms of the development of the pathology in the lung, DTH reaction and sensitivity to disease. Due to the high susceptibility of the guinea pig, a very sensitive read-out of protection can be obtained with a more than 3 log difference in bacterial load between vaccinated and nonvaccinated animals [210], allowing the monitoring of even minor differences in vaccine efficacy. The drawback of the model, however, is the cost and the few immunological reagents available.

Obviously a reliable primate model is needed for testing candidate vaccines which have proven efficacious in the two non-primate models. Attempts have recently been made to develop such a model in *Cynomolgus* monkeys [211]. In this study, monkeys that received moderate doses of *M. tuberculosis* developed a chronic, slowly progressive, localized form of pulmonary tuberculosis. This disease manifestation resembles human disease and the model could constitute an important tool for final evaluation of vaccines before clinical trials in humans.

## Acknowledgements

S.H.E. K. acknowledges financial support from the Sonderforschungsbereich 322 'Lympho-Hemopoiesis', the German Science Foundation, project Ka 573/3-2; the Interdisciplinary Centre for Clinical Research; the BMBF Joint Project 'Mycobacterial Infections', and the German Leprosy Relief Association. P.A. was supported in part by grants from the Danish Association Against Lung Diseases, the World Health Organization Programme for Vaccine Development, the Danish Research Center for Medical Biotechnology and the European Community (project TS3*/CT94/0313). Many thanks to J. Andersen and R. Mahmoudi for excellent secretarial help.

## References

1  Grange JM (ed): Mycobacteria and Human Disease, ed 2. London, Arnold, 1996.
2  Bloom BR, Murray CJL: Tuberculosis: Commentary on reemergent killer. Science 1992;257:1055–1064.
3  Kaufmann SHE, Van Embden JDA: Tuberculosis: A neglected disease strikes back. Trends Microbiol 1993;1:2–5.
4  Davies PDO (ed): Clinical Tuberculosis. London, Chapman & Hall, 1994.
5  Hastings RC (ed): Leprosy, ed 2. Edinburgh, Churchill Livingstone, 1994.
6  Inderlied CB, Kemper CA, Bermudez LE: The *Mycobacterium avium* complex. Clin Microbiol Rev 1993;6:266–310.
7  Brennan PJ, Nikaido H: The envelope of mycobacteria. Annu Rev Biochem 1995;64:29–63.
8  Porcelli SA, Morita CT, Modlin RL: T-cell recognition of non-peptide antigens. Curr Opin Immunol 1996;8:510–516.
9  Kaufmann SHE: Tuberculosis: The role of the immune response. Immunologist 1993;1:109–114.
10 Kaufmann SHE: Cell-mediated immunity; in Hastings RC (ed): Leprosy, ed 2. Edinburgh, Churchill Livingstone, 1993, pp 157–168.

11    Bloom BR, Modlin RL, Salgame P: Stigma variations: Observations on suppressor T cells and leprosy. Annu Rev Immunol 1992;10:453–488.

12    Barnes PF, Modlin RL: Human cellular immune responses to *Mycobacterium tuberculosis*. Curr Top Microbiol Immunol 1996;215:197–220.

13    Small PM, Hopewell PC, Singh SP, Paz A, Parsonnet J, Ruston DC, Schecter GF, Daley CL, Schoolnik GK: The epidemiology of tuberculosis in San Francisco. A population-based study using conventional and molecular methods. N Engl J Med 1994;330:1703–1709.

14    Müller I, Cobbold SP, Waldmann H, Kaufmann SHE: Impaired resistance against *Mycobacterium tuberculosis* infection after selective in-vivo depletion of L3T4+ and Lyt2+ T cells. Infect Immun 1987;55:2037–2041.

15    Orme IM, Collins FM: Adoptive protection of the *Mycobacterium tuberculosis* infected lung: Dissociation between cells that passively transfer protective immunity and those that transfer delayed-type hypersensitivity to tuberculin. Cell Immunol 1984;84:113–120.

16    Flynn JL, Goldstein MM, Triebold KJ, Koller B, Bloom BR: Major histocompatibility complex class I-restricted T cells are required for resistance to *Mycobacterium tuberculosis* infection. Proc Natl Acad Sci USA 1992;89:12013–12017.

17    Turner J, Dockrell HM: Stimulation of human peripheral blood mononuclear cells with live *Mycobacterium bovis* BCG activates cytolytic CD8+ T cells in vitro. Immunology 1996;87:339–342.

18    Rees ADM, Scoging A, Mehlert A, Young DB, Ivanyi J: Specificity of proliferative response of human CD8 clones to mycobacterial antigens. Eur J Immunol 1988;18:1881–1887.

19    Kabelitz D, Bender A, Schondelmaier S, Schoel B, Kaufmann SHE: A large fraction of human peripheral blood $\gamma/\delta^+$ T cells is activated by *Mycobacterium tuberculosis* but not by its 65-kD heat shock protein. J Exp Med 1990;171:667–679.

20    Modlin RL, Pirmez C, Hofmann FM, Torigian V, Uyemura K, Rea TH, Bloom BR, Brenner MB: Lymphocytes bearing antigen-specific $\gamma/\delta$ T-cell receptors accumulate in human infectious disease lesions. Nature 1989;339:544–548.

21    Kaufmann SHE: $\gamma/\delta$ and other unconventional T lymphocytes: What do they see and what do they do? Proc Natl Acad Sci USA 1996;93:2272–2279.

22    Ladel CH, Hess J, Daugelat S, Mombaerts P, Tonegawa S, Kaufmann SHE: Contribution of $\alpha\beta$ and $\gamma/\delta$ T lymphocytes to immunity against *Mycobacterium bovis* bacillus Calmette-Guérin: Studies with T cell receptor-deficient mutant mice. Eur J Immunol 1995;25:838–846.

23    Beckman EM, Porcelli SA, Morita CT, Behar SM, Furlong ST, Brenner MB: Recognition of a lipid antigen by CD1-restricted $\alpha\beta^+$ T cells. Nature 1994;372:691–694.

24    Sieling PA, Chatterjee D, Porcelli SA, Prigozy TI, Mazzaccaro RJ, Soriano T, Bloom BR, Brenner MB, Kronenberg M, Brennan PJ, Modlin RL: CD1-restricted T cell recognition of microbial lipoglycan antigens. Science 1995;269:227–230.

25    Germain RN: MHC-dependent antigen processing and peptide presentation: Providing ligands for T lymphocyte activation. Cell 1994;76:287–299.

26    Kaufmann SHE: CD8+ T lymphocytes in intracellular microbial infections. Immunol Today 1988;9:168–174.

27    Russell DG: Mycobacterium and leishmania: Stowaways in the endosomal network. Trends Cell Biol 1995;5:125–128.

28    McDonough KA, Kress Y, Bloom BR: Pathogenesis of tuberculosis: Interaction of *Mycobacterium tuberculosis* with macrophages. Infect Immun 1993;61:2763–2773.

29    Mor N: Intracellular location of *Mycobacterium leprae* in macrophages of normal and immune-deficient mice and effect of rifampin. Infect Immun 1983;42:802–811.

30    Ladel CH, Daugelat S, Kaufmann SHE: Immune response to *Mycobacterium bovis* bacille Calmette-Guérin infection in major histocompatibility complex class I- and II-deficient knock-out mice: Contribution of CD4 and CD8 T cells to acquired resistance. Eur J Immunol 1995;25:377–384.

31    Jondal M, Schirmbeck R, Reimann J: MHC class I-restricted CTL responses to exogenous antigens. Immunity 1996;5:295–302.

32    Harding CV: Class I MHC presentation of exogenous antigens. J Clin Immunol 1996;16:90–96.

33    Barnes PF, Mistry SD, Cooper CL, Pirmez C, Rea TH, Modlin RL: Compartmentalization of a CD4+ T lymphocyte subpopulation in tuberculous pleuritis. J Immunol 1989;142:1114–1119.

34 Emmrich F, Kaufmann SHE: Human T cell clones with reactivity to *Mycobacterium leprae* as tools for the characterization of candidate vaccines against leprosy. Infect Immun 1986;41:879–883.

35 Orme IM: Characteristics and specificity of acquired immunologic memory to *Mycobacterium tuberculosis* infection. J Immunol 1988;140:3589–3593.

36 Orme IM: The kinetics of emergence and loss of mediator T lymphocytes acquired in response to infection with *Mycobacterium tuberculosis*. J Immunol 1987;138:293–298.

37 Pedrazzini T, Hug K, Louis JA: Importance of L3T4$^+$ and Lyt-2$^+$ cells in the immunologic control of infection with *Mycobacterium bovis* strain bacillus Calmette-Guérin in mice. Assessment by elimination of T cell subsets in vivo. J Immunol 1987;139:2032–2037.

38 Raulet DH: MHC class I-deficient mice. Adv Immunol 1994;55:381–421.

39 Porcelli SA: The CD1 family: A third lineage of antigen-presenting molecules. Adv Immunol 1995; 59:1–98.

40 De Sousa M, Reimao R, Lacerda R, Hugo P, Kaufmann SHE: Iron overload in $\beta_2$-microglobulin-deficient mice. Immunol Lett 1994;39:105–111.

41 O'Brien L, Roberts B, Andrew PW: In vitro interaction of *Mycobacterium tuberculosis* and macrophages: Activation of anti-mycobacterial activity of macrophages and mechanisms of anti-mycobacterial activity. Curr Top Microbiol Immunol 1996;215:97–130.

42 Nabeshima S, Hiromatsu K, Matsuzaki G, Mukasa A, Takada H, Yoshida S, Nomoto K: Infection of *Mycobacterium bovis* bacillus Calmette-Guérin in antibody-mediated $\gamma\delta$ cell-depleted mice. Immunology 1995;84:317–321.

43 Ladel CH, Blum C, Dreher A, Reifenberg K, Kaufmann SHE: Protective role of $\gamma/\delta$ T cells and $\alpha/\beta$ T cells in tuberculosis. Eur J Immunol 1995;25:2877.

44 Falini B, Flenghi L, Pileri S, Pelicci P, Fagioli M, Martelli MF, Moretta L, Ciccone E: Distribution of T cells bearing different forms of the T cell receptor $\gamma/\delta$ in normal and pathological human tissues. J Immunol 1989;143:2480–2488.

45 Tazi A, Fajac I, Soler P, Valeyre D, Battesti JP, Hance AJ: Gamma/delta T lymphocytes are not increased in number in granulomatous lesions of patients with tuberculosis or sarcoidosis. Am Rev Respir Dis 1991;144:1373–1375.

46 Pfeffer K, Schoel B, Gulle H, Kaufmann SHE, Wagner H: Primary responses of human T cells to mycobacteria: A frequent set of $\gamma/\delta$ T cells are stimulated by protease-resistant ligands. Eur J Immunol 1990;20:1175–1179.

47 Constant P, Davodeau F, Peyrat M-A, Poquet Y, Puzo G, Bonneville M, Fournié J-J: Stimulation of human $\gamma\delta$ T cells by nonpeptidic mycobacterial ligands. Science 1994;264:267–270.

48 Tanaka Y, Sano S, Nieves E, De Libero G, Rosa D, Modlin RL, Brenner MB, Bloom BR, Morita CT: Nonpeptide ligands for human $\gamma\delta$ T cells. Proc Natl Acad Sci USA 1994;91:8175–8179.

49 Schoel B, Sprenger S, Kaufmann SHE: Phosphate is essential for stimulation of V$\gamma$9V$\delta$2 T lymphocytes by mycobacterial low molecular weight ligand. Eur J Immunol 1994;24:1886–1892.

50 Tanaka Y, Morita CT, Nieves E, Brenner MB, Bloom BR: Natural and synthetic non-peptide antigens recognized by human $\gamma\delta$ T cells. Nature 1995;375:155–158.

51 Morita CT, Beckman EM, Bukowski JF, Tanaka Y, Band H, Bloom BR, Golan DE, Brenner MB: Direct presentation of nonpeptide prenyl pyrophosphate antigens to human $\gamma\delta$ T cells. Immunity 1995;3:495–508.

52 Boom WH, Balaji KN, Nayak R, Tsukaguchi K, Chervenak KA: Characterization of a 10- to 14-kilodalton protease-sensitive *Mycobacterium tuberculosis* H37Ra antigen that stimulates human $\gamma\delta$ T cells. Infect Immun 1994;62:5511–5518.

53 Munk ME, Elser C, Kaufmann SHE: Human $\gamma/\delta$ T cell response to *Listeria monocytogenes* protein components in vitro. Immunology 1996;87:235.

54 O'Brien RL, Happ MP, Dallas A, Palmer E, Kubo R, Born WK: Stimulation of a major subset of lymphocytes expressing T cell receptor $\gamma/\delta$ by an antigen derived from *Mycobacterium tuberculosis*. Cell 1989;57:667–674.

55 Beckman EM, Melian AM, Behar SM, Sieling PA, Chatterjee D, Matsumoto R, Rosat J-P, Modlin RL, Porcelli SA: CD1c restricts responses of mycobacteria-specific T cells: Evidence for antigen presentation by a second member of the human CD1 family. J Immunol 1996;157:2795–2803.

56    Sugita M, Jackman RM, van Donselaar E, Behar SM, Rogers RA, Peters PJ, Brenner MB, Porcelli SA: Cytoplasmic tail-dependent localization of CD1b antigen-presenting molecules to MIICs. Science 1996;273:349–352.

57    Chan J, Kaufmann SHE. Immune mechanisms of protection; in Bloom BR (ed): Tuberculosis: Pathogenesis, Protection, and Control. Washington, ASM, 1994, pp 389–415.

58    Abbas AK, Murphy KM, Sher A: Functional diversity of helper T lymphocytes. Nature 1996;383: 787–793.

59    Murray HW: Interferon-gamma and host antimicrobial defense: Current and future clinical applications. Am J Med 1994;97:459–467.

60    Trinchieri G: Interleukin–12: A proinflammatory cytokine with immunoregulatory functions that bridge innate resistance and antigen-specific adaptive immunity. Annu Rev Immunol 1995;13:251–276.

61    Zhang M, Gately MK, Wang E, Gong J, Wolf SF, Lu S, Modlin RL, Barnes PF: Interleukin-12 at the site of disease in tuberculosis. J Clin Invest 1994;93:1733–1739.

62    Flynn JL, Chan J, Triebold KJ, Dalton DK, Stewart TA, Bloom BR: An essential role for interferon-γ in resistance to *Mycobacterium tuberculosis* infection. J Exp Med 1993;178:2249–2254.

63    Cooper AM, Dalton DK, Stewart TA, Griffin JP, Russell DG, Orme IM: Disseminated tuberculosis in interferon-γ gene-disrupted mice. J Exp Med 1993;178:2249–2254.

64    Huang S, Hendriks W, Althage A, Hemmi S, Bluethmann H, Kamijo R, Vilcek J, Zinkernagel RM, Aguet M: Immune response in mice that lack the interferon-γ receptor. Science 1993;259:1742–1745.

65    Orme IM, Roberts AD, Griffin JP, Abrams JS: Cytokine secretion by CD4 T lymphocytes acquired in response to *Mycobacterium tuberculosis* infection. J Immunol 1993;151:518–525.

66    Surcel H-M, Troye-Blomberg M, Paulie S, Andersson G, Moreno C, Pasvol G: Th1/Th2 profiles in tuberculosis, based on the proliferation and cytokine response of blood lymphocytes to mycobacterial antigens. Immunology 1994;81:171–176.

67    Hsieh C-S, Macatonia SE, Tripp CS, Wolf SF, O'Garra A, Murphy KM: Development of Th1 CD4+ T cells through IL–12 produced by Listeria-induced macrophages. Science 1993;260:547–549.

68    Del Prete G, De Carli M, Almerigogna F, Daniel CK, D'Elios MM, Zancuoghi G, Vinante F, Pizzolo G, Romagnani S: Preferential expression of CD30 by human CD4+ T cells producing Th2-type cytokines. FASEB J 1995;9:81–86.

69    Munk ME, Kern P, Kaufmann SHE: Human CD30+ T cells are induced by *Mycobacterium tuberculosis* and present in tuberculosis lesions. Int Immunol 1997;9:713–720.

70    Sher A, Coffman RL: Regulation of immunity to parasites by T cells and T cell-derived cytokines. Annu Rev Immunol 1992;10:385–410.

71    Lindblad EB, Elhay MJ, Silva R, Appelberg R, Andersen P: Adjuvant modulation of immune responses to tuberculosis subunit vaccines. Infect Immun 1997;65:623–629.

72    Dinarello CA: Role of interleukin–1 in infectious diseases. Immunol Rev 1992;127:119–146.

73    Akira S, Taga T, Kishimoto T: Interleukin–6 in biology and medicine. Adv Immunol 1993;54:1–78.

74    Tracey KJ, Cerami A: Tumor necrosis factor, other cytokines and disease. Annu Rev Cell Biol 1993; 9:317–343.

75    Law K, Weiden M, Harkin T, Tchou Wong K, Chi C, Rom WN: Increased release of interleukin-1β, interleukin-6, and tumor necrosis factor-α by bronchoalveolar cells lavaged from involved sites in pulmonary tuberculosis. Am J Respir Crit Care Med 1996;153:799–804.

76    Flynn JL, Goldstein MM, Chan J, Triebold KJ, Pfeffer K, Lowenstein CJ, Schreiber R, Mak TW, Bloom BR: Tumor necrosis factor-α is required in the protective immune response against *Mycobacterium tuberculosis* in mice. Immunity 1995;2:561–572.

77    Kindler V, Sappino A-P, Grau Ge, Piquet P-F, Vassalli P: The inducing role of tumor necrosis factor in the development of bactericidal granulomas during BCG infection. Cell 1989;56:731–740.

78    Flesch IEA, Kaufmann SHE: Mechanisms involved in mycobacterial growth inhibition by gamma-interferon activated bone marrow macrophages: Role of reactive nitrogen intermediates. Infect Immun 1991;59:3213–3218.

79    Sampaio EP, Kaplan G, Miranda A, Nery JA, Miguel CP, Viana SM, Sarno EN: The influence of thalidomide on the clinical and immunologic manifestation of erythema nodosum leprosum. J Infect Dis 1993;168:408–414.

80  Tramontana JM, Utaipat U, Molloy A, Akarasewi P, Burroughs M, Makonkawkeyoon S, Johnson B, Klausner JD, Rom W, Kaplan G: Thalidomide treatment reduces tumor necrosis factor alpha production and enhances weight gain in patients with pulmonary tuberculosis. Mol Med 1995;1: 384–397.

81  Sampaio EP, Sarno EN, Galilly R, Cohn ZA, Kaplan G: Thalidomide selectively inhibits tumor necrosis factor-α production by stimulated human monocytes. J Exp Med 1991;173:699–703.

82  Flesch IEA, Kaufmann SHE: Stimulation of antibacterial macrophage activities by B cell stimulatory factor 2/interleukin-6. Infect Immun 1990;58:269–271.

83  Appelberg R, Castro AG, Pedrosa J, Minoprio P: Role of interleukin–6 in the induction of protective T cells during mycobacterial infections in mice. Immunology 1994;82:361–364.

83a Ladel C, Blum C, Dreher A, Reifenberg K, Kopf M, Kaufman SHE: Lethal tuberculosis in interleukin-6-deficient mutant mice. Infect Immun 1997;65:4543–4549.

84  Mackay CR: Chemokine receptors and T cell chemotaxis. J Exp Med 1996;184:799–802.

85  Baggiolini M, Dewald B, Moser B: Interleukin-8 and related chemotactic cytokines – CXC and CC chemokines. Adv Immunol 1994;55:97–179.

86  Rhoades ER, Cooper AM, Orme IM: Chemokine response in mice infected with *Mycobacterium tuberculosis.* Infect Immun 1995;63:3871–3877.

87  Zhang Y, Broser M, Cohen H, Bodkin M, Law K, Reibman J, Rom WN: Enhanced interleukin-8 release and gene expression in macrophages after exposure to *Mycobacterium tuberculosis* and its components. J Clin Invest 1995;95:586–592.

88  Rutledge BJ, Rayburn H, Rosenberg R, North RJ, Gladue RP, Corless CL, Rollins BJ: High level monocyte chemoattractant protein-1 expression in transgenic mice increases their susceptibility to intracellular pathogens. J Immunol 1995;155:4838–4843.

89  Flynn JL, Goldstein MM, Triebold KJ, Sypek J, Wolf S, Bloom BR: IL-12 increases resistance of BALB/c mice to *Mycobacterium tuberculosis* infection. J Immunol 1995;155:2515–2524.

90  Cooper AM, Roberts AD, Rhoades ER, Callahan JE, Getzy DM, Orme IM: The role of interleukin-12 in acquired immunity to *Mycobacterium tuberculosis* infection. Immunology 1995;85:423–432.

91  Frucht DM, Holland SM: Defective monocyte costimulation for IFN-gamma production in familial disseminated *Mycobacterium avium* complex infection: Abnormal IL-12 regulation. J Immunol 1996;157:411–416.

92  Castro AG, Silva RA, Appelberg R: Endogenously produced IL-12 is required for the induction of protective T cells during *Mycobacterium avium* infections in mice. J Immunol 1995;155:2013–2019.

93  Flesch IEA, Hess JH, Huang S, Aguet M, Rothe J, Bluethmann H, Kaufmann SHE: Early interleukin-12 production by macrophages in response to mycobacterial infection depends on interferon-γ and tumor necrosis factor-α. J Exp Med 1995;181:1615–1621.

93a Ladel CH, Szalay G, Riedel D, Kaufmann SHE: Interleukin-12 secretion in *Mycobacterium tuberculosis*-infected macrophages. Infect Immun 1997;65:1936–1938

94  Douvas GS, Looker DL, Vatter AE, Crowle AJ: Gamma interferon activates human macrophages to become tumoricidal and leishmanicidal but enhances replication of macrophage-associated mycobacteria. Infect Immun 1985;50:1–8.

95   Flesch I, Kaufmann SHE: Mycobacterial growth inhibition by interferon-γ activated bone marrow macrophages and differential susceptibility among strains of *Mycobacterium tuberculosis.* J Immunol 1987;138:4408–4413.

96  Denis M: Killing of *Mycobacterium tuberculosis* within human monocytes: Activation by cytokines and calcitriol. Clin Exp Immunol 1991;84:200–206.

97  Rook GA, Steele J, Fraher L, Barker S, Karmali R, O'Riordan J, Stanford J: Vitamin D$_3$, gamma interferon, and control of proliferation of *Mycobacterium tuberculosis* by human monocytes. Immunology 1986;57:159–163.

98  Jouanguy E, Altare F, Lamhamedi S, Revy P, Emile JF, Newport M, Levin M, Blanche S, Seboun E, Fischer A, Casanova J-L: Interferon gamma receptor deficiency in an infant with fatal bacille Calmette-Guérin infection. N Engl J Med 1996;335:1956–1961.

99  Newport MJ, Huxley CM, Huston S, Hawrylowicz CM, Oostra BA, Williamson R, Levin M: A mutation in the interferon-γ-receptor gene and susceptibility to mycobacterial infection. N Engl J Med 1996;335:1941–1949.

100  Sander B, Skansen-Saphir U, Damm O, Hakansson L, Andersson J: Sequential production of Th1 and Th2 cytokines in response to live bacillus Calmette-Guérin. Immunology 1995;86:512–518.
101  Lin Y, Zhang M, Hofman FM, Gong J, Barnes PF: Absence of a prominent Th2 cytokine response in human tuberculosis. Infect Immun 1996;64:1351–1356.
102  Conradt P, Kaufmann SHE: Impact of antigen presenting cells on cytokine profiles of human Th clones established after stimulation with *Mycobacterium tuberculosis* antigens. Infect Immun 1995; 63:2079–2081.
103  Bendelac A: Mouse NK1$^+$ T cells. Curr Opin Immunol 1995;7:367–374.
104  Yoshimoto T, Paul WE: CD4$^{pos}$, NK1.1$^{pos}$ T cells promptly produce interleukin-4 in response to in vivo challenge with anti-CD3. J Exp Med 1994;179:1285–1295.
105  Emoto M, Emoto Y, Kaufmann SHE: IL-4 producing CD4$^+$ TCRα/β$^{int}$ liver lymphocyte: Influence of thymus, β$_2$-microglobulin, and NK1.1 expression. Int Immunol 1995;7:1729–1739.
106  Emoto M, Emoto Y, Kaufmann SHE: Bacille Calmette-Guérin and interleukin-12 down-modulate interleukin-4-producing CD4$^+$ NK1$^+$ T lymphocytes. Eur J Immunol 1997;27:183–188.
107  Wahl SM: Transforming growth factor β: The good, the bad, and the ugly. J Exp Med 1994;180: 1587–1590.
108  Dahl KE, Shiratsuchi H, Hamilton BD, Ellner JJ, Toossi Z: Selective induction of transforming growth factor beta in human monocytes by lipoarabinomannan of *Mycobacterium tuberculosis*. Infect Immun 1996;64:399–405.
109  Hirsch CS, Hussain R, Toossi Z, Dawood G, Shahid F, Ellner JJ: Cross-modulation by transforming growth factor beta in human tuberculosis: Suppression of antigen-driven blastogenesis and interferon gamma production. Proc Natl Acad Sci USA 1996;93:3193–3198.
110  DeLibero G, Flesch I, Kaufmann SHE: Mycobacteria reactive Lyt2$^+$ T cell lines. Eur J Immunol 1988;18:59–66.
111  Kumararatne DS, Pithie AS, Drysdale P, Gaston JS, Kiessling R, Iles PB, Ellis CJ, Innes J, Wise R: Specific lysis of mycobacterial antigen-bearing macrophages by class II MHC-restricted polyclonal T cell lines in healthy donors or patients with tuberculosis. Clin Exp Immunol 1990;80:314–323.
112  Mustafa AS, Godal T: BCG induced CD4$^+$ cytotoxic T cells from BCG vaccinated healthy subjects: Relation between cytotoxicity and suppression in vitro. Clin Exp Immunol 1987;69:255–262.
113  McDonough KA, Kress Y: Cytotoxicity for lung epithelial cells is a virulence-associated phenotype of *Mycobacterium tuberculosis*. Infect Immun 1995;63:4802–4811
114  Chan J, Fujiwara T, Brennan P, McNeil M, Turco SJ, Sibille JC, Snapper M, Aisen P, Bloom BR: Microbial glycolipids: Possible virulence factors that scavenge oxygen radicals. Proc Natl Acad Sci USA 1989;86:2453–2457.
115  Kägi D, Ledermann B, Bürki K, Hengartner H, Zinkernagel RM: CD8$^+$ T cell-mediated protection against an intracellular bacterium by perforin-dependent cytotoxicity. Eur J Immunol 1994;24: 3068–3072.
116  Laochumroonvorapong P, Wang J, Liu C-C, Ye W, Moreira A, Elkon K, Freedman VH, Kaplan G: Perforin, a cytotoxic molecule which mediates cell necrosis, is not required for the early control of mycobacterial infection in mice. Infect Immun 1997;65:127–132.
117  Cerottini JC, MacDonald HR: The cellular basis of T-cell immunology. Annu Rev Immunol 1989; 7:77–89.
118  Constant S, Zain M, West J, Pasqualini T, Ranney P, Bottomly K: Are primed CD4$^+$ T lymphocytes different from unprimed cells? Eur J Immunol 1994;24:1073–1079.
119  Mackay CR: T-cell memory: The connection between function, phenotype and migration pathways. Immunol Today 1991;12:189–192.
120  Bradley LM, Duncan DD, Yoshimoto K, Swain SL: Memory effectors: A potent, IL-4-secreting helper T cell population that develops in vivo after restimulation with antigen. J Immunol 1993; 150:3119–3130.
121  Lefford MJ, McGregor DD: Immunological memory in tuberculosis. I. Influence of persisting viable organisms. Cell Immunol 1974;14:417–428.
122  North RJ: Nature of 'memory' in T-cell-mediated antibacterial immunity: Anamnestic production of mediator T cells. Infect Immun 1975;12:754–760.

123  Andersen P, Andersen AB, Sorensen AL, Nagai S: Recall of long-lived immunity to *Mycobacterium tuberculosis* infection in mice. J Immunol 1995;154:3359–3372.

124  Dianzani U, Luqman M, Rojo J, Yagi J, Baron JL, Woods A, Janeway CA, Bottomly K: Molecular associations on the T cell surface correlate with immunological memory. Eur J Immunol 1990;20: 2249–2257.

125  Griffin JP, Harshan KV, Born WK, Orme IM: Kinetics of accumulation of gamma delta receptor-bearing T lymphocytes in mice infected with live mycobacteria. Infect Immun 1991;59:4263–4265.

126  Bell EB, Sparshott SM: Interconversion of CD45R subsets of CD4 T cells in vivo. Nature 1990; 348:163–166.

127  Sprent J, Tough DF: Lymphocyte life-span and memory. Science 1994;265:1395–1400.

128  Michie CA, McLean A, Alcock C, Beverley PC: Lifespan of human lymphocyte subsets defined by CD45 isoforms. Nature 1992;360:264–265.

129  Tough DF, Sprent J: Turnover of naive- and memory-phenotype T cells. J Exp Med 1994;179: 1127–1135.

130  Brandt L, Oettinger T, Holm A, Andersen P: Key epitopes on the ESAT-6 antigen recognized in mice during the recall of protective immunity to *Mycobacterium tuberculosis*. J Immunol 1996;157: 3527–3533.

131  Andersen P, Heron I: Specificity of a protective memory immune response against *Mycobacterium tuberculosis*. Infect Immun 1993;61:844–851.

132  Closs O, Harboe M, Axelsen NH, Bunch-Christensen K, Magnusson M: The antigens of *Mycobacterium bovis*, strain BCG, studied by crossed immunoelectrophoresis: A reference system. Scand J Immunol 1980;12:249–263.

133  Bergh S, Cole ST: MycDB: An integrated mycobacterial database. Mol Microbiol 1994;12:517–534.

134  Andersen P: Host responses and antigens involved in protective immunity to *Mycobacterium tuberculosis*. Scand J Immunol 1997;45:115–131.

135  Andersen P, Askgaard D, Ljungqvist L, Bennedsen J, Heron I: Proteins released from *Mycobacterium tuberculosis* during growth. Infect Immun 1991;59:1905–1910.

136  Daugelat S, Gulle H, Schoel B, Kaufmann SH: Secreted antigens of *Mycobacterium tuberculosis*: Characterization with T lymphocytes from patients and contacts after two-dimensional separation. J Infect Dis 1992;166:186–190.

137  Lee BY, Hefta SA, Brennan PJ: Characterization of the major membrane protein of virulent *Mycobacterium tuberculosis*. Infect Immun 1992;60:2066–2074.

138  Nagai S, Wiker HG, Harboe M, Kinomoto M: Isolation and partial characterization of major protein antigens in the culture fluid of *Mycobacterium tuberculosis*. Infect Immun 1991;59:372–382.

139  Kadival GV, Chaparas SD, Hussong D: Characterization of serologic and cell-mediated reactivity of a 38-kDa antigen isolated from *Mycobacterium tuberculosis*. J Immunol 1987;139:2447–2451.

140  Young RA, Bloom BR, Grosskinsky CM, Ivanyi J, Thomas D, Davis RW: Dissection of *Mycobacterium tuberculosis* antigens using recombinant DNA. Proc Natl Acad Sci USA 1985;82:2583–2587.

141  Mustafa AS, Oftung F, Deggerdal A, Gill HK, Young RA, Godal T: Gene isolation with human T lymphocyte probes. Isolation of a gene that expresses an epitope recognized by T cells specific for *Mycobacterium bovis* BCG and pathogenic mycobacteria. J Immunol 1988;141:2729–2733.

142  Boesen H, Jensen BN, Wilcke T, Andersen P: Human T-cell responses to secreted antigen fractions of *Mycobacterium tuberculosis*. Infect Immun 1995;63:1491–1497.

143  Kawamura I, Yang J, Takaesu Y, Fujita M, Nomoto K, Mitsuyama M: Antigen provoking gamma interferon production in response to *Mycobacterium bovis* BCG and functional difference in T-cell responses to this antigen between viable and killed BCG-immunized mice. Infect Immun 1994;62: 4396–4403.

144  Ben-Nun A, Mendel I, Sappler G, Kerlero-de-Rosbo N: A 12-kDa protein of *Mycobacterium tuberculosis* protects mice against experimental autoimmune encephalomyelitis. Protection in the absence of shared T cell epitopes with encephalitogenic proteins. J Immunol 1995;154:2939–2948.

145  Roche PW, Winter N, Triccas JA, Feng CG, Britton WJ: Expression of *Mycobacterium tuberculosis* MPT64 in recombinant *Mycobacterium smegmatis*: Purification, immunogenicity and application to skin tests for tuberculosis. Clin Exp Immunol 1996;103:226–232.

146  Herrmann JL, O'Gaora PO, Gallagher A, Thole JER, Young DB: Bacterial glycoproteins: A link between glycosylation and proteolytic cleavage of a 19 kDa antigen from *Mycobacterium tuberculosis*. EMBO J 1996;15:3547–3554.

147  Young DB, Lamb JR: T lymphocytes respond to solid-phase antigen: A novel approach to the molecular analysis of cellular immunity. Immunology 1986;59:167–171.

148  Mehra V, Bloom BR, Torigian VK, Mandich D, Reichel M, Young SM, Salgame P, Convit J, Hunter SW, McNeil M, Brennan PJ, Rea TH, Modlin RL: Characterization of *Mycobacterium leprae* cell wall-associated proteins with the use of T lymphocyte clones. J Immunol 1989;142:2873–2878.

149  Torres M, Mendez-Sampeiro P, Jimenez-Zamudio L, Teran L, Camarena A, Quezada R, Ramos E, Sada E: Comparison of the immune response against *Mycobacterium tuberculosis* antigens between a group of patients with active pulmonary tuberculosis and healthy household contacts. Clin Exp Immunol 1994;96:75–78.

150  Andersen P, Askgaard D, Gottschau A, Bennedsen J, Nagai S, Heron I: Identification of immunodominant antigens during infection with *Mycobacterium tuberculosis*. Scand J Immunol 1992;36:823–831.

151  Gulle H, Schoel B, Kaufmann SH: Direct blotting with viable cells of protein mixtures separated by two-dimensional gel electrophoresis. J Immunol Methods 1990;133:253–261.

152  Andersen P, Heron I: Simultaneous electroelution of whole SDS-polyacrylamide gels for the direct cellular analysis of complex protein mixtures. J Immunol Methods 1993;161:29–39.

153  Schoel B, Gulle H, Kaufmann SH: Heterogeneity of the repertoire of T cells of tuberculosis patients and healthy contacts to *Mycobacterium tuberculosis* antigens separated by high-resolution techniques. Infect Immun 1992;60:1717–1720.

154  Hasløv K, Andersen A, Nagai S, Gottschau A, Sorensen T, Andersen P: Guinea pig cellular immune responses to proteins secreted by *Mycobacterium tuberculosis*. Infect Immun 1995;63:804–810.

154a  Pollock JM, Andersen P: The potential of the ESAT-6 antigen secreted by virulent mycobacteria for specific diagnosis of tuberculosis. J Infect Dis 1997;175:1251–1254.

154b  Pollock JM, Andersen P: Predominant recognition of the ESAT-6 in the first phase of infection with *Mycobacterium bovis* in cattle. Infect Immun 1997;65:2587–2592.

155  Sorensen AL, Nagai S, Houen G, Andersen P, Andersen AB: Purification and characterization of a low-molecular-mass T-cell antigen secreted by *Mycobacterium tuberculosis*. Infect Immun 1995;63:1710–1717.

156  Alavi MR, Affronti LF: Induction of mycobacterial proteins during phagocytosis and heat shock: A time interval analysis. J Leukoc Biol 1994;55:633–641.

157  Lee BY, Horwitz MA: Identification of macrophage and stress-induced proteins of *Mycobacterium tuberculosis*. J Clin Invest 1995;96:245–249.

158  Tascon RE, Colston MJ, Ragno S, Stavropoulos E, Gregory D, Lowrie DB: Vaccination against tuberculosis by DNA injection. Nat Med 1996;2:888–892.

159  Hess J, Gentschev I, Miko D, Welzel M, Ladel C, Goebel W, Kaufmann SH: Superior efficacy of secreted over somatic antigen display in recombinant Salmonella vaccine induced protection against listeriosis. Proc Natl Acad Sci USA 1996;93:1458–1463.

159a  Hess J, Dietrich G, Gentschev I, Miko D, Goebel W, Kaufmann SHE: Protection against murine listeriosis by an attenuated recombinant *Salmonella typhimurium* vaccine secreting the naturally somatic antigen superoxide dismutase. Infect Immun 1997;65:1286–1292.

160  Smith DW: Protective effect of BCG in experimental tuberculosis. Adv Tuberc Res 1985;22:1–97.

161  Fine PE: The BCG story: Lessons from the past and implications for the future. Rev Infect Dis 1989;11(suppl 2):353–359.

162  Fine PE: Variation in protection by BCG: Implications of and for heterologous immunity. Lancet 1995;346:1339–1345.

163  Hart PD, Sutherland I: BCG and vole bacillus vaccines in the prevention of tuberculosis in adolescence and early adult life. Br Med J 1977;ii:293–295.

164 Dahlstrom G: Tuberculosis in BCG vaccinated and non-vaccinated young adults. A comparative prognostic study. Acta Tuberc Scand 1953;suppl 32.

165 Colditz GA, Berkey CS, Mosteller F, Brewer TF, Wilson ME, Burdick E, Fineberg HV: The efficacy of bacillus Calmette-Guérin vaccination of newborns and infants in the prevention of tuberculosis: Meta-analyses of the published literature. Pediatrics 1995;96:29–35.

166 al-Kassimi FA, al-Hajjaj MS, al-Orainey IO, Bamgboye EA: Does the protective effect of neonatal BCG correlate with vaccine-induced tuberculin reaction? Am J Respir Crit Care Med 1995;152: 1575–1578.

167 Stanford JL, Shield MJ, Rook GA: How environmental mycobacteria may predetermine the protective efficacy of BCG. Tubercle 1981;62:55–62.

168 Rook GA, Bahr GM, Stanford JL: The effect of two distinct forms of cell-mediated response to mycobacteria on the protective efficacy of BCG. Tubercle 1981;62:63–68.

169 Palmer CE, Long MW: Effects of infection with atypical mycobacteria on BCG vaccination and tuberculosis. Am Rev Respir Dis 1966;94:553–568.

170 Harboe M, Oettinger T, Wiker HG, Rosenkrands I, Andersen P: Evidence for occurrence of the ESAT-6 protein in *Mycobacterium tuberculosis* and virulent *Mycobacterium bovis* and for its absence in *Mycobacterium bovis* BCG. Infect Immun 1996;64:16–22.

171 Ravn P, Boesen H, Pedersen BK, Andersen P: Human T cell responses induced by vaccination with *M. bovis* bacillus Calmette-Guérin. J Immunol 1997;58:1949–1955.

172 Ribi E, Larson C, Wicht W, List R, Goode G: Effective nonliving vaccine against experimental tuberculosis in mice. J Bacteriol 1966;91:975–983.

173 Ribi E, Anacker RL, Brehmer W, Goode G, Larson CL, List RH, Milner KC, Wicht WC: Factors influencing protection against experimental tuberculosis in mice by heat-stable cell wall vaccines. J Bacteriol 1966;92:869–879.

174 Masihi KN, Brehmer W, Azuma I, Lange W, Muller S: Stimulation of chemiluminescence and resistance against aerogenic influenza virus infection by synthetic muramyl dipeptide combined with trehalose dimycolate. Infect Immun 1984;43:233–237.

175 Masihi KN, Lange W, Brehmer W, Ribi E: Immunobiological activities of nontoxic lipid A: Enhancement of nonspecific resistance in combination with trehalose dimycolate against viral infection and adjuvant effects. Int J Immunopharmacol 1986;8:339–345.

176 Mackaness GB: The relationship of delayed hypersensitivity to acquired cellular resistance. Br Med Bull 1967;23:52–54.

177 Orme IM: Induction of nonspecific acquired resistance and delayed-type hypersensitivity, but not specific acquired resistance in mice inoculated with killed mycobacterial vaccines. Infect Immun 1988;56:3310–3312.

178 Orme IM, Andersen P, Boom WH: T cell response to *Mycobacterium tuberculosis*. J Infect Dis 1993;167:1481–1497.

179 Andersen P: Effective vaccination of mice against *Mycobacterium tuberculosis* infection with a soluble mixture of secreted mycobacterial proteins. Infect Immun 1994;62:2536–2544.

180 Horwitz MA, Lee BW, Dillon BJ, Harth G: Protective immunity against tuberculosis induced by vaccination with major extracellular proteins of *Mycobacterium tuberculosis*. Proc Natl Acad Sci USA 1995;92:1530–1534.

181 Roberts AD, Sonnenberg MG, Ordway DJ, Furney SK, Brennan PJ, Belisle JT, Orme IM: Characteristics of protective immunity engendered by vaccination of mice with purified culture filtrate protein antigens of *Mycobacterium tuberculosis*. Immunology 1995;85:502–508.

182 Hubbard RD, Flory CM, Collins FM: Immunization of mice with mycobacterial culture filtrate proteins. Clin Exp Immunol 1992;87:94–98.

183 Pal PG, Horwitz MA: Immunization with extracellular proteins of *Mycobacterium tuberculosis* induces cell-mediated immune responses and substantial protective immunity in a guinea pig model of pulmonary tuberculosis. Infect Immun 1992;60:4781–4792.

184 Bomford R: The comparative selectivity of adjuvants for humoral and cell-mediated immunity. II. Effect on delayed-type hypersensitivity in the mouse and guinea pig, and cell-mediated immunity to tumour antigens in the mouse of Freund's incomplete and complete adjuvants, alhydrogel, *Corynebacterium parvum*, *Bordetella pertussis*, muramyl dipeptide and saponin. Clin Exp Immunol 1980;39:435–441.

185  Bomford R: The comparative selectivity of adjuvants for humoral and cell-mediated immunity. I. Effect on the antibody response to bovine serum albumin and sheep red blood cells of Freund's incomplete and complete adjuvants, alhydrogel, *Corynebacterium parvum, Bordetella pertussis,* muramyl dipeptide and saponin. Clin Exp Immunol 1980;39:426–434.

186  Heeg K, Kuon W, Wagner H: Vaccination of class I major histocompatibility complex (MHC)-restricted murine CD8$^+$ cytotoxic T lymphocytes towards soluble antigens: Immunostimulating-ovalbumin complexes enter the class I MHC-restricted antigen pathway and allow sensitization against the immunodominant peptide. Eur J Immunol 1991;21:1523–1527.

187  Snapper SB, Lugosi L, Jekkel A, Melton RE, Kieser T, Bloom BR, Jacobs WR: Lysogeny and transformation in mycobacteria: Stable expression of foreign genes. Proc Natl Acad Sci USA 1988; 85:6987–6991.

188  Husson RN, James BE, Young RA: Gene replacement and expression of foreign DNA in mycobacteria. J Bacteriol 1990;172:519–524.

189  Aldovini A, Young RA: Humoral and cell-mediated immune responses to live recombinant BCG-HIV vaccines. Nature 1991;351:479–482.

190  Connell ND, Medina-Acosta E, McMaster WR, Bloom BR, Russell DG: Effective immunization against cutaneous leishmaniasis with recombinant bacille Calmette-Guérin expressing the Leishmania surface proteinase gp63. Proc Natl Acad Sci USA 1993;90:11473–11477.

191  Li H, Ulstrup JC, Jonassen TO, Melby K, Nagai S, Harboe M: Evidence for absence of the MPB64 gene in some substrains of *Mycobacterium bovis* BCG. Infect Immun 1993;61:1730–1734.

192  Mahairas GG, Sabo PJ, Hickey MJ, Singh DC, Stover CK: Molecular analysis of genetic differences between *Mycobacterium bovis* BCG and virulent *M. bovis.* J Bacteriol 1996;178:1274–1282.

193  Murray PJ, Aldovini A, Young RA: Manipulation and potentiation of antimycobacterial immunity using recombinant bacille Calmette-Guérin strains that secrete cytokines. Proc Natl Acad Sci USA 1996;93:934–939.

194  Khan CM, Villarreal-Ramos B, Pierce RJ, Demarco-de-Hormaeche R, McNeill H, Ali T, Chatfield S, Capron A, Dougan G, Hormaeche CE: Construction, expression, and immunogenicity of multiple tandem copies of the *Schistosoma mansoni* peptide 115–131 of the P28 glutathione S-transferase expressed as C-terminal fusions to tetanus toxin fragment C in a live aro-attenuated vaccine strain of Salmonella. J Immunol 1994;153:5634–5642.

195  Khan CM, Villarreal-Ramos B, Pierce RJ, Riveau G, Demarco-de-Hormaeche R, McNeill H, Ali T, Fairweather N, Chatfield S, Capron A, Dougan G, Hormaeche CE: Construction, expression, and immunogenicity of the *Schistosoma mansoni* P28 glutathione S-transferase as a genetic fusion to tetanus toxin fragment C in a live Aro attenuated vaccine strain of Salmonella. Proc Natl Acad Sci USA 1994;91:11261–11265.

196  Lyons J, Sinos C, Destree A, Caiazzo T, Havican K, McKenzie S, Panicali D, Mahr A: Expression of *Mycobacterium tuberculosis* and *Mycobacterium leprae* proteins by vaccinia virus. Infect Immun 1990;58:4089–4098.

197  Baumgart KW, McKenzie KR, Radford AJ, Ramshaw I, Britton WJ: Immunogenicity and protection studies with recombinant mycobacteria and vaccinia vectors coexpressing the 18-kilodalton protein of *Mycobacterium leprae.* Infect Immun 1996;64:2274–2281.

198  Curtiss R III: Attenuated *Salmonella* strains as live vectors for the expression of foreign antigens; in Woodrow GC, Levine MM (eds): New Generation Vaccines. New York, Dekker, 1990, pp 161–188.

199  Norman E, Dellagostin OA, McFadden J, Dale JW: Gene replacement by homologous recombination in *Mycobacterium bovis.* Mol Microbiol 1995;16:755–760.

200  Balasubramanian V, Pavelka MS, Bardarov SS, Martin J, Weisbrod TR, McAdam RA, Bloom BR, Jacobs WR: Allelic exchange in *Mycobacterium tuberculosis* with long linear recombination substrates. J Bacteriol 1996;178:273–279.

201  Reyrat JM, Berthet FX, Gicquel B: The urease locus of *Mycobacterium tuberculosis* and its utilization for the demonstration of allelic exchange in *Mycobacterium bovis* bacillus Calmette-Guérin. Proc Natl Acad Sci USA 1995;92:8768–8772.

202  McAdam RA, Weisbrod TR, Martin J, Scuderi JD, Brown AM, Cirillo JD, Bloom BR, Jacobs WR: In vivo growth characteristics of leucine and methionine auxotrophic mutants of *Mycobacterium bovis* BCG generated by transposon mutagenesis. Infect Immun 1995;63:1004–1012.

203  Guleria I, Teitelbaum R, McAdam RA, Kalpana G, Jacobs WR, Bloom BR: Auxotrophic vaccines for tuberculosis. Nat Med 1996;2:334–337.

204  Montgomery DL, Shiver JW, Leander KR, Perry HC, Friedman A, Martinez D, Ulmer JB, Donnelly JJ, Liu MA: Heterologous and homologous protection against influenza A by DNA vaccination: Optimization of DNA vectors. DNA Cell Biol 1993;12:777–783.

205  Ulmer JB, Donnelly JJ, Parker SE, Rhodes GH, Felgner PL, Dwarki VJ, Gromkowski SH, Deck RR, DeWitt CM, Friedman A, Hawe LA, Leander KR, Martinez D, Perry HC, Shiver JW, Montgomery DL, Liu MA: Heterologous protection against influenza by injection of DNA encoding a viral protein. Science 1993;259:1745–1749.

206  Donnelly JJ, Ulmer JB, Liu MA: Immunization with DNA. J Immunol Methods 1994;176:145–152.

207  Huygen K, Content J, Denis O, Montgomery DL, Yawman AM, Deck RR, DeWitt CM, Orme IM, Baldwin S, D'Souza C, Drowart A, Lozes E, Vandenbussche P, Van-Vooren JP, Liu MA, Ulmer JB: Immunogenicity and protective efficacy of a tuberculosis DNA vaccine. Nat Med 1996;2:893–898.

208  Barry MA, Lai WC, Johnston SA: Protection against mycoplasma infection using expression-library immunization. Nature 1995;377:632–635.

209  Collins FM: Protection against mycobacterial disease by means of live vaccines tested in experimental animals; in Kubica GP, Wayne LG (eds.): The Mycobacterial Sourcebook. New York, Dekker, 1984, pp 787–840.

210  Smith DW, Wiegeshaus EH: What animal models can teach us about the pathogenesis of tuberculosis in humans. Rev Infect Dis 1989;11(suppl 2):385–393.

211  Walsh GP, Tan EV, de la Cruz EC, Abalos RM, Villahermosa LG, Young LJ, Cellona RV, Nazareno JB, Horwitz MA: The Philippine cynomolgus monkey (*Macaca fasicularis*) provides a new nonhuman primate model of tuberculosis that resembles human disease. Nat Med 1996;2:430–436.

212  Young DB, Garbe TR: Heat shock proteins and antigens of *Mycobacterium tuberculosis*. Infect Immun 1991;59:3086–3093.

213  Young D, Lathigra R, Hendrix R, Sweetser D, Young RA: Stress proteins are immune targets in leprosy and tuberculosis. Proc Natl Acad Sci USA 1988;85:4267–4270.

214  Peake PW, Britton WJ, Davenport MP, Roche PW, McKenzie KR: Analysis of B-cell epitopes in the variable C-terminal region of the *Mycobacterium leprae* 70-kilodalton heat shock protein. Infect Immun 1993;61:135–141.

215  Shinnick TM, Vodkin MH, Williams JC: The *Mycobacterium tuberculosis* 65-kilodalton antigen is a heat shock protein which corresponds to common antigen and to the *Escherichia coli* GroEL protein. Infect Immun 1988;56:446–451.

216  Rinke de Wit TF, Bekelie S, Osland A, Miko TL, Hermans PW, van Soolingen D, Drijfhout JW, Schoningh R, Janson AA, Thole JE: Mycobacteria contain two groEL genes: The second *Mycobacterium leprae* groEL gene is arranged in an operon with groES. Mol Microbiol 1992;6:1995–2007.

217  Clemens DL, Lee BY, Horwitz MA: Purification, characterization, and genetic analysis of *Mycobacterium tuberculosis* urease, a potentially critical determinant of host-pathogen interaction. J Bacteriol 1995;177:5644–5652.

218  Harth G, Clemens DL, Horwitz MA: Glutamine synthetase of *Mycobacterium tuberculosis*: Extracellular release and characterization of its enzymatic activity. Proc Natl Acad Sci USA 1994;91:9342–9346.

219  Romain F, Augier J, Pescher P, Marchal G: Isolation of a proline-rich mycobacterial protein eliciting delayed-type hypersensitivity reactions only in guinea pigs immunized with living mycobacteria. Proc Natl Acad Sci USA 1993;90:5322–5326.

220  Romain F, Laqueyrerie A, Militzer P, Pescher P, Chavarot P, Lagranderie M, Auregan G, Gheorghiu M, Marchal G: Identification of a *Mycobacterium bovis* BCG 45/47-kilodalton antigen complex, an immunodominant target for antibody response after immunization with living bacteria. Infect Immun 1993;61:742–750.

221  Dobos KM, Khoo KH, Swiderek KM, Brennan PJ, Belisle JT: Definition of the full extent of glycosylation of the 45-kilodalton glycoprotein of *Mycobacterium tuberculosis*. J Bacteriol 1996;178:2498–2506.

222   Andersen AB, Andersen P, Ljungqvist L: Structure and function of a 40,000-molecular-weight protein antigen of *Mycobacterium tuberculosis*. Infect Immun 1992;60:2317–2323.
223   Andersen AB, Ljungqvist L, Olsen M: Evidence that protein antigen b of *Mycobacterium tuberculosis* is involved in phosphate metabolism. J Gen Microbiol 1990;136:477–480.
224   Young DB, Garbe TR: Lipoprotein antigens of *Mycobacterium tuberculosis*. Res Microbiol 1991; 142:55–65.
225   Wiker HG, Harboe M: The antigen 85 complex: A major secretion product of *Mycobacterium tuberculosis*. Microbiol Rev 1992;56:648–661.
226   Belisle JT, Sievert T, Takayana K, Besra GS: Identification of a mycolyltransferase from *Mycobacterium tuberculosis* and the coincident definition of the physiological function of antigen 85B. In program of the 30th Joint Conference on Tuberculosis and Leprosy. US-Japan Cooperative Medical Science Program. NIAID. Fort Collins, NIH, 1995, pp 212–216.
227   Abou-Zeid C, Garbe T, Lathigra R, Wiker HG, Harboe M, Rook GA, Young DB: Genetic and immunological analysis of *Mycobacterium tuberculosis* fibronectin-binding proteins. Infect Immun 1991;59:2712–2718.
228   Menozzi FD, Rouse JH, Alavi M, Laude-Sharp M, Muller J, Bischoff R, Brennan P, Locht C: Identification of a heparin-binding hemagglutinin present in mycobacteria. J Exp Med 1996;184: 993–1001.
229   Wiker HG, Nagai S, Harboe M, Ljungqvist L: A family of cross-reacting proteins secreted by *Mycobacterium tuberculosis*. Scand J Immunol 1992;36:307–319.
230   Kusunose E, Ichihara K, Noda Y, Kusunose M: Superoxide dismutase from *Mycobacterium tuberculosis*. J Biochem Tokyo 1976;80:1343–1352.
231   Garbe T, Harris D, Vordermeier M, Lathigra R, Ivanyi J, Young D: Expression of the *Mycobacterium tuberculosis* 19-kilodalton antigen in *Mycobacterium smegmatis*: Immunological analysis and evidence of glycosylation. Infect Immun 1993;61:260–267.
232   Verbon A, Hartskeerl RA, Schuitema A, Kolk AH, Young DB, Lathigra R: The 14,000-molecular-weight antigen of *Mycobacterium tuberculosis* is related to the alpha-crystallin family of low-molecular-weight heat shock proteins. J Bacteriol 1992;174:1352–1359.
233   Chang Z, Primm TP, Jakana J, Lee IH, Serysheva I, Chiu W, Gilbert HF, Quiocho FA: *Mycobacterium tuberculosis* 16-kDa antigen (Hsp 16.3) functions as an oligomeric structure in vitro to supress thermal aggregation. J Biol Chem 1996;271:7218–7223.
234   Mehra V, Bloom BR, Bajardi AC, Grisso CL, Sieling PA, Alland D, Convit J, Fan XD, Hunter SW, Brennan PJ, Rea TH, Modlin RL: A major T cell antigen of *Mycobacterium leprae* is a 10-kD heat-shock cognate protein. J Exp Med 1992;175:275–284.
235   Mande SC, Mehra V, Bloom BR, Hol WG: Structure of the heat shock protein chaperonin-10 of *Mycobacterium leprae*. Science 1996;271:203–207.

Prof. Dr. S.H.E. Kaufmann, Department of Immunology, University of Ulm,
D–89070 Ulm (Germany)
Tel. +49 731 502 3361 or 3360, fax +49 731 502 3367,
e-mail stefan.kaufmann@medizin.uni-ulm.de

Liew FY, Cox FEG (eds): Immunology of Intracellular Parasitism.
Chem Immunol. Basel, Karger, 1998, vol 70, pp 60–80

..........................

# Experimental Cutaneous Leishmaniasis: Induction and Regulation of T Cells following Infection of Mice with *Leishmania major*

*Phillip Scott, Jay P. Farrell*

Department of Pathobiology, School of Veterinary Medicine, University of
Pennsylvania, Philadelphia, Pa., USA

## Introduction

Leishmaniasis is a widespread and debilitating protozoal disease of humans and animals. Kala-azar, or visceral leishmaniasis, is often fatal in the absence of drug treatment. Cutaneous leishmaniasis, while not fatal, can leave disfiguring scars upon healing or, alternatively, lead to long-term chronic infections, such as diffuse cutaneous leishmaniasis (DCL), mucocutaneous leishmaniasis (MCL) or leishmaniasis recidivans (also called tuberculoid or lupoid leishmaniasis). Some of the more common species of *Leishmania* causing cutaneous disease include *L. major* and *L. tropica* in the Old World, and *L. mexicana, L. amazonensis* and *L. braziliensis* in the New World. In all cases, these organisms are transmitted by a sandfly, which inoculates the promastigote stage of the parasite into the host. These promastigotes rapidly infect macrophages, transform to amastigote forms and multiply within the phagolysosome. After several cycles of replication, the organisms rupture the macrophage and reinvade other macrophages. Immunologic control of the disease is believed to be primarily through the generation of T cells that produce IFN-$\gamma$, which activates macrophage leishmanicidal activity. This chapter focuses on the events involved in the differentiation and regulation of Th cell subsets following experimental infection of mice with *L. major*. Several additional reviews that cover various aspects of the immunology of leishmaniasis have been published in the last several years [1–3].

Because patients exhibit a spectrum of clinical presentations correlating with their degree of cell-mediated immunity, leishmaniasis has been characterized as a spectral disease [4]. For example, patients with DCL fail to mount a cell-mediated immune response following infection, and thus are unable to control parasite proliferation. These patients are of great interest and highlight the importance of cell-mediated immunity in controlling this disease. Other patients develop a cell-mediated immune response and yet are still unable to heal. For example, MCL patients exhibit a very strong cell-mediated immune response, and eliminate most of the parasites from their lesions. However, in spite of their ability to control the parasites, these patients apparently are unable to down-regulate their immune response, and hence fail to heal. Leishmaniasis recidivans is an immunologically similar nonhealing form of cutaneous leishmaniasis characterized by persisting primary lesions with few if any parasites, and a persisting inflammatory response [5]. At present, we have no understanding of the mechanism of pathogenesis in MCL of leishmaniasis recidivans patients, and drug treatment in patients with any of these chronic forms of leishmaniasis is often unsuccessful.

Experimental infections with *Leishmania* in mice can mimic several forms of human cutaneous leishmaniasis. Some strains of mice, such as BALB/c, are highly susceptible to *L. major* infection and fail to develop a cell-mediated response to the parasite. Since these animals develop metastatic lesions, they are often considered as a model for DCL. In contrast, other strains of mice, such as C3H, C57BL/6 and 129, develop self-healing lesions associated with a strong cell-mediated immunity [3, 6, 7]. The course of infection in these animals is similar to that observed in patients with self-healing lesions. Murine infections with other species of *Leishmania* may lead to a somewhat different pattern of resistance and susceptibility. For example, mice that are resistant to *L. major* develop nonhealing lesions following infection with *L. amazonensis* [8–10], suggesting that parasite-specific factors have an important role to play in disease outcome.

Studies in the early 1980s were crucial in establishing the usefulness of this murine model both for understanding human leishmaniasis and for dissecting the immune system. Thus, Howard et al. [11] found that the extreme susceptibility of BALB/c mice to *L. major* could be abrogated if the animals were sublethally irradiated. Furthermore, these authors found that the induction of resistance could be overcome by transfer of normal CD4+ T cells back into the mice, while transfer of CD4+ T cells from animals that had healed enhanced resistance. Such studies were interpreted according to the understanding of the immune system at the time, namely that *L. major* infection in BALB/c mice preferentially induced a radiation-sensitive T-suppressor cell population. A series of experiments then demonstrated that CD4+ T cells could promote both resistance and susceptibility. More recently, these studies were refined using knockout mice, where it was found that resistance occurred in the absence of CD8+ T cells, but not in the absence of Class II-restricted T cells [12].

When our understanding of T-cell biology shifted in the late 1980s, so too did our interpretation of the experiments described above. Thus, the suppressor cells of the 1980s became the Th2 cells of the 1990s, and it was shown by adoptive transfer of Th1 and Th2 cell lines that Th1 cells mediate resistance, while Th2 cells mediate susceptibility [13]. Furthermore, it was shown that infection in susceptible mice was associated with the preferential production of IL-4, while cells from animals that were resistant to *L. major* produced high levels of IFN-γ and little IL-4 [14–16]. Thus, experimental murine leishmanial infections provided one of the first examples of the importance of Th1 and Th2 cell subsets in disease. Because of the clear differential development of Th1 and Th2 cells in mice infected with *L. major*, this model has been used to define the factors that control the development of CD4+ T cell subsets, and regulate those subsets once they have developed [3, 6, 7].

## Initiation of the Immune Response to *L. major*

Studies of the events leading to Th1 and Th2 cell development in *L. major*-infected animals have shown that IL-4 is important for Th2 cell development, while IL-12 and IFN-γ promote Th1 cell development. For example, depletion of either IL-12 or IFN-γ prior to infection of normally resistant mice abrogates Th1 cell development, leading to Th2 cell dominance and susceptibility [15, 17]. Conversely, neutralization of IL-4 in susceptible BALB/c mice blocks Th2 cell development and such mice develop a Th1 response and self-heal [14]. These results are consistent with in vitro studies unrelated to leishmaniasis demonstrating a role for IL-4 in Th2 cell differentiation and IL-12 in Th1 cell differentiation [18]. Thus, at present the simple model for both in vitro and in vivo Th cell subset development would be that the presence of IL-4 promotes Th2 development, while the presence of IL-12 promotes Th1 cell development.

If cytokines determine which T-cell subsets develop, they must be present soon after infection in order to mediate their influence. A comparison of the early immune responses associated with *L. major* infection in the susceptible BALB/c and resistant C3H mouse can be used to illustrate how the innate immune response contributes to the adaptive immune response. *L. major* infection in both of these mouse strains leads to a rapid enlargement of the lymph nodes draining the site of parasite inoculation. During the first few days of infection, lymph node cells from C3H mice produce IFN-γ, but no IL-4, while cells from BALB/c mice produce less IFN-γ, and substantial amounts of IL-4 [15]. NK cells are the source of the IFN-γ produced at this early stage of infection in C3H mice. NK cell activity is higher in resistant C3H mice than in susceptible BALB/c mice and removal of NK cells reduces IFN-γ production, increases IL-4 production, and decreases parasite clearance [19, 20].

There is by now a long list of studies demonstrating that IL-12 initiates cell-mediated immunity and Th1 cell development during the immune response to many pathogens. In leishmaniasis, *L. major* infection in C3H mice is associated with increased levels of IL-12 production [17]. Neutralization of IL-12 with mAb treatment demonstrated that this early IL-12 is required both for NK cell activation and Th1 cell development. Thus, when C3H mice were treated with anti-IL-12, the mice failed to develop an NK cell response. Furthermore, these mice exhibited enhanced IL-4 production, and a dominant Th2 response at 2 weeks of infection [17]. Consistent with these results are findings demonstrating that treatment of *L. major*-infected BALB/c mice with IL-12, given at the time of infection, enhances Th1 cell development and healing [21, 22], and that IL-12 can facilitate Th1 cell development in a vaccine model for *L. major* [23]. The efficacy of exogenous IL-12 contrasts with IFN-γ, which is unable to permanently induce a Th1 response [24]. Thus, Th1 cell development in C3H mice occurs via a pathway involving IL-12, which subsequently activates NK cells to produce IFN-γ, and both IL-12 and IFN-γ are required for the development of the Th1 response. A likely role for IFN-γ at this early stage of infection is to act on macrophages to up-regulate IL-12 production, which is consistent with the observations that the early kinetics of IL-12 and IFN-γ production are very similar. Finally, the most stringent test for the importance of IL-12 comes from studies with IL-12 p40 knockout mice, which have been shown to be susceptible to *L. major* [25].

The source of the IL-12 produced in vivo after *L. major* infection has not been established. The simplest model would be that IL-12 is produced by macrophages following *L. major* infection. However, macrophages infected in vitro with *L. major* promastigotes fail to produce IL-12 [26, P. Scott and J.P. Farrell, unpubl. data]. This observation suggests that *L. major* silently infects the host [26], although the rapid increase in the size of the lymph nodes draining the site of infection, accompanied by enhanced cytokine production including IL-12, suggests that this is not the case. One explanation for these contradictory results is that the in vitro culture conditions do not adequately mimic conditions in vivo. In this regard, it was found that macrophages infected in vivo with *L. major*, and removed at 24 h, produced IL-12 in vitro [27]. A protein from *L. major*, termed Leif, has been described that stimulates IL-12 production by human monocytes, and could be responsible for the induction of IL-12 [28]. However, it has also been suggested that amastigotes, rather than promastigotes, induce IL-12 production by macrophages [26]. Alternatively, the in vivo source of IL-12 may be another cell type, such as dendritic cells or neutrophils. Finally, another possibility is that macrophages (and/or dendritic cells) are stimulated to produce IL-12 due to the stimulation of the cells by CD40-CD40L interactions, rather than due to parasite molecules. The importance of CD40 and CD40L in the development of resistance was recently demonstrated by experimental infections of mice lacking either CD40 or CD40L [29–31]. *L. major* infection in CD40L knockout mice on a genetically resistant background led to the development of a Th2 response and susceptibility. However, administration of IL-12 at the initiation of the infection completely abrogated this susceptibility [29]. These results suggest that IL-12 production following *L. major* infection is dependent upon up-regulation of CD40L on T cells, and stimulation of CD40 expressing cells (such as macrophages and dendritic cells) to produce IL-12. In summary, the source of the IL-12 following *L. major* infection may not be clear, but the importance of the IL-12 in the development of resistance is well established.

Following infection of BALB/c mice a completely different set of events occurs, highlighted by an early burst of IL-4 production. The source of the early IL-4 has been of great interest, since its presence influences the outcome of infection. Experiments with purified populations of CD4+ T cells indicated that the primary source was CD4+ T cells, although whether this was a unique CD4+ T-cell population was unclear. While the CD4+ NK1.1 T cell has been shown to be a major source of IL-4 under certain circumstances, several studies have indicated that these cells are not required for the early IL-4 burst associated with *L. major* infection in BALB/c mice [32, 33]. Interestingly, however, recent data suggest that a particular parasite antigen may be the principal one recognized by the CD4+ T cells that produce the early IL-4. This antigen, known as LACK, is recognized by a Th1 T-cell clone that transferred protective immunity to BALB/c mice [34, 35]. Originally the rationale for defining the antigen recognized by this clone was that it might be a protective antigen. Indeed, immunization with LACK and IL-12 induced significant protection [35]. What was surprising, however, was that the ablation of the response to LACK could completely reverse susceptibility of BALB/c mice. Thus, transgenic mice carrying a truncated LACK cDNA driven by the MHC class II I-E promoter, which resulted in the expression of LACK in several organs including the thymus, failed to exhibit an IL-4 burst and were more resistant than controls [36]. Thus, LACK appears to be a parasite protein that normally elicits an IL-4 response in BALB/c mice, although under certain circumstances (e.g. immunization) it can expand a population of Th1 cells.

Indeed, expansion of T cells bearing the Va8Vb4 TCR – which is associated with recognition of LACK – is a characteristic of both susceptible and resistant mice [37]. Overall, these data suggest that strong responses to a particular parasite antigen may influence the outcome of infection. They leave unanswered the issues of why such a strong T-cell response occurs to LACK, why it is biased towards IL-4 production, and whether the cells responding are conventional T cells.

While the results obtained by comparing C3H and BALB/c mice present a clear picture of the dual role that IL-4 and IL-12 (and IFN-γ) play in determining Th cell development following infection, a more complicated picture emerges when one examines L. major infections in the resistant C57BL/6 mouse strain. These mice, although ultimately resistant, develop larger lesions with more parasites during the early stage of infection, when compared to C3H mice [19, 20]. Associated with the lack of early resistance is the absence of an NK cell response, and the lack of IFN-γ or IL-12 production during the first week of infection. Moreover, during the first few days of infection, C57BL/6 mice exhibit an IL-4 burst that is similar to that observed in BALB/c mice. Nevertheless, by 7–14 days of infection, IL-12 production is initiated and the IL-4 response is lost [26]. Similarly, early immune responses in CB6F$_1$ mice (a cross between BALB/c and C57BL/6) are characterized by high production of IL-4, yet the mice eventually develop predominantly Th1-type responses and heal [38]. Together, these results are particularly informative since they demonstrate that the presence of IL-4 or IL-12 immediately after infection may not always be predictive of the outcome [39].

The question remains as to what determines the outcome of infection with L. major infection. While all of the data would indicate that IL-4 and IL-12 levels are critical, which of these is the ultimate factor in determining whether Th1 or Th2 cells predominate after L. major infection is unclear. On the one hand, depletion of IL-4 in BALB/c mice promotes Th1 cell development and resistance [14], suggesting that the presence of IL-4 determines susceptibility. On the other hand, depletion of IL-12 in normally resistant mice promotes Th2 development, suggesting that IL-12 determines resistance. Thus, are BALB/c mice susceptible because they produce IL-4 early after infection, or because they fail to produce, or are unresponsive to, IL-12? Several observations suggest the latter. First, it appears that the presence of IL-4 does not predict that animals will be, or remain, susceptible to L. major infection. For example, BALB/c and C57BL/6 mice exhibit similar levels of IL-4 during the first few days of infection, although only BALB/c mice will develop a Th2 response [26, 39]. However, once C57BL/6 mice begin to produce IL-12, which occurs between 7 and 14 days after infection, the animals stop producing IL-4 and develop Th1 cells [26, 39]. This is in contrast to BALB/c mice, in which administration of IL-12 after the initiation of the infection fails to promote Th1 cell development, suggesting a difference in the ability of T cells to respond to IL-12 in these two different mouse strains [21, 22]. Interestingly, it has been shown that T cells cultured in vitro exhibit a genetically based difference in their responsiveness to IL-12, with T cells from BALB/c mice rapidly losing their ability to respond to IL-12 compared with T cells from B10 mice [40]. Further support for the hypothesis that IL-12 dominates over IL-4 comes from studies in C3H or C57BL/6 mice treated with anti-IL-12 mAb. Thus, while genetically resistant mice treated with anti-IL-12 mAb develop a Th2 response and large lesions [17], the maintenance of this Th2 response is dependent upon continued administration of anti-IL-12 mAb. If anti-IL-12 treatment is stopped, mice can revert to a Th1 phenotype and heal [B. Hondo-wicz et al., in press]. Thus, in these mice high levels of IL-4 are not sufficient to maintain a Th2 response, implying that Th1 cells can develop in spite of levels of IL-4 equal to that observed in BALB/c mice. Nevertheless, how does one reconcile these observations with the clear finding that IL-4 plays a central role in Th2 cell development and susceptibility in BALB/c mice, as indicated by anti-IL-4 mAb treatment [14]. One possibility is that the response to IL-4, potentially at the level of IL-12 responsiveness, differs between mice of different backgrounds. Thus, one could argue that in BALB/c mice IL-4 rapidly down-regulates IL-12 receptor expression (either directly or indirectly), while IL-4 does not have the same effect on T cells from C57BL/6 mice. In such a scenario, IL-4 would be involved in maintaining a Th2-dominant response in BALB/c mice, but might be less important in resistant strains, such as C3H and C57BL/6.

This leaves the issue of how to interpret recent controversial studies done with IL-4 knockout mice, where it was reported in one laboratory that IL-4 knockout mice on a BALB/c background still fail to heal after *L. major* infection [41], while results from another laboratory showed that similar mice infected with *L. major* were able to heal [42]. The reasons for the differences in these results have not been explained. One difference between the studies was the parasite strain used. However, while *L. major* strains do exhibit distinct degrees of virulence in mice, and thus might play a role in the differences observed, it is unlikely to be the whole story, since anti-IL-4 treatment has been shown to induce resistance in BALB/c mice with all of the *L. major* strains tested. To best understand this issue, it may be useful to remember that what determines which Th cell subset dominates after *Leishmania* infec-tion, and whether mice are ultimately able to heal, may at times differ. Thus, the long-term outcome of infection may depend on many factors, only one of which is a dominant Th2 response. Furthermore, it is important to note that the terms resistance and susceptibility are rather vague. In experimental leishmaniasis, all animals are susceptible, since they all develop an infection, however there are several degrees of resistance, ranging from control of lesion size to complete healing. Parasite strain, dose and site of parasite inoculation can all alter the relative resistance observed in mice [J. Li, T.J. Nolan, J.P. Farrell, submitted, 38, 43, 44].

Although altering cytokine levels at the initiation of the infection has been the most informative way to define the factors contributing to Th cell differentiation, other experiments also provide insights into the development of Th cell subsets after *L. major* infection. One of the first experiments to show that the outcome of *L. major* infection in BALB/c mice could be altered was done by exposing mice to a sublethal dose of irradiation [11]. When such animals were infected, they were able to heal their infections. However, when the animals were reconstituted with normal spleen cells this resistance was lost. One interpretation of this result is that the magnitude of the initial immune response influences the outcome of infection. Consistent with this interpretation are the results of several other experiments. For example, transfer of low numbers of CD4+ T cells in BALB/c nude or SCID mice renders the animals resistant to *L. major* infection, while transfer of high numbers reconstitutes the susceptibility that is normally seen in BALB/c mice [45, 46]. Similarly, transient treatment of BALB/c mice with anti-CD4 mAb or anti-IL-2 mAb, both of which block the early immune response, leads to the development of resistance [47, 48]. A related observation is that very low doses of parasites can lead to a healing infection in BALB/c mice [43]. The most straightforward way to explain these results is to postulate that in order to achieve sufficient levels of IL-4 to promote Th2 cell development, the initial immune response must be of a certain magnitude, which would depend upon both antigen dose and the presence of sufficient T cells to generate the response.

If the magnitude of the initial immune response influences Th cell differentiation, then it could be postulated that blocking costimulatory molecules might alter the outcome of the infection. Indeed, administration of CTLA4-Ig fusion protein, which blocks CD28-B7 interactions, enhances resistance in BALB/c mice [49]. Associated with this alteration in the outcome of the infection is a loss of the early IL-4 burst normally seen in *L. major*-infected BALB/c mice. Based on these results, one could expect that mice lacking CD28 might have a course of infection substantially different from wild-type littermates. Surprisingly, however, this was not the case, since CD28 knockout mice bred onto either the BALB/c or C57BL/6 background exhibited a course of *L. major* infection similar to the wild-type control mice [50]. While several possible explanations can be provided for the discrepancy between the CTLA4-Ig treatment and infection of CD28 knockout mice, no conclusive evidence has been presented to support any one particular explanation. Recent experiments do suggest, however, that the virulence of the organisms – or the magnitude of the antigen challenge – may determine whether a particular response is CD28 dependent, and thus differences in parasite virulence and dose might influence the results obtained [51]. One of the challenges in this field will be to integrate the increasing amount of information on the role that costimulatory molecules play in T-cell proliferation and apoptosis into our models of Th cell development in experimental leishmaniasis.

### Regulation of Established Immune Responses to *L. major*

Although the mechanisms which control the initial differentiation of naive CD4 + T cells into either Th1- or Th2-type effector cells have been extensively studied, less is known about how T-cell populations are regulated during chronic stages of an *L. major* infection. However, there is considerable evidence from in vitro studies that a variety of factors have the potential to regulate the effector function of differentiated T-helper cell subsets. For example, IFN-γ has been shown to inhibit the growth of Th1 clones and IL-10 will inhibit cytokine production by Th1 cells, suggesting that Th1 and Th2 cells may cross-regulate each other during an immune response [52, 53]. This concept of reciprocal regulation of effector cell populations was originally put forward in the now classic experiments by Parish and his colleagues [reviewed in 54], which defined many of the parameters of 'immune deviation' and demonstrated that once DTH or antibody production was elicited in immunized mice, it was nearly impossible to induce the reciprocal response in individual animals. These studies also suggest that under appropriate conditions, immunization could 'lock in' a CMI versus humoral response. That humoral and cell-mediated responses may be mutually exclusive was first shown to apply to leishmanial infections in a series of pioneering studies by Liew and Howard [55], which demonstrated that CD4 + cells from nonhealing BALB/c mice infected with *L. major* could suppress the generation of DTH responses to leishmanial antigens following transfer to naive mice.

Much of what we currently know about the stability of effector cell responses in *L. major*-infected animals has come from studies directed at understanding how various immunological manipulations alter the initial development of Th1- or Th2-type responses in susceptible or resistant strains of mice. For example, nonspecific treatments of susceptible BALB/c mice with sublethal irradiation, or with administration of cyclosporin A, or with antibody to CD4, will all induce healing [11, 47, 56]. In addition, treatment with recombinant IL-12, CTLA4-Ig or an antibody to IL-2, IL-4, or TGF-β will also promote healing in BALB/c mice [22–24, 49, 57–59]. Importantly, most if not all of these treatments must be administered to mice either prior to, or at the time of, infection, suggesting that they function to influence events in initial T-cell differentiation, rather than function to reverse established T-cell responses. The failure of various cytokine or anticytokine therapies to alter either the course of disease or the phenotype of the immune response when treatment is delayed until the 2nd or 3rd week of infection suggests that once established, polarized Th2-type responses may be much less amenable to immune manipulation.

Although BALB/c mice infected for several weeks with *L. major* have polarized Th2-type responses, they do appear to harbor a small, but significant population of IFN-γ-producing Th1 cells. Low levels of IFN-γ production by antigen-stimulated lymph node cells can be detected through at least day 28 of infection in BALB/c mice [15], and limiting dilution analysis has demonstrated that a significant number of CD4+ cells from BALB/c mice produce IFN-γ through at least 8 weeks of infection [60]. More recently, it has been shown that a CD45RB$^{high}$ subset of CD4+ cells from infected BALB/c mice contain a population of Th1-type cells. These cells produce IFN-γ in vitro and transfer resistance to infection in C.B-17 SCID mice [61]. Thus, a population of Th1 cells develops in mice with polarized Th2-type responses, but are functionally suppressed within the Th2-dominant in vivo environment. These studies raise interesting questions about the mechanisms by which the proliferation and/or effector functions of coexisting populations of Th1 and Th2 cells are regulated during the course of an infectious disease.

The mechanism by which cells from *L. major*-infected mice can be induced to switch from a dominant Th2 to Th1 population, or vice versa, was addressed by measuring the capacity of exogenous IL-4, IFN-γ and IL-12 to alter patterns of cytokine production in vitro. A Th2-dominant population of CD4+ cells from infected BALB/c mice, when cultured for 7 days with antigen presenting cells and leishmanial antigen, produced high levels of IL-4, but low levels of IFN-γ upon restimulation [62]. The addition of IFN-γ and/or IL-12 to these cultures increased IFN-γ production, but had little effect on the ability of the cultured cells to produce IL-4. Even the further addition of anti-IL-4 antibody to cultures treated with IFN-γ and IL-12 did not induce a dramatic Th2 to Th1 switch, despite the fact that these treatments induced a significant increase in IFN-γ production. In contrast, addition of IL-4 to a Th1-dominant population from resistant C57BL/6 mice induced a rapid increase in both IL-4 and IL-10 production and a decrease in IFN-γ production. Thus, IL-4 appears capable of switching a polarized Th1- to a Th2-type population [62]. The capacity of IL-4 to promote a Th1 to Th2 switch in vitro is in keeping with its known ability to promote naive CD4+ T cells to differentiate into Th2 effector cells and its capacity to suppress IFN-γ production by Th1 cell populations [63]. Whether these studies also suggest that Th1 populations may be more amenable to regulation than Th2 populations during infection, or whether additional factors other than those tested regulate the stability of Th2-dominant cell populations, is currently unclear.

An alternative approach to understanding how differentiated CD4+ cells are regulated during infection has been to examine their effector function following transfer into SCID mice. As mentioned above, identification of CD45RB[high] CD4+ cells from chronically infected BALB/c mice as a source of IFN-γ-producing cells, and CD45RB[low] cells as a source of IL-4-producing cells, provided a method to enrich for antigen-specific Th1- and Th2-type cell populations [61]. The CD45RB[high] population transferred resistance to C.B-17 SCID mice, while CD45RB[low] cells transferred enhanced susceptibility to a *L. major* infection. The resistance or susceptibility to infection transferred by the two cell populations can be reversed by treating CD45RB[high] cell recipients with antibody to IFN-γ, and CD45RB[low] cell recipients with antibody to IL-4. Interestingly, SCID mice which received mixtures of the two cell populations failed to resolve their infections suggesting that the Th1-type population was functionally suppressed by the Th2 cells. This in vivo inhibition of Th1 cell function by Th2-type cells was shown to occur via an IL-4-dependent mechanism [61]. Since there is little evidence to suggest that fully differentiated Th1 or Th2 cells can reverse their pattern of cytokine production, it is likely that the cell populations used in these transfer studies were not pure Th1 or Th2 effector cells, but were heterogeneous with respect to either their cytokine production or state of activation. However, the fact that mice receiving a Th2-dominant cell population can be manipulated by anti-IL-4 treatment to expand a population of cells capable of IFN-γ production is clearly evidence that it is possible to switch a Th2-type response to a protective Th1 response.

Although anti-IL-4 antibody treatment can lead to cure of C.B-17 SCID mice following transfer of a Th2-dominant cell population, suggesting that IL-4 is required to maintain a Th2-type response in vivo, anti-IL-4 antibody treatment, as mentioned above, does not consistently induce cure of an active *L. major* infection in intact BALB/c mice. Treatment with high doses of anti-IL-4 antibody initiated after 2 weeks of infection has been shown in one study to dramatically slow lesion development, but not induce a Th2 to Th1 switch [16]. However, another similar study demonstrated that anti-IL-4 treatment may induce cure of infected BALB/c mice when mice were infected with a much lower parasite inoculum [64]. Differences in the response of infected mice to IL-4 treatment may possibly be due to differences in the degree of Th2-type polarization at the time of anti-IL-4 administration, which would probably be greater at week 2 of infection in mice given higher parasite inocula. It is also possible that higher levels of infection elicit other in vivo changes which may influence the response of mice to anti-IL-4 antibody treatment.

Several studies suggest that in vivo infection levels may markedly influence the response of CD4+ subsets to immunological manipulation. Chronically infected BALB/c mice treated with anti-IL-4 antibody at a dose which has no apparent effect on the course of disease or immune response, will resolve their infections and develop Th1-type response if treated simultaneously with an antileishmanial drug such as sodium stibogluconate [64]. Since short-term drug treatment, alone, will reduce parasite numbers, but not induce cure, these results suggest that reductions in infection levels in some way influence the capacity of CD4+ cells to respond to immunotherapy. Even more dramatic evidence that polarized Th2 responses may be switched to protective Th1-type response comes from a study examining the effects of combined chemotherapy and IL-12 in *L. major*-infected BALB/c mice [65]. IL-12 treatment, initiated at 3 weeks of infection to mice with clearly defined Th2-type responses, had marginal effects on the subsequent course of disease or on the levels of IL-4 and IFN-$\gamma$ production by cells from infected mice. However, combined treatment with IL-12 and sodium stibogluconate over a 2-week period induced healing and a clear switch from a Th2- to a Th1-type response. Importantly, healed mice were resistant to reinfection showing that therapy had elicited a switch to a stable Th-type response. Given the capacity of IL-12 to promote naive CD4+ cells to differentiate into Th1 cells and to enhance proliferation and IFN-$\gamma$ production by effector T cells, it is possible that reductions in infection levels create an environment conducive to either the induction of Th1 cell differentiation or the expansion of a small number of pre-existing Th1-type cells which are normally present in these mice. In a similar study, we have also shown that IFN-$\gamma$ treatment may also promote cure of infected BALB/c mice when administered with an antileishmanial drug. In this experiment the development of a protective Th1-type response in these mice required the production of endogenous IL-12 [J. Li, S. Sutterwala, J.P. Farrell, submitted]. Although IFN-$\gamma$ can directly activate macrophage microbicidal functions, the fact that IFN-$\gamma$ therapy has little effect in anti-IL-12 treated mice suggests that it may act, instead, to either suppress Th2 cell functions or enhance Th1 cell development, possibly by acting to enhance IL-12 production.

If high levels of infection in vivo preferentially drive Th2-type responses, reducing infection levels should eventually lead to a reduction in Th2-associated cytokine production and possibly up-regulation of a Th1-type response. This has, indeed, been shown to occur. When *L. major*-infected BALB/c mice were treated with sodium stibogluconate for 12 continuous weeks beginning at 3 weeks of infection, approximately 55% of the mice gave evidence of cure as assessed by their failure to relapse within 5–6 weeks after cessation of treatment [66]. Cytokine analysis showed that these cured mice exhibited a Th1-type response. When challenged, all exhibited positive DTH reactions, and were resistant to reinfection. Thus, in this system, reducing parasite numbers and maintaining them at low numbers for a prolonged period establishes an in vivo environment favorable to expansion of an existing Th1 population or induction of newly derived Th1 cells from a population of naive CD4+ cells.

The observation that prolonged exposure of a drug-treated BALB/c mouse to low levels of infection may induce a Th2 to Th1 switch may have parallels to the studies of Bretscher et al. [43], who have shown that the inoculation of low numbers of *L. major* promastigotes ($1-3 \times 10^2$) into naive BALB/c mice leads to a stable Th1 response, whereas inoculation of higher numbers of promastigotes ($>10^3$) results in the activation of a Th2-type response and progressive disease. It has been suggested that the threshold for Th2 activation may be lower in BALB/c mice than in healing strains, and that a stable CMI response is generated in this strain only by inoculation of very low numbers of parasites [43]. This hypothesis is consistent with earlier studies demonstrating 'immune deviation' in which immunization with low amounts of antigen elicited stable DTH responses and low antibody production, whereas higher antigen doses induced antibody production, but no DTH reactivity as discussed earlier [54, 67, 68]. The early cytokine response to low dose *Leishmania* infections has yet to be analyzed; however, it might be predicted that low parasite inocula may not elicit the early burst in IL-4 production required for Th2 development. If IL-4 production gradually wanes in infected mice treated for a prolonged period of time with antiparasite drugs, it is possible that low levels of infection may preferentially lead to the activation of a Th1 response analogous to that seen in naive mice infected with low numbers of parasites.

An important question relative to the induction of a Th2 to Th1 switch during infection is whether the expanded Th1-type population which develops in healing mice derives from a pre-existing population of Th1 effector cells or is derived from a pool of naive CD4+ cells. Although this question has not been addressed experimentally, there is some evidence to suggest that a pool of pre-existing Th1 cells may facilitate a Th2 to Th1 switch during infection. Long-term drug therapy, which leads to cure of a majority of *L. major*-infected BALB/c mice, leads to cure in less than 10% of mice treated with anti-IFN-γ antibody prior to infection. Anti-IFN-γ treatment of BALB/c mice prior to infection results in reduced IFN-γ production and the development of a more highly polarized Th2-type response compared to that which develops normally [66]. Thus, mice which appear to develop a smaller pool of antigen-specific Th1 cells and exhibit a more polarized Th2-type response prior to drug treatment are far less likely to undergo a Th2 to Th1 switch during prolonged antiparasite chemotherapy. These observations raise obvious questions about treatment of nonhealing forms of human leishmaniasis. A majority of patients with visceral leishmaniasis are cured following several weeks of conventional drug therapy with antimony-based compounds such as sodium stibogluconate. These cured individuals develop positive DTH responses to leishmanial antigens and their cells produce IFN-$\gamma$ following in vitro stimulation [69]. Although there is evidence that patients with nonhealing leishmaniasis exhibit some characteristics of Th2-type responses, including the presence of IL-4 and IL-10 transcripts within parasitized lesions and the production of these cytokines by their peripheral blood cells, there is considerable patient-to-patient variability and it is difficult to compare their responses to those seen in *L. major*-infected BALB/c mice [70–75]. Still, it is tempting to speculate that most individuals with visceral leishmaniasis have less polarized responses, which may be shifted towards Th1 dominance following short-term therapy, while individuals with diffuse cutaneous leishmaniasis, which is notoriously resistant to drug therapy, may have more polarized Th2-type responses.

The observation that treatment of infected BALB/c mice with IL-12, IFN-$\gamma$, or antibody to IL-4 facilitates a Th2 to Th1 switch only when combined with drug therapy suggests that reducing infection levels is a critical step in this process. It is possible that drug treatment reduces the overall level of parasite antigen required to expand a developing Th2-type population. However, it is also possible that drug treatment reduces numbers of parasitized macrophages and that parasitized macrophages function to create a cytokine environment which helps to regulate T-helper cell function. Macrophages may produce IL-10 and TGF-$\beta$ which can, in turn, inhibit the production of IFN-$\gamma$ by T cells or the production of IL-12 and nitric oxide by macrophages [53, 76, 77]. Although anti-IL-10 treatment has not been shown to modify an *L. major* infection in mice, anti-TGF-$\beta$ treatment prior to infection with *L. amazonensis* will promote healing in BALB/c mice [59]. Both IL-10 and TGF-$\beta$ are produced during infection and may be present in high levels in susceptible strains of mice [78, 79]. Although there is little published evidence to suggest that IL-10 and TGF-$\beta$ directly influence the response to therapy, it has been noted that lesion transcript levels for TGF-$\beta$, but not IL-10, are sharply decreased in *L. major*-infected CB6F1 mice induced to heal following treatment with a combination of IL-12 and antibody to IL-4, while TGF-$\beta$ transcript levels remained unchanged in BALB/c mice which failed to heal following similar treatment [79]. Similarly, TGF-$\beta$ transcripts are reduced within lesions of infected BALB/c mice following sodium stibogluconate treatment. Recent studies from this laboratory show that treatment with anti-TGF-$\beta$ may result in a rapid decrease in infection levels in CB6F$_1$ mice without markedly altering the production of IL-4 and IFN-$\gamma$, suggesting that TGF-$\beta$

may inhibit microbicidal functions such as the production of nitric oxide [J. Li, C. Hunter, J.P. Farrell, in preparation]. Whether TGF-β, or other macrophage products, can directly influence a response to immunotherapy and whether drug treatment functions to down-regulate the production of macrophage-derived cytokines as well as reduce parasite numbers has yet to be determined.

The role that T cells play in the resolution of leishmanial lesions may not only be confined to the production of cytokines that activate or deactivate macrophages, since resolution of leishmanial lesions depends upon both elimination of the parasites as well as elimination of the T cells that have infiltrated the lesion site. One major way in which T cells may be eliminated is by programmed cell death, or apoptosis. Two principal mechanisms important for apoptosis of T cells involve fas-fasL and TNF receptor signalling, and interesting results have been obtained pertinent to both apoptosis pathways. Thus, *L. major* infection in fas-deficient mice (lpr/lpr) on an MRL background exhibit increased lesion size, the development of metastatic lesions and increased parasite numbers compared to controls [80, B. Hondowicz, S. Kanaly, M. Nashleanas, P. Scott, in preparation]. The enhanced susceptibility does not appear to be due to the preferential development of Th2 cells, suggesting that apoptosis may contribute to parasite elimination. However, the influence that the lymphoproliferative disease that occurs in these mice might have on leishmaniasis is difficult to assess.

Unexpected results have also been obtained in mice that lack one of the two major TNF receptors. Mice have been developed that lack either the p55 receptor (TNFRp55−/−) [81, 82], p75 receptor (TNFRp75−/−) [83], or both receptors (TNFRp55p75−/−) [unpubl. data]. These mice have been useful in delineating some of the unique functions that these receptors play. The notable characteristics of the mice lacking the p55 receptor are that they are relatively resistant to endotoxin-induced shock, and are relatively susceptible to *Listeria monocytogenes* or *Mycobacterium tuberculosis* [81, 82, 84]. Similarly, we found that TNFRp55−/− mice developed much larger *L. major* lesions, with more parasites, than control animals [85]. However, these animals eventually eliminated the parasites from their lesions, suggesting that TNF signalling via the TNFRp55 is not required for parasite control. Even more unexpected was the finding that in spite of eliminating the parasites, the lesions failed to heal [85]. These nonhealing lesions were composed of large numbers of lymphocytes, suggesting that a defect in lymphocyte apoptosis might be responsible for the maintenance of the lesions. This hypothesis is consistent with several recent studies, which suggest that in certain circumstances TNF may play a role in apoptosis of peripheral lymphocytes. For example, it is known that lpr mice develop a lymphoproliferative disease after 10–12 weeks of age, which is presumed to be due to defective fas-dependent T-cell deletion.

However, when lpr mice were crossed with TNFRp55−/− mice the animals developed lymphoproliferative disease significantly earlier. One possible interpretation of these results is that TNF signalling became important for cell deletion in the absence of fas [86]. Other studies have been done with lpr mice that have been crossed with an influenza hemagglutinin (HA) TCR transgenic mouse, producing an animal in which the influence of fas on both thymic and peripheral antigen-specific T-cell deletion can be assessed [87]. Thus, injection of TCR-specific antigen into a TCR transgenic mouse leads to deletion of both thymic and peripheral T cells. Using the TCR transgenic/lpr mouse, it was found that injection of HA could still induce apoptosis of peripheral T cells, suggesting that fas was not required for T-cell apoptosis. However, when animals were treated with a neutralizing anti-TNF mAb, apoptosis of T cells was abrogated, suggesting that TNF contributes to T-cell apoptosis. It should be pointed out, however, that in animals that have fas, anti-TNF mAb did not abrogate apoptosis, and that in other TCR transgenic/lpr mice a defect in apoptosis was seen without injecting anti-TNF mAb [88]. Nevertheless, these results argue that under certain circumstances, TNF may contribute to peripheral T-cell deletion. The finding that lpr and TNFR receptor knockout mice infected with *L. major* have a defective healing response provides the basis for further exploration of the events involved in controlling and downregulating *L. major*-induced inflammation.

## Conclusions

*L. major* infections have been especially useful for studies of how T-cell responses are regulated in vivo. The fact that different inbred strains of mice develop highly divergent patterns of cutaneous disease which correlate with the differential activation of Th1 or Th2 CD4+ T-cell subsets has enabled investigators to assess the function of multiple cytokines in directing the early stages of Th1 and Th2 cell differentiation, as well as to examine how cytokines regulate the function of established Th1- and Th2-type effector cell populations. Studies using this model were some of the first to demonstrate an in vivo role for IL-4 and IL-12 in Th cell subset development, and have led to an understanding of the importance of the innate immune response in determining the adaptive immune response. However, we are just beginning to understand all of the components that are involved in the development of resistance following *L. major* infection. Many important issues have yet to be resolved, some of which include the relative importance of IL-4 and IL-12 in Th cell development, the role that costimulatory molecules play in the innate immune response, and the role that responses to specific parasite antigens (such as Leif or LACK) play in determining the immune response. New areas of understanding are also beginning to emerge regarding the regulation of established T-cell responses. It has now been shown that the immune response during an established *L. major* infection in BALB/c mice, often used as a prime example of a Th2 response, can be switched to a Th1 response and lead to a healing infection. Recent studies also demonstrate that healing of lesions may require TNF, possibly to induce a signal for apoptosis of T cells within lesions. The mechanism(s) involved in Th cell subset development, in the ability to switch an established immune response, or to down-regulate the inflammatory response associated with leishmaniasis, may not yet be completely understood. However, it is clear that there are clinical ramifications to the information already accumulated. Thus, our current understanding of T-cell function in leishmaniasis has provided information that provides the impetus to develop new prophylactic and therapeutic vaccines that incorporate cytokines, leading to the ability to direct the immune response in ways that were never possible in the past.

## Acknowledgements

Grant support: P.S. is supported by NIH AI35914 and AI41880 and is a recipient of a Burroughs Wellcome Award in Molecular Parasitology. J.P.F. is supported by NIH AI-27828.

## References

1    Liew FY, O'Donnell CA: Immunology of leishmaniasis. Adv Parasitol 1993;32:162–259.
2    Bogdan C, Gessner A, Rollinghoff M: Cytokines in leishmaniasis: A complex network of stimulatory and inhibitory interactions. Immunobiology 1993;189:356–396.
3    Reiner SL, Locksley RM: The regulation of immunity to *Leishmania major*. Annu Rev Immunol 1995;13:151–177.
4    Turk JL, Bryceson ADM: Immunologic phenomena in leprosy and related diseases. Adv Immunol 1971;13:209–266.
5    Wyler DJ, Marsden PD: Leishmaniasis; in Warren KS, Mahmoud AAF (eds): Tropical and Geographical Medicine. New York, McGraw-Hill, 1984, pp 270–280.
6    Locksley RM, Scott P: Helper T-cell subsets in mouse leishmaniasis: Induction, expansion and effector function. Immunol Today 1991;12:A58–A61.
7    Scott P: Th cell development and regulation in experimental cutaneous leishmaniasis; in Romagnani S (ed): Th1 and Th2 Cells in Health and Disease. Chem Immunol. Basel, Karger, 1995, vol 63, pp 98–114.
8    Grimaldi G Jr, Moriearty PL, Hoff R: *Leishmania mexicana*: Immunology and histopathology in C3H mice. Exp Parasitol 1980;50:45–56.
9    Barral A, Petersen EA, Sacks DL, Neva FA: Late metastatic leishmaniasis in the mouse. A model for mucocutaneous disease. Am J Trop Med Hyg 1983;32:277–285.
10   Afonso LCC, Scott P: Immune responses associated with the susceptibility of C57BL/10 mice to *Leishmania amazonensis*. Infect Immun 1993;61:2952–2959.

11    Howard JG, Hale C, Liew FY: Immunologic regulation of experimental cutaneous leishmaniasis. IV. Prophylactic effect of sublethal irradiation as a result of abrogation of suppressor T cell generation in mice genetically susceptible to *Leishmania tropica*. J Exp Med 1981;153:557–568.

12    Locksley RM, Reiner SL, Hatam F, Littman DR, Killeen N: Helper T cells without CD4: Control of leishmaniasis in CD4-deficient mice. Science 1993;261:1448–1451.

13    Scott P, Natovitz P, Coffman RL, Pearce E, Sher A: Immunoregulation of cutaneous leishmaniasis. T cell lines that transfer protective immunity or exacerbation belong to different T helper subsets and respond to distinct parasite antigens. J Exp Med 1988;168:1675–1684.

14    Heinzel FP, Sadick MD, Holaday BJ, Coffman RL, Locksley RM: Reciprocal expression of interferon-gamma or IL-4 during the resolution or progression of murine leishmaniasis. Evidence for expansion of distinct helper T cell subsets. J Exp Med 1989;169:59–72.

15    Scott P: IFN-gamma modulates the early development of Th1 and Th2 responses in a murine model of cutaneous leishmaniasis. J Immunol 1991;147:3149–3155.

16    Chatelain R, Varkila K, Coffman RL: IL-4 induces a Th2 response in *Leishmania major*-infected mice. J Immunol 1992;148:1182–1187.

17    Scharton-Kersten T, Afonso LCC, Wysocka M, Trinchieri G, Scott P: IL-2 is required for natural killer cell activation and subsequent T helper 1 cell development in experimental leishmaniasis. J Immunol 1995;154:5320–5330.

18    O'Garra A, Murphy K: Role of cytokines in determining T-lymphocyte function. Curr Opin Immunol 1994;6:458–466.

19    Scharton TM, Scott P: Natural killer cells are a source of IFN-γ that drives differentiation of CD4 + T cell subsets and induces early resistance to *Leishmania major* in mice. J Exp Med 1993;178:567–577.

20    Scharton-Kersten T, Scott P: The role of the innate immune response in Th1 cell development following *Leishmania major* infection. J Leukoc Biol 1995;57:515–522.

21    Heinzel FP, Rerko RM, Ahmed F, Pearlman E: Endogenous IL-12 is required for control of Th2 cytokine responses. J Immunol 1995;155:730–739.

22    Sypek JP, Chung CL, Mayor SEH, Subramanyam JM, Goldman SJ, Sieburth DS, Wolf SF, Schaub RG: Resolution of cutaneous leishmaniasis: Interleukin-12 initiates a protective Th1 immune response. J Exp Med 1993;177:1797–1802.

23    Afonso LCC, Scharton TM, Vieira LQ, Wysocka M, Trinchieri G, Scott P: The adjuvant effect of interleukin-12 in a vaccine against *Leishmania major*. Science 1994;263:235–237.

24    Sadick MD, Heinzel FP, Holaday BJ, Pu RT, Dawkins RS, Locksley RM: Cure of murine leishmaniasis with anti-interleukin-4 monoclonal antibody. Evidence for a T cell-dependent, interferon-gamma-independent mechanism. J Exp Med 1990;171:115–127.

25    Mattner F, Magram J, Ferrante J, Launois P, Di Padova K, Behin R, Gately MK, Louis JA, Alber G: Genetically resistant mice lacking interleukin-12 are susceptible to infection with *Leishmania major* and mount a polarized Th2 cell response. Eur J Immunol 1996;26:1553–1559.

26    Reiner SL, Zheng S, Wang Z-E, Stowring L, Locksley RM: Leishmania promastigotes evade interleukin-12 induction by macrophages and stimulate a broad range of cytokines from CD4 + T cells during initiation of infection. J Exp Med 1994;179:447–456.

27    Vieira LQ, Hondowicz BD, Afonso LCC, Wysocka M, Trinchieri G, Scott P: Infection with *Leishmania major* induces interleukin-12 production in vivo. Immunol Letters 1994;40:157–161.

28    Skeiky YA, Guderian JA, Benson DR, Bacelar O, Carvalho EM, Kubin M, Badaro R, Trincheiri G, Reed SG: A recombinant *Leishmania* antigen that stimulates human peripheral blood mononuclear cells to express a Th1-type cytokine profile and to produce interleukin-12. J Exp Med 1995; 181:1527–1537.

29    Campbell KA, Ovendale PJ, Kennedy MK, Fanslow WC, Reed SG, Maliszewski CR: CD40 ligand is required for protective cell-mediated immunity to *Leishmania major*. Immunity 1996;4:283–290.

30    Soong L, Su J-C, Grewal IS, Kima P, Sun J, Longley BJ, Ruddle NH, McMahon-Pratt D, Flavell RA: Disruption of CD40-CD40 ligand interactions results in enhanced susceptibility to *Leishmania amazonensis* infection. Immunity 1996;4:263–274.

31    Kamanaka M, Yu P, Yasui T, Yoshida K, Kawabe T, Horii T, Kishimoto T, Kikitana H: Protective role of CD40 in *Leishmania major* infection at two distinct phases of cell-mediated immunity. Immunity 1996;4:275–282.

32  Launois P, Ohteki T, Swihart K, MacDonald HR, Louis JA: In susceptible mice, *Leishmania major* induce very rapid interleukin-4 production by CD4+ T cells which are NK1.1⁻. Eur J Immunol 1996;25:3298–3307.

33  Brown DR, Fowell DJ, Corry DB, Wynn TA, Moskowitz NH, Cheever AW, Locksley RM, Reiner SL: β₂-Microglobulin-dependent NK1.1⁺ T cells are not essential for T helper cell 2 immune responses. J Exp Med 1996;184:1295–1304.

34  Scott P, Caspar P, Sher A: Protection against *Leishmania major* in BALB/c mice by adoptive transfer of a T cell clone recognizing a low molecular weight antigen released by promastigotes. J Immunol 1990;144:1075–1079.

35  Mougneau E, Altare F, Wakil AE, Zheng S, Coppola T, Wang LE, Waldmann R, Locksley RM, Glaichenhaus N: Expression cloning of a protective *Leishmania* antigen. Science 1995;268:563–566.

36  Julia V, Rassoulzadegan M, Glaichenhaus N: Resistance to *Leishmania major* induced by tolerance to a single antigen. Science 1996;274:421–423.

37  Reiner SL, Wang Z-E, Hatam F, Scott P, Locksley RM: Common lineage of Th1 and Th2 subsets in leishmaniasis. Science 1993;259:1457–1460.

38  Nabors GS, Nolan T, Croop W, Li J, Farrell JP: The influence of the site of parasite inoculation on the development of Th1 and Th2 type immune responses in (BALB/c × C57BL/6)F₁ mice infected with *Leishmania major*. Parasite Immunol 1995;17:569–579.

39  Scott P, Eaton A, Gause WC, Zhou XD, Hondowicz B: Early IL-4 production does not predict susceptibility to *Leishmania major*. Exp Parasitol 1996;84:178–187.

40  Guler ML, Gorham JD, Hsieh C-S, Mackey AJ, Steen RG, Dietrich WF, Murphy KM: Genetic suscep- tibility to *Leishmania*: IL-12 responsiveness in Th1 cell development. Science 1996;271:984–986.

41  Noben-Trauth N, Kropf P, Muller I: Susceptibility to *Leishmania major* infection in interleukin-4- deficient mice. Science 1996;271:987–990.

42  Kopf M, Brombacher F, Kohler G, Kienzle G, Widmann K-H, Lefrang K, Humborg C, Ledermann B, Solbach W: IL-4 deficient BALB/c mice resist infection with *Leishmania major*. J Exp Med 1996; 184:1127–1136.

43  Bretscher PA, Wei G, Menon JN, Bielefeldt-Ohmann H: Establishment of stable, cell-mediated immunity that makes 'susceptible' mice resistant to *Leishmania major*. Science 1992;257:539–542.

44  Nabors GS, Farrell JP: Site-specific immunity to *Leishmania major* in SWR mice: The site of infection influences susceptibility and expression of the antileishmanial immune response. Infect Immun 1994;62:3655–3662.

45  Mitchell GF, Curtis JM, Scollay RG, Handman E: Resistance and abrogation of resistance to cutaneous leishmaniasis in reconstituted BALB/c nude mice. Aust J Exp Med Biol Sci 1981;59: 539–554.

46  Varkila K, Chatelain R, Leal LMCC, Coffman RL: Reconstitution of C.B-17 SCID mice with BALB/c T cells initiates a T helper type-1 response and renders them capable of healing *Leishmania major* infection. Eur J Immunol 1993;23:262–268.

47  Titus RG, Ceredig R, Cerottini JC, Louis JA: Therapeutic effect of anti-L3T4 monoclonal antibody GK1.5 on cutaneous leishmaniasis in genetically-susceptible BALB/c mice. J Immunol 1985;135: 2108–2114.

48  Heinzel FP, Rerko RM, Hatam R, Locksley RM: IL-2 is necessary for the progression of leishmani- asis in susceptible murine hosts. J Immunol 1993;150:3924–3931.

49  Corry DB, Reiner SL, Linsley PS, Locksley RM: Differential effects of blockade of CD28-B7 on the development of Th1 or Th2 effector cells in experimental leishmaniasis. J Immunol 1994;153: 4142–4148.

50  Brown DR, Green JM, Moskowitz NH, Davis M, Thompson CB, Reiner SL: Limited role of CD28- mediated signals in T helper subset differentiation. J Exp Med 1996;184:803–810.

51  Kundig TM, Shahinian A, Kawai K, Mittrucker H-W, Sebzda E, Bachmann MF, Mak TW, Ohashi PS: Duration of TCR stimulation determines costimulatory requirement of T cells. Immunity 1996; 5:41–52.

52  Gajewski TF, Fitch FW: Anti-proliferative effect of IFN-γ in immune regulation. I. IFN-γ inhibits the proliferation of Th2 but not Th1 murine helper T lymphocyte clones. J Immunol 1988;140: 4245–4252.

53 Fiorentino DF, Zlotnik A, Vieira P, Mosmann TR, Howard M, Moore KW, O'Garra AJ: IL-10 acts on the antigen-presenting cell to inhibit cytokine production by Th1 cells. J Immunol 1991; 146:3444–3451.

54 Parish CR: Immune deviation: A historical perspective. Immunol Cell Biol 1996;74:449–456.

55 Liew FY, Hale C, Howard JG: Immunologic regulation of experimental cutaneous leishmaniasis. V. Characterization of effector and specific suppressor T cells. J Immunol 1982;128:1917–1922.

56 Solbach W, Forberg K, Rollinghoff M: Effect of T-lymphocyte suppression on parasite burden in *Leishmania major*-infected, genetically susceptible BALB/c mice. Infect Immun 1986;54:909–912.

57 Heinzel FP, Schoenhaut DS, Rerko RM, Rosser LE, Gately MK: Recombinant interleukin-12 cures mice infected with *Leishmania major*. J Exp Med 1993;177:1505–1509.

58 Bryceson ADM: Therapy in man; in Killick-Kendrick R, Peters W (eds): The Leishmaniases in Biology and Medicine. London, Academic Press, 1987, pp 848–907.

59 Barral-Netto M, Barral A, Brownell CE, Skeiky YAW, Ellingsworth LR, Twardzik DR, Reed SG: Transforming growth factor-β in leishmanial infection: A parasite escape mechanism. Science 1992; 257:545–548.

60 Morris L, Troutt AB, Handman E, Kelso A: Changes in the precursor frequencies of IL-4 and IFN-γ secreting CD4+ cells correlate with resolution of lesions in murine cutaneous leishmaniasis. J Immunol 1992;149:2715–2721.

61 Powrie F, Correa-Oliveira R, Mauze S, Coffman RL: Regulatory interactions between CD45RB[high] and CD45RB[low] CD4+ T cells are important for the balance between protective and pathogenic cell-mediated immunity. J Exp Med 1994;179:589–600.

62 Mocci S, Coffman RL: Induction of a Th2 population from a polarized *Leishmania*-specific Th1 population by in vitro culture with IL-4. J Immunol 1995;154:3779–3787.

63 Powrie F, Menon S, Coffman RL: Interleukin-4 and interleukin-10 synergize to inhibit cell-mediated immunity in vivo. Eur J Immunol 1993;23:3043–3049.

64 Nabors GS, Farrell JP: Depletion of interleukin-4 in BALB/c mice with established *Leishmania major* infections increases the efficacy of antimony therapy and promotes Th1-like responses. Infect Immun 1994;62:5498–5504.

65 Nabors GS, Afonso LCC, Farrell JP, Scott P: Switch from a type 2 to a type 1 T helper cell response and cure of established *Leishmania major* infection in mice is induced by combined therapy with interleukin-12 and pentostam. Proc Natl Acad Sci USA 1995;92:3142–3146.

66 Nabors GS, Farrell JP: Successful chemotherapy in experimental leishmaniasis is influenced by the polarity of the T cell response before treatment. J Infect Dis 1996;173:979–986.

67 Lagrange PH, MacKaness GB, Miller TE: Influence of dose and route of antigen injection on the immunological induction of T cells. J Exp Med 1974;139:528–542.

68 Parish CR: The relationship between humoral and cell-mediated immunity. Transplant Rev 1972; 13:35–66.

69 Carvalho EM, Bacellar O, Brownell C, Regis T, Coffman RL, Reed SG: Restoration of IFN-gamma production and lymphocyte proliferation in visceral leishmaniasis. J Immunol 1994;152:5949–5956.

70 Kemp M, Hey AS, Kurtzhals JAL, Christensen CBV, Gaafar A, Mustafa MD, Kordofani AAY, Ismail A, Kharazmi A, Theander TG: Dichotomy of the human T cell response to *Leishmania* antigens. I. Th1-like response to *Leishmania major* promastigote antigens in individuals recovered from cutaneous leishmaniasis. Clin Exp Immunol 1994;96:410–415.

71 Caceres-Dittmar G, Tapia FJ, Sanchez MA, Yamamura M, Uyemura K, Modlin RL, Bloom BR, Convit J: Determination of the cytokine profile in American cutaneous leishmaniasis using the polymerase chain reaction. Clin Exp Immunol 1993;91:500–505.

72 Melby P, Andrade-Narvaez FJ, Darnell BJ, Valencia-Pacheco G, Tryon V, Palomo-Cetina A: Increased expression of proinflammatory cytokines in chronic lesions of human cutaneous leishmaniasis. Infect Immun 1994;62:837–842.

73 Zwingenberger K, Harms G, Pedrosa C, Omena S, Sandkamp B, Neifer S: Determinants of the immune response in visceral leishmaniasis: Evidence for predominance of endogenous interleukin-4 over interferon-gamma production. Clin Immunol Immunopathol 1990;57:242–249.

74  Holaday BJ, Pompeu MM, Jeronimo S, Texeira MJ, Sousa A, Vasconcelos AW, Pearson RD, Abrams JS, Locksley RM: Potential role for interleukin-10 in the immunosuppression associated with kala-azar. J Clin Invest 1993;92:2626–2632.

75  Ghalib HW, Piuvezam MR, Skeiky Y, Siddig M, Hashim FA, el-Hassan AM, Russo DM, Reed SG: Interleukin-10 production correlates with pathology in human *Leishmania donovani* infections. J Clin Invest 1993;92:324–329.

76  Bogdan C, Nathan C: Modulation of macrophage function by transforming growth factor beta, interleukin-4 and interleukin-10. Ann NY Acad Sci 1993;685:713–739.

77  D'Andrea A, Ma X, Aste-Amezaga M, Paganin C, Trinchieri G: Stimulatory and inhibitory effects of IL-4 and IL-13 on the production of cytokines by human peripheral blood mononuclear cells: Priming for IL-12 and tumor necrosis factor-α production. J Exp Med 1995;181:537–546.

78  Stenger S, Thruing H, Rollinghoff M, Bogdan C: Tissue expression of inducible nitric oxide synthase is closely associated with resistance to *Leishmania major*. J Exp Med 1994;180:783–793.

79  Li J, Scott P, Farrell JP: In vivo alterations in cytokine production following interleukin-12 and anti-interleukin-4 antibody treatment of CB6F$_1$ mice with chronic cutaneous leishmaniasis. Infect Immun 1996;64:5248–5254.

80  Boyer MH, Jaffe CL: Increased susceptibility to *Leishmania tropica* infection in autoimmune MRL/ MpJ-lpr mice. J Parasitol 1984;70:145–146.

81  Pfeffer K, Matsuyama T, Kundig TM, Wakeham A, Kishihara K, Shahinian A, Weignmann K, Ohashi PS, Kronte M, Mak TW: Mice deficient for the 55 kD tumor necrosis factor receptor are resistant to endotoxic shock, yet succumb to *L. monocytogenes* infection. Cell 1993;73:457–467.

82  Rothe J, Lesslauer W, Loetscher H, Lang Y, Koebel P, Koentgen F, Althage A, Zinkernagel R, Steinmetz M, Bluethmann H: Mice lacking the tumor necrosis receptor 1 are resistant to TNF-mediated toxicity but highly susceptible to infection by *Listeria monocytogenes*. Nature 1993;364: 798–800.

83  Erickson SL, de Sauvage FJ, Kikly K, Carver-Moore K, Pitts-Meek S, Gillet N, Sheehan KCF, Schreiber RD, Goeddel DV, Moore MW: Decreased sensitivity to tumor-necrosis factor but normal T-cell development in TNF receptor-2-deficient mice. Nature 1994;372:560–563.

84  Flynn JL, Goldstein MM, Chan J, Triebold KJ, Pfeffer K, Lowenstein CJ, Schreiber R, Mak TW, Bloom BR: Tumor necrosis factor-α is required for the protective immune response against *Mycobacterium tuberculosis* in mice. Immunity 1995;2:561–572.

85  Vieira LQ, Goldschmidt M, Nashleanas M, Pfeffer K, Mak T, Scott P: Mice lacking the TNF receptor p55 fail to resolve lesions caused by infection with *Leishmania major*, but control parasite replication. J Immunol 1996;157:827–835.

86  Zhou T, Edwards CK, Yang P, Wang Z, Bluethmann H, Mountz JD: Greatly accelerated lymph-adenopathy and autoimmune disease in lpr mice lacking tumor necrosis factor receptor. I. J Immunol 1996;156:2661–2665.

87  Sytwu H-K, Liblau RS, McDevitt HO: The role of Fas/APO-1 (CD95) and TNF in antigen-induced programmed cell death in T cell receptor transgenic mice. Immunity 1996;5:17–30.

88  Singer GG, Abbas AK: The fas antigen is involved in peripheral but not thymic deletion of T lymphocytes in T cell receptor transgenic mice. Immunity 1994;1:365–371.

Phillip Scott, Department of Pathobiology, School of Veterinary Medicine,
University of Pennsylvania, 3800 Spruce Street, Philadelphia, PA, 19104 (USA)
e-mail pscott@phl.vet.upenn.edu, fax +1 215-573-7023

Liew FY, Cox FEG (eds): Immunology of Intracellular Parasitism.
Chem Immunol. Basel, Karger, 1998, vol 70, pp 81–102

..........................

# Immunoregulation during Toxoplasmosis

*James Alexander*[a], *Christopher A. Hunter*[b]

[a] Department of Immunology, University of Strathclyde, Glasgow, UK and
[b] Department of Pathobiology, School of Veterinary Medicine, University of
Pennsylvania, Philadelphia, Pa., USA

## Introduction

Toxoplasmosis is of major clinical and veterinary importance being a
cause of congenital disease and abortion in humans and domestic animals.
*Toxoplasma gondii* has a global distribution, infects approximately 30% of the
world's human population and has a high incidence in most warm-blooded
vertebrates [1]. The sexual stage of the life cycle takes place in the intestine
of the definitive host, the cat. Transmission to the intermediate host may be
brought about by ingesting infective sporulated oocysts released in cat faeces.
Alternatively, transmission can take place directly from one intermediate host
to another by the ingestion of meat containing the long-lived cyst stage. Despite
a sexual life cycle stage in cats, only three major clonal lineages have been
identified with little of the recombination one would expect if these animals
fed on prey that had succumbed to more than one *T. gondii* infection [2, 3].
These findings indicate that, under normal conditions, the protective immune
response generated following infection with *T. gondii* is effective and long-
lasting and prevents infection of animals with multiple strains of *T. gondii*.

In immunocompetent individuals, infection with *T. gondii* normally results
in an early mild to subclinical phase of infection, associated with the rapidly
dividing tachyzoite stage of the life cycle. Following recovery from this stage
of the infection individuals are thought to harbour cysts, which contain the
bradyzoite stage of the parasite, particularly within skeletal and heart muscle
and the central nervous system (CNS) for life. This results in a state of immunity
to reinfection which is presumed to be lifelong. However, in patients who
develop defects in T-cell function, toxoplasmosis can cause significant disease.
This group of susceptible individuals includes organ transplant recipients,

patients with certain cancers and patients with AIDS where *T. gondii* is the single largest cause of cerebral mass lesions. In these patients, it appears that the reactivation of latent tissue cysts, rather than recently acquired infection, is the cause of disease [4, 5]. Clinical toxoplasmosis is a consequence of tachyzoite replication and this stage of the parasite can be effectively treated with pyrimethamine and sulphadiazine. However, the bradyzoite stage, found within the tissue cysts and associated with the chronic stage of infection, is generally refractory to treatment. Thus, even after treatment the cyst stage persists and is responsible for the high incidence of relapses observed in AIDS patients with toxoplasmic encephalitis.

The present report reviews our current knowledge of the various factors, in particular immunological mechanisms, which determine the outcome of infection. Recent studies have given an insight into the events that occur when protective immunity breaks down, how these protective responses can be detrimental to the host, and how our knowledge of the immune response to *T. gondii* affects the prospects for successful vaccination strategies.

## Host and Parasite Factors Affecting Susceptibility to *T. gondii*

The severity of disease resulting from infection with *T. gondii* is under the influence of various parasite- and host-related factors. The recognition that the three major clonal lineages of *T. gondii* correlated with virulence of the parasite was an important step in our understanding of the role of parasite-derived factors in the pathogenesis of this infection. The type 1 lineage is associated with acute virulence in mice [6], whereas the type 2 lineage induces chronic pathology in susceptible strains of mice and the type 3 lineage is the least virulent [2, 7]. In addition, acute virulence in mice is associated in part with polymorphisms on the major tachyzoite surface antigen SAG1 [7, 8]. In humans, the type 1 lineage is most frequently associated with congenital infection whereas the type 2 lineage is more common in patients in whom the disease has reactivated [2]. Additional parasite factors involved in the outcome of infection include the fact that oocysts produce more virulent infections than tissue cysts [1], while the frequency of tissue cyst passage can also affect virulence as can the inoculum size of the initial infection [9]. Although only an experimental phenomenon, the route of infection can also greatly alter disease severity [10, 11]. Of particular interest are recent reports that *T. gondii* has superantigen activity, the first parasite for which this phenomenon has been demonstrated [12–14]. There is the intriguing possibility that different clonal lineages of *T. gondii* may differ in their ability to act as superantigens and so provide a basis for the differences in virulence.

Numerous host factors have been described which influence the severity of infection. The influence of human genes in controlling *T. gondii* infection is demonstrated by the variation in disease susceptibility in different ethnic groups and different HLA haplotypes, as well as concordance of disease manifestations in monozygotic, but not dizygotic twins, following congenital infection [reviewed in 15]. Studies in mice, using inbred congenic and recombinant mouse strains, have characterized the contribution of host genetics to different facets of infection. In contrast to humans, where the development of toxoplasmic encephalitis (TE) is associated most commonly with a loss of T-cell function, susceptibility to progressive TE in immunocompetent mice is genetically based rather than due to a lack of T cells. At least five genes including linkages with H-2 have been shown to determine survival during acute infection. Interestingly, different genes influence the cyst burden that develops in the brain during subacute infection [10, 16]. Both mice resistant and susceptible to TE initially develop encephalitis of similar severity but resistant mice are able to resolve the encephalitis while mice susceptible to TE develop a progressive encephalitis which results in death 2–3 months after infection [17, 18] (fig. 1). Analysis of the genetic basis of resistance to development of TE has revealed that differences in the genes within the H-2D region correlate with resistance or susceptibility to development of TE and that resistance to TE, in mice infected with the Me49 strain, is correlated absolutely with the $L^d$ gene [17]. That resistance maps to this MHC class I gene suggests that it is a defect in the CD8+ T-cell response that results in susceptibility to TE. Interestingly, Remington and colleagues [19] have correlated the HLA phenotype of patients with AIDS with susceptibility to TE.

In addition to the class I $L^d$ gene, MHC class II genes [11] and the *Nramp* gene also influence cyst burden [16, 20]. Mortality during chronic infection would appear to be under still further controls [16]. Work by Deckert-Schluter et al. [21, 22] comparing the same MHC haplotypes on two different genetic backgrounds demonstrates clearly that non-MHC genes can have a marked influence on survival, parasite burden and encephalitis. Other well-documented factors that can profoundly influence disease outcome include host age, sex hormones, pregnancy [23] and immunological status [4, 5].

## NK Cells and Innate Resistance to *T. gondii*

In murine models, activation of NK cells (as measured by NK cell cytolysis of tumor target cells), is one of the first events to occur following infection with *T. gondii* [24, 25]. Although human IL-2-activated NK cells have been reported to lyse targets infected with *T. gondii* [26] this does not appear to be

A

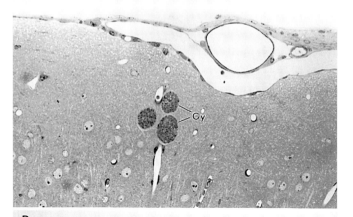

B

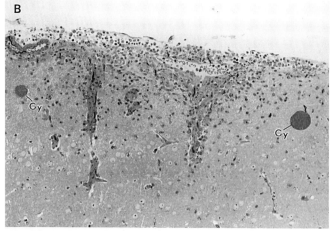

C

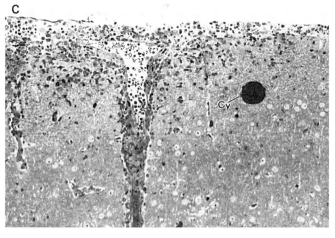

the case with murine NK cells [27]. Instead, it is the ability of NK cells to produce IFN-γ early in the course of infection that results in resistance to *T. gondii* [28–31].

Direct evidence of a role for NK cells during *T. gondii* infection was provided by studies in which severe combined immunodeficient (SCID) mice, which lack T and B lymphocytes but have normal NK cell responses [32], were shown to have a T-cell-independent mechanism of parasite control. Although the mice eventually succumb to disease, NK cell production of IFN-γ leads to resistance during the acute phase of infection with *T. gondii* [33–35]. This model has proved useful in defining the role of IL-12 in stimulating NK cells to produce IFN-γ during infection with *T. gondii*. Gazzinelli and Sher [36, 37] demonstrated that activated macrophages stimulated with live or dead tachyzoites of *T. gondii*, produced high levels of IL-12 which in turn stimulated NK cells to produce IFN-γ [36, 37]. The importance of IL-12 in resistance to *T. gondii* was demonstrated by studies in SCID mice in which administration of IL-12 resulted in a remarkable delay in time to death [37] while treatment with anti-IL-12 resulted in early mortality following infection [27, 38].

Live parasites are not required to induce the activation of NK cells. Antigen preparations of *T. gondii* can activate murine NK cells in vivo [39] and stimulate human and mouse NK cells to produce IFN-γ in vitro [36, 40]. This is likely due to the ability of activated macrophages to respond to antigen preparations of *T. gondii* and produce different monokines. Studies on the molecular basis for these events suggest that distinct parasite glycoproteins stimulate macrophage production of different monokines (IL-1, IL-12, TNF-α). Moreover, the ability of different parasite glycoproteins to stimulate monokine production is reflected in their biochemical properties and the types of intracellular signalling pathways that they stimulate [41].

While IL-12 alone can stimulate NK cells to produce low levels of IFN-γ, its ability to stimulate the production of high levels of IFN-γ is dependent on additional co-factors. For example, the ability of *T. gondii* to stimulate splenocytes from SCID mice to produce IFN-γ (from NK cells) is dependent not only on IL-12 but also on TNF-α and IL-1 [36, 42]. However, neither TNF-α nor IL-1 alone can stimulate NK cell production of IFN-γ [27, 36, 42]. Thus, although IL-12 is a critical regulator of NK cell production of IFN-γ its effect on NK cells is at least partially dependent upon other cytokines. The

*Fig. 1.* Light micrographs of brain tissue (1-μm plastic sections stained with azure A) from Strathclyde A strain outbred mice 3 months after infection with *T. gondii* (Beverley strain). The mice which are genetically heterogeneous show different degrees of susceptibility to TE – with little to no inflammation (*A*) through to increased inflammatory cell infiltration into the meninges (*B, C*). Cysts (Cy) are present in all mice irrespective of presence or absence of TE. × 350. (These micrographs were kindly provided by Dr. David Ferguson.)

CD28/B7 interaction also has a role in the regulation of NK cell responses during toxoplasmosis. Recent studies have shown that infection of SCID mice with *T. gondii* results in increased expression of CD28 by NK cells. The ability of these NK cells to interact with CD80 or CD86 (the ligands for CD28) can amplify IL-12-driven NK cell production of IFN-γ. The relevance of these results to the in vivo situation was shown by studies in which blocking of the CD28/B7 interaction in SCID mice infected with *T. gondii* led to decreased NK cell responses, a reduction in serum levels of IFN-γ and enhanced parasite replication [43].

While activation of NK cells occurs early in the course of infection with *T. gondii*, this is followed by a fall in NK cell activity shortly after the initial peak of activation [24, 25]. This observation indicates that there is a mechanism(s) to switch off the NK cell response. At least two cytokines, IL-10 and TGF-β, have been shown to antagonize NK cell responses during experimental toxoplasmosis. Following infection of SCID mice with *T. gondii*, the levels of these cytokines are up-regulated and treatment with neutralizing antibodies specific for IL-10 or TGF-β delays the time to death of these mice [36, 44]. These findings correlate with the ability of these antibodies to enhance the production of IFN-γ by splenocytes from infected SCID mice stimulated with *T. gondii*. However, IL-10 and TGF-β affect NK cell activation in different ways; whereas TGF-β has a direct inhibitory effect on NK cell production of IFN-γ [44, 45] this is not observed with IL-10 [46]. Rather, it is likely that the ability of IL-10 to antagonize macrophage functions, specifically macrophage production of TNF-α, IL-1 and IL-12 [47–49] that leads to an inhibition of NK cell responses.

**T Cells and the Adaptive Immune Response**

The early response to *T. gondii* infection is also driven by the recently described superantigen activity of the parasite [12–14]. This is manifest as an expansion of CD8 + Vβ5 + T cells and enhanced IFN-γ production during early infection [12] followed by nonresponsiveness of this T-cell population during chronic infection [13]. Expansion of the CD8 + population is CD4 + T-cell-dependent and the expansion is greatest in those mouse strains which express highest levels of Vβ5 + [14]. Surprisingly these strains also have the highest mortality levels [12–14]. The proinflammatory cytokines associated with the early response, IL-12 [50, 51] and IFN-γ [52], have also been clearly demonstrated as playing influential roles in the development of adaptive immune response. IL-12 and IFN-γ trigger the expansion of the Th1 subset of CD4 + lymphocytes which in turn produce IL-2 which drives the expansion of CD8 lymphocytes [53], perhaps in conjunction with macrophage-derived IL-15 [54]. IL-12 has also been shown to promote type 1 (IFN-$\gamma$-producing) cytolytic CD8 + T-cell development [55], again emphasizing the important role of the innate immune system in directing the evolution of the adaptive immune response. Adoptive transfer and in vivo depletion studies in various mouse strains confirm the paramount importance of CD8 + T cells in mediating immunity, not only during acute infection but also in preventing high cyst burdens and toxoplasmic encephalitis [56–60].

It has been suggested that CD8 + T cells may mediate their effect through IFN-$\gamma$ production [61]. A role for CD8 + T cells in class 1 restricted cytolytic responses has also been demonstrated in humans [62] and mice [53]. Furthermore, CD8 + T cells appear to have direct tachyzoite cytolytic activity [63]. However, a role for the CD4 + lymphocyte population cannot be discounted as MHC-controlled cytolytic activity has also been demonstrated by human CD4 + T-cell clones [64], and the Th1 subset has been implicated as playing a synergistic role in CD8 + T-cell-mediated protective immunity in mice [57, 59]. While CD4 + NK1.1 + cells may be a further source of IL-2, independent of MHC class II, in priming CD8 + T cells [65] paradoxically the CD4 + NK1.1 + population is probably also an early source of IL-4 production [66]. Generally, however, the role of the CD4 + populations during *T. gondii* infection remains controversial. Depletion of CD4 + cell populations in vivo has been reported to exacerbate disease, increase cyst burdens and promote recrudescence of latent infection [67, 68]. Nevertheless, further studies indicate that CD8 + cell depletion is necessary to reactivate latent infection while CD4 + cell depletion actually reduces brain inflammation [69]. Furthermore, the Th1 cell population may have detrimental effects if expanded in certain tissues. Thus IFN-$\gamma$-producing CD4 + $\alpha\beta$ T cells are associated with the development of necrotic lesions in the ilea of susceptible mice [70]. Significantly, this and other studies [71] demonstrated that protective responses in the gut-associated lymphoid tissue are related to the expansion of CD8 + $\alpha\beta$ T cells which are also capable of high IFN-$\gamma$ release and cytolytic activity for enterocytes. However, the co-production of significant quantities of Th2-type cytokines in gut-associated lymphoid tissue may be essential to limit this pathological response [72]. With particular relevance to gut involvement, protection against *T. gondii* has also been associated with the expansion $\gamma\delta$ T cells [73] though the mechanisms await clarification.


### Parasite Killing and Tachyzoite to Bradyzoite Transformation

Following acute disease the subacute phase of infection is associated with both the killing of tachyzoites and their conversion to cyst-forming bradyzoites.

*Table 1.* Comparison of the percentage survival plus brain cyst burden between cytokine or cytokine receptor-deficient mice and their wild-type counterparts

| Cytokine/cytokine receptor | Mouse strain | % survival | | Cyst burden ± SE | |
|---|---|---|---|---|---|
| | | +/+ | −/− | +/+ | −/− |
| IL-4 | B6/129 | 70 | 25 | 16,264 ± 2,998 | 7,244 ± 1,071 |
| IL-6 | 129 SVJ | 85 | 30 | 1,355 ± 59 | 10,450 ± 3,350 |
| INF-γR | 129 SVeV | 85 | 0 | ND | ND |
| TNF-αR-1 | 129 SVJ | 85 | 0 | ND | ND |

All measurements were 28 days postinfection with 20 tissue cysts *T. gondii* perorally. ND = Not done.

In vitro and in vivo studies have shown IFN-γ to be of paramount importance in the control of infection, although other cytokines such as TNF-α and IL-12 may play influential roles in this process [29, 61, 73] IFN-γ probably in synergy with TNF-α is thought to mediate killing through the production of oxygen metabolites and nitric oxide (NO) [28, 29, 74]. IFN-γ induces indoleamine 2,3-dioxygenase in human nonphagocytic cells thus starving the parasites of tryptophan [30, 31]. In addition to these antiparasite properties, IFN-γ may promote the expression of bradyzoite antigens [75] as well as preventing cyst rupture [76]. NO also plays a major role in the transformation of tachyzoites to bradyzoites probably by inhibition of mitochondrial respiration [77]. IL-6 has also been shown to increase cyst formation in vitro by as yet unknown mechanisms [78] and it is significant that IL-6-deficient mice on a resistant 129 SVJ background are extremely susceptible to infection as measured by mortality and brain cyst burden (table 1). Several other studies have indicated that tachyzoite multiplication can be inhibited by a variety of alternative mechanisms. Thus in IRF−/− mice (interferon regulatory factor negative), the control of parasite growth is mediated by IL-12 perhaps acting through CD4+ cells and has been reported to be independent of IFN-γ and NO production [79]. In addition, both CD4+ [64] and CD8+ [53, 62, 63] cells as well as human platelets [80] have been shown to have cytolytic activity against both parasitized cells and, on occasions, the parasites directly [63]. Human platelets do this via thomboxane production [80]. *T. gondii* growth can also be limited by antibodies which have been shown not only to inhibit uptake into the host cells [81] but when ingestion takes place they facilitate phagosome/lysosome fusion and parasite killing [82].

## Toxoplasmosis and the Brain

Although toxoplasmosis may have a multiorgan involvement (eye, lung, heart, intestine, lymph nodes, liver), it is the brain in human cases that is most frequently affected [83, 84]. The limited access of the immune system to the brain may, in part, explain the persistence of the cyst stage in the brain and the frequent neurological involvement in congenital toxoplasmosis and in immune-compromised patients in which this infection reactivates. The unique immune status of the brain is a consequence of a number of factors, in particular, the presence of the blood-brain barrier which inhibits the ability of antibodies and cytokines to access the brain [84, 85] and the reported ability of glial cells to suppress T-cell responses [86, 87]. In addition, the CNS lacks a lymphatic system and there are only low levels of endogenous MHC expression compared to other tissues [88, 89]. Thus, it may be easier for *T. gondii* to evade the full consequences of the host immune system in this site.

Although TE is the most common manifestation of clinical toxoplasmosis, there is evidence for a specific antiparasite effector mechanism within the brain. This is clearly shown by studies with mice but most notably by the lack of clinical disease in immune-competent individuals infected with *T. gondii*. The critical role of T cells as mediators of protective immunity against latent *T. gondii* infection in the brain in humans is illustrated by the correlation of fall in peripheral T-cell numbers with the development of TE in AIDS patients [90]. At the time these patients present with clinical TE they almost invariably have CD4+ T-cell counts that have fallen to less than $100/mm^3$ with a corresponding reduction in CD8+ T cells [90, 91]. Since cell-mediated immunity is required for resistance to *T. gondii* and control of this infection within the brain, a loss of this response would account for the recrudescence of this infection and development of TE. This hypothesis is supported by studies which demonstrated that HIV infection in patients infected with *T. gondii* results in a suppression of type 1 lymphokine and IL-12 responses to *T. gondii* but fails to inhibit the synthesis of other parasite-induced monokines [92]. In addition, macrophages from HIV-infected individuals have a reduced ability to inhibit parasite replication [93, 94] and infection of macrophages with HIV inhibits their ability to kill *T. gondii* [95]. Thus, infection with HIV suppresses the production of cytokines involved in resistance to *T. gondii* and inhibits the effector functions of macrophages important for killing *T. gondii*. Furthermore, a direct link between replication of *T. gondii* and increased viral load is suggested by studies in which infection of HIV-1 transgenic mice with *T. gondii* stimulated proviral transcription in macrophages in vivo [96]. Thus, infection with *T. gondii* might increase the rate of viral replication, hasten the decline in T-cell numbers, and so allow development of TE.

Murine models of toxoplasmosis have proven useful for the study of the pathogenesis of TE. The critical role for T cells in resistance to *T. gondii* in the brain is illustrated by several studies using these models. For example, infection of SCID mice with *T. gondii* results in CNS lesions that are a consequence of essentially unrestricted parasite replication leading to the development of large necrotic lesions with parasites demonstrable at the periphery. In addition there is a lack of an obvious inflammatory response and these lesions resemble in many ways those observed in AIDS patients [33, 35, 97]. However, in immunocompetent mice, even those highly susceptible to TE, there are T cells scattered throughout the parenchyma and inflammatory lesions composed of CD4+ and CD8+ T cells and macrophages while large areas of necrosis are rarely observed (fig. 1). The importance of T cells in this response was shown by studies in which the depletion of both CD4+ and CD8+ T-cell populations resulted in the development of severe toxoplasmic encephalitis accompanied by increased mortality [98, 99]. Conversely, it was shown that reconstitution of SCID mice with naive or immune T cells protected SCID mice from toxoplasmic encephalitis [100].

Previous studies in which the production of cytokines in the brains of mice infected with *T. gondii* was analyzed indicated that the outcome of the encephalitis was dependent on the differential production of cytokines by Th1 and Th2 cells [22, 101, 102]. IFN-γ appears to be the most important cytokine in this respect since administration of anti-IFN-γ to chronically infected mice results in increased severity of an established encephalitis [103]. Furthermore, treatment with IFN-γ reduces the severity of established TE although the disease will reactivate when treatment is discontinued [104]. In murine models, the mechanism of IFN-γ-dependent resistance within the brain is likely to be a consequence of the ability of IFN-γ to activate macrophages to inhibit parasite replication through increased production of NO. This idea is supported by studies in which elevated levels of transcripts for inducible NO synthase (iNOS) as well as protein [Hunter, unpubl. observations] were detected in the brains of mice with TE [102]. Moreover, administration of aminoguanidine (an inhibitor of iNOS) to mice resulted in increased severity of TE [105].

Other cytokines have also been shown to have an important role in resistance to TE. In particular, neutralization of endogenous TNF-α results in decreased levels of iNOS mRNA within the brain, and increased severity of TE and early mortality of infected mice [102]. These data are consistent with a role for TNF-α as an important co-factor for the IFN-γ-induced activation of antiparasite effector mechanisms within the brain. The role of IL-6 in TE is less clear. Studies in which mice with an established encephalitis were treated with anti-IL-6 showed a reduction in brain inflammation, a decrease in the numbers of parasite cysts within the brain and reduced serum levels of IFN-γ [106]. However, the administration of anti-IL-6 actually results in an increase in serum levels of IL-6 (perhaps a consequence of cytokine-antibody complexes). Significantly, therefore, we have found IL-6-deficient mice to be more susceptible to TE than their immunocompetent counterparts [unpubl. data] and to develop higher cyst burdens (table 1).

The role of the Th2-type cytokines IL-4 and IL-10 in TE is also uncertain. Several studies detected the presence of elevated levels of IL-4 and IL-10 mRNA [22, 101], as well as protein for IL-10 [18] in the brains of mice with TE. The ability of these cytokines to inhibit cell-mediated immune responses suggested that their production during TE would antagonize the protective immune response and would enhance the development of progressive TE [107]. Studies with mice deficient in IL-4 or IL-10 demonstrated that these mice were more susceptible to acute infection than wild-type mice [108, 109] (table 1) but that IL-4-deficient mice were resistant to TE unlike immunocompetent controls [108] (table 1). Subsequent studies reported that IL-4-deficient mice were more susceptible to TE and this was associated with decreased production of IFN-γ by T cells from infected IL-4-deficient mice stimulated with parasite antigen [110]. The differences between these two studies may be related to the strains of parasite used or the different genetic backgrounds of the mice. Alternatively, these results may be an example of a phenotype related to a developmental problem with T cells in IL-4-deficient mice since studies using lineage ablation have shown that effector cells producing either IL-4 or IFN-γ have a common precursor, which expresses the IL-4 gene [111]. Thus, mice deficient in IL-4 may have a defect in the ability of their T cells to produce IFN-γ.

The role of the resident glial cell populations in resistance to *T. gondii* is still uncertain. While macrophages from the peripheral immune system can infiltrate the brain during TE, histological evidence has shown that TE results in activation of both astrocytes and microglia which suggests a role for these cells in the pathogenesis of toxoplasmic encephalitis [101, 112]. In vitro studies have shown that murine microglia can be stimulated by IFN-γ, in combination with TNF-α, to inhibit the replication of intracellular *T. gondii* in an NO-dependent manner [113–115]. However, IFN-γ alone or in combination with TNF-α was unable to inhibit parasite replication in murine astrocytes [114]. The situation in human glial cells appears to be slightly different and it has been shown that human microglia lack an NO-dependent mechanism of killing of *T. gondii* [113] but astrocytes do have this mechanism [116]. Moreover, the ability of IFN-γ to induce the enzyme indolamine oxygenase (the enzyme responsible for tryptophan starvation) inhibits parasite replication in a human glioblastoma [31].

## Parasite Control versus Host Pathogenesis

More than any other pathogen studied to date, the control of *T. gondii* infection during both the acute and chronic phases of disease appears to be a delicate balance between the production of proinflammatory and regulatory cytokines. Inhibition of proinflammatory cytokines such as IFN-γ, TNF-α and IL-12 [27, 28, 33, 38, 117], using neutralizing antibodies or ablating iNOS activity with metabolic inhibitors [105], results in increased mortality during infection. Conversely, treatment with neutralizing antibodies for IL-10 and TGF-β (two inhibitors of cell-mediated immunity) delay time to death [34, 44] of infected mice. Similarly, administration of rIFN-γ [76, 117], rIL-12 [34, 37] though not rTNF-α [117, 118] can increase the survival of infected SCID as well as immunocompetent mice while administration of TGF-β [44], which down-modulates IL-12 activity results in more rapid death. Furthermore, IFN-γR and TNF-αR-1 gene-deficient mice on a resistant 129 background rapidly die following infection [117, 119] (table 1). While the production of IL-12, IFN-γ, TNF-α and NO are important in protective immunity, their overproduction can also be deleterious to the host [120]. Thus, mouse strains producing the highest levels of IFN-γ have the highest mortality levels [12, 14]. In addition, administration of rTNF-α results in earlier mortality in both SCID and immunocompetent mice [117, 118]. Furthermore, mice deficient in IL-10 (an antagonist of cell-mediated immunity) die during the acute stage of infection due to the overproduction of IL-12 and subsequent CD4+ T-cell production of high levels of IFN-γ [109, 121]. Similarly, mice deficient in IL-4, which down-regulates IFN-γ activity, have significantly increased mortality [108, 110]. In addition to IL-10, NO [122] has been identified as playing an important regulatory role limiting cachexia and reducing tissue damage and death during early *T. gondii* infection. IL-10 and NO do this by inhibiting IL-2 and IFN-γ production and inducing lymphocyte hyporesponsiveness 7 days postinfection [122–124]. Nevertheless, administration of rIL-7 which reverses the inhibition of IL-2, a cytokine associated with protection [125], as well as IFN-γ protects mice during acute parasite challenge [126].

Thus, subtle shifts in the kinetics and magnitude of proinflammatory and regulatory cytokine production can markedly alter parasite growth and disease outcomes. Therefore, for example, we and others have shown that male mice are more resistant than females to moderate infection with *T. gondii*, both in terms of mortality and cyst burdens [23, 127, 128] and this resistance is associated with more rapid production of IL-12 and IFN-γ [128] as well as greater production of TNF-α [23, 127] and NO in males [unpubl. data]. However, IL-10 is produced in similar quantities at the same time in both males and females [23, 127]. Thus, the more rapid and greater proinflammatory response of males allows increased parasite control. Nevertheless, increasing the virulence of the challenge infection in SCID mice results in a more severe cachexic response and increased mortality in males compared to female mice [unpubl. data]. Thus, a balanced interaction between proinflammatory and regulatory cytokines is essential at all stages of a *T. gondii* infection in order to most effectively control parasite growth with minimal host tissue damage.

Th1/Th2-associated cytokine production might not only differ with the life cycle development of the parasite within the host [14] but the functional and effective equilibrium at any one time may be different in different host tissues [72]. This might explain why cyst formation occurs at different rates in different tissues and why the early immune response to *T. gondii* in the mesenteric lymph nodes is predominantly Th2-like while there is a shift to a predominant Th1 phenotype in the spleen late in infection.

## Vaccination

A vaccine consisting of live attenuated tachyzoites that successfully prevents abortion in sheep is already commercially available in several countries [129]. While this demonstrates the potential for successful vaccination against *T. gondii*, and a similar vaccine has been shown to limit experimental infections in pigs [130, 131], it is unlikely that a live vaccine would ever be approved for use in humans. Furthermore, vaccinating sheep fails to prevent vertical disease transmission and the development of cysts in lambs [132]. Thus, the resultant food source will continue to present a potential large reservoir of parasite material for subsequent disease transmission to the consumer. Thus an ideal vaccine should comprise either defined parasite subunits, recombinant antigens or synthetic peptides and be capable of not only preventing abortion or foetal damage but also of limiting cyst formation in intermediate hosts and oocyst shedding in cats. Current evidence suggests that the outcome of vaccination will be dependent on several factors including the route of administration of the vaccine, the life cycle stage or antigens comprising the vaccine and the adjuvant or immunopotentiators included in the vaccine formulation [119].

The normal portal of entry of *T. gondii* is via the gut mucosa. Surprisingly, therefore, despite it being well documented that the susceptibility to infection is significantly altered using different routes of parasite infection [10], numerous experimental studies circumvent this tissue when initiating disease. Furthermore, it has recently been demonstrated that the intestine is a major site of severe to life-threatening pathology in susceptible mice mediated by CD4+ cells secreting IFN-γ [70]. However, it should be noted that, to the best of our knowledge, this type of pathology is not observed in humans with recently acquired toxoplasmosis. Protective responses may also be operating in these tissues. Thus, intraepithelial IFN-$\gamma$-producing CD8 + T cells cytolytic for parasitized enterocytes are generated following infection [71, 72], while IgA may protect mucosal surfaces from parasite invasion following oral vaccination with SAG1 [81]. Unfortunately, conventional parenterally administered vaccines do not generally induce mucosal immune responses and the most successful method to induce this type of response has been to administer vaccines orally [133]. Thus, it is in retrospect not surprising that intraintestinal immunization of mice with the temperature-sensitive mutant TS-4 but not subcutaneous immunization was effective in reducing the incidence of congenital toxoplasmosis [134]. More recently it has been shown that nasal vaccination with SAG1 lined to cholera toxin reduces cyst burden following oral infection [135]

Over recent years a number of *Toxoplasma* antigens, SAG1, ROP1, GRA1, 2 and 4, and peptides derived from them have been shown to be recognized by murine and human T cells and have been suggested as vaccine candidates [136]. While vaccine formulations based on these antigens have resulted in reduced mortality, in those studies where brain cyst burdens have also been quantified only a reduction has been achieved with no sterile immunity observed. What may be significant is that these antigens are either tachyzoite specific, e.g. SAG1, or shared, e.g. GRA 1, 2 and 4, while none are bradyzoite specific. Similar incomplete protection has also resulted when attenuated or 'crude' tachyzoite antigen preparations have constituted the vaccine [129, 137]. What could be of significance in this respect is that serological studies in *T. gondii* infected humans [138, 139] as well as mice have indicated that recognition is generally of immunodominant stage-specific antigens with little recognition of shared antigens. This would imply a requirement for additional antigens to those expressed in tachyzoites for complete protection following vaccination and a series of experimental studies highlight this probability. For example, we have recently demonstrated that a parenteral mixed tachyzoite/cyst antigen vaccine was more effective at limiting cyst burdens in mice following challenge than either preparation alone [119]. In addition, while oral and intraduodenal immunization with tissue cysts or bradyzoites of the non-oocyst-forming mutant T-263 protected cats totally against oocyst shedding following challenge, vaccination by either route with T-263 tachzyoites was only partially protective [140]. In a similar manner, immunizing mice with tachyzoite antigens in ISCOMs protected against challenge against this life cycle stage and oocysts but not tissue cysts [141].

Antigens may, however, not be inherently protective or exacerbative but it is rather how they are presented to the immune response that can determine the outcome of challenge infections. Thus while vaccination with lipid vesicle entrapped STAg [137] or SAG1 [142] has been shown to limit *T. gondii*-induced murine abortion and mortality respectively, vaccination with unadjuvanted STAg increased foetal death [137] and with SAG1 [143] emulsified in Freund's complete adjuvant (FCA) increased mortality following infection. These results may arise as a result of the ability of lipid vesicle adjuvants to stimulate, in addition to Th1 cells, CD8+ cytolytic T-cell responses [144]. There is little evidence that soluble antigen preparations or FCA have this ability despite the fact that STAg is a potent inducer of IFN-γ production [reviewed in 14] and FCA of Th1 activation [119]. As CD8+ T cells have been well characterized as comprising the protective adaptive response [56–60], it has been suggested by ourselves and others that vaccines formulated with cytokines such as IL-12 and IL-2 could be used to enhance CD8+ T-cell activity and thus protection in a controlled manner [119]. This exciting possibility has recently been demonstrated in an elegant study by Khan and Kasper [54] using IL-15 as the immunopotentiator. This cytokine, which signals through IL-2R [145], administered with STAg stimulated complete protection against lethal infection. Neither the cytokine nor the antigen alone had a protective effect. Immunity was associated with increased serum IFN-γ levels. Protection could be adoptively transferred with CD8+ cells but not CD4+ cells. In addition, CD8+ T cells proliferated on exposure to antigen and demonstrated CTL activity against infected target cells.

On the whole the prospects for developing new improved vaccines against *T. gondii* remain good. Live attentuated vaccines are already available or about to become available to limit infections in cats and domestic live-stock. The existence of only three major clonal lineages [2] removes the problem of antigenic heterogenicity and variation posed by other parasites. However, there is the possibility that the effectiveness of nonlive vaccines could be limited as they may be unable to maintain the anamnestic response induced by a latent infection. This problem may be circumvented by the use of DNA vaccines.


## Conclusion

By any stretch of the imagination, *T. gondii* has to be acknowledged as a very successful parasite. It not only parasitizes all warm-blooded vertebrates but can invade all nucleated cells and tissues within the host. Infection is also lifelong but generally only life-threatening in immune-compromised patients. In order to control such a uniquitous parasite it has become apparent that many elements of the immune response (innate and adaptive, proinflammatory and regulatory) must be integrated to prevent clinical disease. As infection proceeds from the acute through to the chronic phase of infection the inflammatory mediators, which are essential to control parasite growth, must be counterbalanced by the production of regulatory cytokines to prevent the development of a pathogenic immune response. Thus, recent studies using *T. gondii* have contributed greatly to our general understanding of the role of cytokines in protective immunity and their relationship to disease pathogenesis.

## References

1   Jackson MH, Hutchison WM: The prevalence and source of *Toxoplasma* infection in the environment. Adv Parasitol 1989;28:55–105.
2   Sibley LD, Howe DK: Genetic basis of pathogenicity in toxoplasmosis. Curr Top Microbiol Immunol 1996;219:3–16.
3   Darde ML: Biodiversity in *Toxoplasma gondii*. Curr Top Microbiol Immunol 1996;219:27–41.
4   Luft BJ, Remington JS: Toxoplasmic encephalitis in AIDS. Clin Infect Dis 1992;15:211–222.
5   Ambroise-Thomas P, Pelloux H: Toxoplasmosis – Congenital and in immuno-compromised patients: A parallel. Parasitol Today 1993;9:61–62.
6   Sibley LD, Boothroyd JC: Virulent strains of *Toxoplasma gondii* comprise a single clonal lineage. Nature 1992;350:82–85.
7   Howe DK, Sibley LD: *Toxoplasma gondii* is comprised of 3 clonal lineages: Correlation of parasite genotype with human disease. J Infect Dis 1995;13:322–356.
8   Rinder H, Thomschkle A, Darde ML, Loscher T: Specific DNA polymorphisms discriminate between virulence and non-virulence to mice in nine *Toxoplasma gondii* isolates. Mol Biochem Parasitol 1995;69:123–126.
9   Araujo FG, Williams DM, Grumet FC, Remington JS: Strain dependent differences in murine susceptibility to *Toxoplasma gondii*. Infect Immun 1976;13:1528–1530.
10  Blackwell JM, Roberts CW, Alexander J: Influence of genes within the MHC on mortality and brain cyst development in mice infected with *Toxoplasma gondii*: Kinetics of immune regulation in BALB H-2 congenic mice. Parasit Immunol 1993;15:317–324.
11  Brown CR, McLeod R: Mechanisms of survival of mice during acute and chronic *Toxoplasma gondii* infection. Parasitol Today 1994;10:290–292.
12  Denkers EY, Caspar P, Sher A: *Toxoplasma gondii* possesses a super antigen that selectively expands murine T cell receptor Vβ5-bearing CD8+ lymphocytes. J Exp Med 1994;180:985–994.
13  Denkers EY, Caspar P, Hieny S, Sher A: *Toxoplasma gondii* infection induces specific nonresponsiveness in lymphocytes bearing the Vβ5 chain of the mouse T cell receptor. J Immunol 1996;156: 1089–1094.
14  Denkers EY: A *Toxoplasma gondii* superantigen. Biological effects and implications for the host-parasite interaction. Parasitol Today 1996;12:362–366.
15  McLeod R, Johnson J, Estes R, Mack D: Immunogenetics in pathogenesis and protection against toxoplasmosis. Curr Top Microbiol Immunol 1996;219:95–112.
16  McLeod R, Skamene E, Brown CR, Eisenhauer PB, Mack DG: Genetic regulation of early survival and cyst number after peroral *Toxoplasma gondii* infection of AxB/BxA recombinant inbred and B10 congenic mice. J Immunol 1989;143:3031–3034.
17  Brown CR, Hunter CA, Estes RG, Beckmann J, Forman J, David C, Remington JS, McLeod R: Definitive identification of a gene that confers resistance against *Toxoplasma* cyst burden and encephalitis. Immunology 1995;85:419–428.
18  Hunter CA, Litton MJ, Remington JS, Abrams JS: Immunocytochemical detection of cytokines in the lymph nodes and brains of mice resistant or susceptible to toxoplasmic encephalitis. J Infect Dis 1994;170:939–945.
19  Suzuki Y, Wong SY, Grumet FC, Fessel J, Montoya JG, Zolopa AR, Patmore A, Schumacher-Perdreau F, Schrappe M, Koppen S, Ruf B, Brown BW, Remington JS: Evidence for genetic regulation of susceptibility to toxoplasmic encephalitis in AIDS patients. J Infect Dis 1996;173: 265–268.

20   Blackwell JM, Roberts CW, Roach TI, Alexander J: Influence of macrophage resistance gene Lsh/Ity/Bcg (candidate) NRamp on *Toxoplasma gondii* infection in mice. Clin Exp Immunol 1994;97: 107–112.

21   Deckert-Schluter M, Schluter D, Schmidt D, Schwendmann G, Wiestler OD, Hof H: *Toxoplasma encephalitis* in congenic B10 and BALB mice: Impact of genetic factors on the immune response. Infect Immun 1994;62:221–228.

22   Deckert-Schluter M, Albrecht S, Hof H, Wiestler OD, Schluter D: Dynamics of the intracerebral and splenic cytokine mRNA production in *Toxoplasma gondii*-resistant and -susceptible congenic strains of mice. Immunology 1995;85:408–418.

23   Roberts CW, Satoskar A, Alexander J: The influence of sex steroids and pregnancy associated hormones on the development and maintenance of immunity to parasite infection. Parasitol Today 1996;12:382–388.

24   Goyal M, Ganguly NK, Mahajan RC: Natural killer cell cytotoxicity against *Toxoplasma gondii* in acute and chronic toxoplasmosis. Med Sci Res 1988;16:375–377.

25   Hauser WE, Sharma SD, Remington JS: Natural killer cells induced by acute and chronic *Toxoplasma* infection. Cell Immunol 1982;69:330–346.

26   Subauste CS, Dawson L, Remington JS: Human lymphokine-activated killer cells are cytotoxic against cells infected with *Toxoplasma gondii*. J Exp Med 1992;176:1511–1519.

27   Hunter CA, Subauste CS, Van Cleave VH, Remington JS: Production of gamma interferon by natural killer cells from *Toxoplasma gondii*-infected SCID mice: Regulation by interleukin-10, interleukin-12, and tumor necrosis factor alpha. Infect Immun 1994;62:2818–2824.

28   Suzuki Y, Orelana MA, Schreiber RD, Remington JS: Interferon-γ: The major mediator of resistance against *Toxoplasma gondii*. Science 1988;240:516–518.

29   Sibley LD, Adams LB, Fukutomi Y, Krahenbuhl JL: Tumor necrosis factor-α triggers antitoxoplasmal activity of IFN-γ primed macrophages. J Immunol 1991;147:2340–2345.

30   Pfefferkorn ER, Eckel M, Rebhun S: Interferon-γ suppresses the growth of *Toxoplasma gondii* in human fibroblasts through starvation for tryptophan. Mol Biochem Parasitol 1986;20:215–224.

31   Daubener W, Remscheid C, Nockemann S, Pilz K, Seghrouchini S, Mackenzie C, Hadding U: Antiparasite effector mechanism in human brain tumor cells: Role of interferon-γ and tumor necrosis factor-α. Eur J Immunol 1996;26:487–492.

32   Bosma GC, Custer RP, Bosma MJ: A severe combined immunodeficiency mutation in the mouse. Nature 1983;301:527–531.

33   Johnson LL: SCID mouse models of acute and relapsing chronic *Toxoplasma gondii* infections. Infect Immun 1992;60:3719–3724.

34   Hunter CA, Abrams JS, Beaman MH, Remington JS: Cytokine mRNA in the central nervous system of SCID mice infected with *Toxoplasma gondii*: Importance of T-cell-independent regulation of resistance to *T. gondii*. Infect Immun 1993;61:4038–4044.

35   Schluter D, Deckert-Schluter M, Schwendemann G, Brunner H, Hof H: Expression of major histocompatability complex class II antigens and levels of interferon-γ, tumor necrosis factor, and interleukin-6 in cerebrospinal fluid and serum in *Toxoplasma gondii*-infected SCID and immunocompetent C.B-17 mice. Immunology 1993;78:430–435.

36   Sher A, Oswald IP, Hieny S, Gazzinelli R: *Toxoplasma gondii* induces a T-independent IFN-γ response in natural killer cells that requires both adherent accessory cells and tumor necrosis factor-α. J Immunol 1993;150:3982–3989.

37   Gazzinelli RT, Hieny S, Wynn TA, Wolf S, Sher A: Interleukin-12 is required for the T-lymphocyte-independent induction of interferon-γ by an intracellular parasite and induces resistance in T-cell-deficient hosts. Proc Natl Acad Sci USA 1993;90:6115–6119.

38   Gazzinelli RT, Wysocka M, Hayashi S, Denkers EY, Hieny S, Caspar P, Trinchieri G, Sher A: Parasite-induced IL-12 stimulates early IFN-γ synthesis and resistance during acute infection with *Toxoplasma gondii*. J Immunol 1994;153:2533–2543.

39   Hauser WE, Sharma SD, Remington JS: Augmentation of NK cell activity by soluble and particulate fractions of *Toxoplasma gondii*. J Immunol 1983;131:458–463.

40   Sharma SD, Verhoef J, Remington JS: Enhancement of human natural killer cell activity by subcellular components of *Toxoplasma gondii*. Cell Immunol 1986;86:317–326.

41 Grunvald E, Chiaramonte M, Hieny S, Wysocka M, Trinchieri G, Vogel S, Gazzinelli R, Sher A: Biochemical characterization and protein kinase C dependency of monokine-inducing activities of *Toxoplasma gondii*. Infect Immun 1996;64:2010–2018.

42 Hunter CA, Chizzonite R, Remington JS: Interleukin-1β is required for the ability of IL-12 to induce production of IFN-γ by NK cells: A role for IL-1β in the T cell independent mechanism of resistance against intracellular pathogens. J Immunol 1995;155:4347–4354.

43 Hunter CA, Ellis-Neyer L, Gabriel K, Kennedy M, Linsley P, Remington JS: The role of the CD28/B7 interaction in the regulation of NK cell responses during infection with *Toxoplasma gondii*. J Immunol 1997;158:2285–2293.

44 Hunter CA, Bermudez L, Beernink H, Waegell W, Remington JS: Transforming growth factor-β inhibits interleukin-12-induced production of interferon-γ by natural killer cells: A role for transforming growth factor-β in the regulation of T-cell independent resistance to *Toxoplasma gondii*. Eur J Immunol 1995;25:994–1000.

45 Bellone G, Aste-Amezaga M, Trinchieri G, Rodeck U: Regulation of NK cell functions by TGF-β1. J Immunol 1995;155:1066–1073.

46 Tripp CS, Wolf SF, Unanue ER: Interleukin-12 and tumor necrosis factor-α are costimulators of interferon-γ production by natural killer cells in severe combined immunodeficiency mice with listeriosis, and interleukin-10 is a physiological antagonist. Proc Natl Acad Sci USA 1993;90:3725–3729.

47 D'Andrea A, Aste-Amezaga M, Valiante NM, Ma X, Kubin M, Trinchieri G: Interleukin-10 inhibits human lymphocyte interferon-γ production by suppressing natural killer cell stimulatory factor/IL-12 synthesis in accessory cells. J Exp Med 1993;178:1041–1048.

48 Rennick D, Berg D, Holland G: Interleukin-10: An overview. Prog Growth Factor Res 1992;4: 207–227.

49 Fiorentino DF, Zlotnik A, Mosmann TR, Howard M, O'Garra A: IL-10 inhibits cytokine production by activated macrophages. J Immunol 1991;146:3815–3822.

50 Hsieh CS, Macatonia SE, Tripp CS, Wolf S, O'Garra A, Murphy KM: Development of Th1 CD4+ T cells through IL-12 produced by *Listeria*-induced macrophages. Science 1993;260:547–549.

51 Scott P: IL-12: Initiation cytokine for cell-mediated immunity. Science 1993;260:496–497.

52 Gajewski TF, Fitch FW: Differential activation of murine Th1 and Th2 clones. Res Immunol 1991; 142:19–23.

53 Denkers EY, Sher A, Gazzinelli RT: T cell interactions with *Toxoplasma gondii*: Implications for processing of antigen for class I-restricted recognition. Res Immunol 1993;14:51–57.

54 Khan IA, Kasper LH: IL-15 augments CD8+ T cell-mediated immunity against *Toxoplasma gondii* infection in mice. J Immunol 1996;157:2103–2108.

55 Croft M, Carter L, Swain SL, Dutton RW: Generation of polarised antigen-specific CD8 effector populations: Reciprocal action of interleukin (IL)-4 and IL-12 in promoting type 2 versus type 1 cytokine profiles. J Exp Med 1994;180:1715–1728.

56 Brown CR, McLeod R: Class I MHC genes and CD8+ T cells determine cyst number in *Toxoplasma gondii* infection. J Immunol 1990;145:3438–3441.

57 Gazzinelli RT, Hakim FT, Hieny S, Shearer GM, Sher A: Synergistic role of CD4+ and CD8+ lymphocytes in IFN-γ production and protective immunity induced by an attenuated *Toxoplasma gondii* vaccine. J Immunol 1991;146:286–292.

58 Khan IA, Ely KH, Kasper LH: A purified parasite antigen (P30) mediates CD8+ T cell immunity against fatal *Toxoplasma gondii* infection in mice. J Immunol 1991;47:3501–3506.

59 Parker SJ, Roberts CW, Alexander J: CD8+ T cells are the major lymphocyte subpopulation involved in the protective immune response to *Toxoplasma gondii* in mice. Clin Exp Immunol 1991; 84:207–212.

60 Subuaste CS, Koniaris AH, Remington JS: Murine CD8+ cytotoxic T lymphocytes lyse *Toxoplasma gondii*-infected cells. J Immunol 1991;147:3955–3959.

61 Gazzinelli RT, Denkers EY, Sher A: Host resistance to *Toxoplasma gondii*: Model for studying the selective induction of cell-mediated immunity by intracellular parasites. Infect Agents Dis 1993;2:139–149.

62 Yano A, Aosai F, Ohta M, Hasekura H, Sugana K, Hayashi S: Antigen presentation by *Toxoplasma gondii*-infected cells to CD4+ proliferative T cells and CD8+ cytotoxic cells. J Parasitol 1989;75: 411–416.

63  Khan IA, Smith KA, Kasper LH: Induction of antigen-specific parasiticidal cytotoxic T cell spleno-cytes by a major membrane protein (p30) of *Toxoplasma gondii*. J Immunol 1988;141:3600–3605.

64  Curiel TJ, Krug EC, Purner MB, Poignard P, Berens RL: Cloned human CD4+ cytotoxic T lymphocytes specific for *Toxoplasma gondii* lyse tachyzoite-infected target cells. J Immunol 1993; 151:2024–2031.

65  Denkers EY, Scharton Kersten T, Barbieri S, Caspar P, Sher A: A role for CD4+NK1.1+ T lymphocytes as major histocompatibility complex class II independent helper cells in the generation of CD8+ effector function against intracellular infection. J Exp Med 1996;184:131–139.

66  Denkers EY, Gazzinelli RT, Martin D, Sher A: Emergence of NK1.1+ cells as effectors of immunity to *Toxoplasma gondii* in MHC class I-deficient mice. J Exp Med 1993;178:1465–1472.

67  Araujo FS: Depletion of L3T4+ (CD+) T lymphocytes prevent the development of resistance to *Toxoplasma gondii* in mice. Infect Immun 1991;59:1614–1619.

68  Vollmer TL, Waldour MK, Steinman L, Conley FK: Depletion of T-4+ lymphocytes with mono-clonal antibody reactivates toxoplasmosis in the central nervous system: A model of superinfection in AIDS. J Immunol 1987;138:3737–3741.

69  Remington JS: Treatment with anti-L3T4 (CD4) monoclonal antibody reduces the inflammatory response in toxoplasmic encephalitis. J Immunol 1989;142:954–958.

70  Liesenfeld O, Kosek J, Remington JS, Suzuki Y: Mice definition in α/β CD4 T cells did not develop necrosis in the ilea but mice deficient in γ/δ or CD8+ T cells did. J Exp Med 1996;184:597–607.

71  Chardes T, Buzoni-Gatel D, Lepage A, Bernard F, Bout D: *Toxoplasma gondii* oral infection induces specific cytotoxic CD8α/β Thy-1+ gut intraepithelial lymphocytes, lytic for parasite-infected enterocytes. J Immunol 1994;153:4596–4603.

72  Chardes T, Velge-Roussel F, Mevelec P, Mevelec M-N, Buzoni-Gatei D, Bout D: Mucosal and systemic cellular immune responses induced by *Toxoplasma gondii* antigens in cyst orally infected mice. Immunology 1993;78:421–429.

73  Hisaeda H, Nagasawa H, Maeda K, Maekawa Y, Ishikawa H, Ito Y, Good RA, Himeno K: γδ T cells play an important role in hsp65 expression and in acquiring protective immune responses against infection with *Toxoplasma gondii*. J Immunol 1995;154:244–251.

74  Langermans JAM, Van der Hulst MEB, Nibbering PH, Hiemstra PS, Fransen L, Van Furth R: IFN-γ induced L-arginine-dependent toxoplasmastatic activity in murine peritoneal macrophages is mediated by endogenous tumor necrosis factor-α. J Immunol 1992;148:568–574.

75  Bohne W, Heesemann J, Gross U: Induction of bradyzoite-specific *Toxoplasma gondii* antigens in gamma interferon-treated mouse macrophages. Infect Immun 1993;61:1141–1145.

76  McCabe RE, Luft BJ, Remington JS: Effect of murine interferon gamma on murine toxoplasmosis. J Infect Dis 1984;150:961–962.

77  Bohne W, Heesemann J, Gross U: Reduced replication of *Toxoplasma gondii* is necessary for induction of bradyzoite specific antigens: A possible role for nitric oxide in triggering stage conversion. Infect Immun 1994;62:1761–1767.

78  Weiss LM, Laplace D, Takvorian PM, Tanowitz HP, Cali A, Wittner M: A cell culture system for study of the development of *Toxoplasma gondii* bradyzoites. J Eukaryot Microbiol 1995;42:150–157.

79  Khan IA, Matsuura T, Fonseka S, Kasper LH: Production of nitric oxide is not essential for protection against acute *Toxoplasma gondii* infection in IRF-1−/− mice. J Immunol 1996;156: 636–646.

80  Yong EC, Chi EY, Fritsche TR, Henderson WR: Human platelet-mediated cytotoxicity against *Toxoplasma gondii*: Role of thromboxane. J Exp Med 1991;173:65–78.

81  Mineo JR, McLeod R, Mack D, Smith J, Khan IA, Ely KH, Kasper LH: Antibodies to *Toxoplasma gondii* major surface protein (SAG1 P30) inhibit infection of host cells and are produced in murine intestine after peroral infection. J Immunol 1993;150:3951–3964.

82  Jones TC, Len L, Hirsch JG: Assessment in vitro of immunity against *Toxoplasma gondii*. J Exp Med 1975;141:466–482.

83  Luft BJ, Remington JS: Toxoplasmic encephalitis. J Infect Dis 1988;157:1–6.

84  Luft BJ, Hafner R, Korzun AH, Leport C, Antoniskis D, Bosler EM, Bourland DD, Uttamchandani R, Fuhrer J, Jacobson J, Morlat P, Vilde JL, Remington JS: Toxoplasmic encephalitis in patients with the acquired immunodeficiency syndrome. N Engl J Med 1993;329:995–1000.

85   Cserr HF, Knopf PM: Cervical lymphatics, the blood-brain barrier and the immunoreactivity of the brain: A new view. Immunol Today 1993;13:507–510.
86   Benveniste EN: Lymphokine and monokines in the neuroendocrine system. Prog Allergy 1988;43: 84–120.
87   Fontana A, Frei K, Bodmer S, Hofer E: Immune-mediated encephalitis: On the role of antigen-presenting cells in brain tissue. Immunol Rev 1987;100:185–201.
88   Fabry Z, Raine CS, Hart MN: Nervous tissue as an immune compartment: The dialect of the immune response in the CNS. J Immunol 1994;15:218–224.
89   Werkle H: Lymphocyte traffic to the brain; in Partridge WM (ed): The Blood Brain Barrier. New York, Raven Press, 1993, pp 67–85.
90   Israelski DM, Remington JS: AIDS associated toxoplasmosis; in Sande MA, Volderding PA (eds): The Medical Management of AIDS, ed 3. Philadelphia, Saunders, 1992, pp 319–345.
91   Clerici M, Shearer GM: A Th1-Th2 switch is a critical step in the etiology of HIV infection. Immunol Today 1993;14:107–111.
92   Gazzinelli RT, Bala S, Stevens R, Baseler M, Wahl L, Kovacs J, Sher A: HIV infection suppresses type 1 lymphokine and IL-12 responses to *Toxoplasma gondii* but fails to inhibit the synthesis of other parasite-induced monokines. J Immunol 1995;155:1565–1574.
93   Delemarre FGA, Stevenhagen A, Kroon FP, Van Eer MY, Meenhorst PL, Van Furth R: Effect of IFN-$\gamma$ on the proliferation of *Toxoplasma gondii* in monocytes and monocyte-derived macrophages from AIDS patients. Immunology 1995;83:646–650.
94   Delemarre FGA, Stevenhagen A, Kroon FP, Van Eer MY, Meenhorst PL, van Furth R: Reduced toxoplasmastatic activity of monocytes and monocyte derived macrophages from AIDS patients is mediated via prostaglandin E$_2$. AIDS 1995;9:441–445.
95   Biggs B-A, Hewish M, Kent S, Hayes K, Crowe SM: HIV-1 infection of human macrophages impairs phagocytosis and killing of *Toxoplasma gondii*. J Immunol 1995;154:6132–6139.
96   Gazzinelli RT, Sher A, Cheever A, Gerstberger S, Martin M, Dickie P: Infection of human immunodeficiency virus 1 transgenic mice with *Toxoplasma gondii* stimulates proviral transcription in macrophages in vivo. J Exp Med 1996;183:1645–1655.
97   Hunter CA, Roberts CW, Murray M, Alexander J: Detection of cytokine mRNA in the brains of mice with toxoplasmic encephalitis. Parasite Immunol 1992;14:405–413.
98   Gazzinelli R, Xu Y, Hieny S, Cheever A, Sher A: Simultaneous depletion of CD4+ and CD8+ T lymphocytes is required to reactivate chronic infections with *Toxoplasma gondii*. J Immunol 1992;149:175–180.
99   Suzuki Y, Remington JS: Dual regulation of resistance against *Toxoplasma gondii* infection by Lyt-2+ and Lyt-1+, L3T4 T cells in mice. J Immunol 1988;140:3943–3946.
100  Beaman MH, Araujo FG, Remington JS: Protective reconstitution of the SCID mouse against reactivation of *Toxoplasmic encephalitis*. J Infect Dis 1994;169:375–383.
101  Hunter CA, Roberts CW, Alexander J: Kinetics of cytokine mRNA production in the brains of mice with progressive toxoplasmic encephalitis. Eur J Immunol 1992;22:2317–2322.
102  Gazzinelli RT, Eltoum I, Wynn TA, Sher A: Acute cerebral toxoplasmosis is induced by in vivo neutralization of TNF-$\alpha$ and correlates with the down-regulated express of inducible nitric oxide synthase and other markers of macrophage activation. J Immunol 1993;151:3672–3681.
103  Suzuki Y, Conley FK, Remington JS: Importance of endogenous IFN-$\gamma$ for prevention of toxoplasmic encephalitis in mice. J Immunol 1989;143:2045–2050.
104  Suzuki Y, Conley FK, Remington JS: Treatment of toxoplasmic encephalitis in mice with recombinant gamma interferon. Infect Immun 1990;58:3050–3055.
105  Hayashi S, Chan C-C, Gazzinelli R, Roberge FC: Contribution of nitric oxide to the host parasite equilibrium in toxoplasmosis. J Immunol 1996;156:1476–1481.
106  Suzuki Y, Yang Q, Conley FK, Abrams JS, Remington JS: Antibody against interleukin-6 reduces inflammation and numbers of cysts in brains of mice with toxoplasmic encephalitis. Infect Immun 1994;62:2773–2778.
107  Hunter CA, Remington JS: Immunopathogenesis of toxoplasmic encephalitis. J Infect Dis 1994; 170:1057–1067.
108  Roberts CW, Ferguson DJP, Jebbari J, Satoskar A, Bluethmann H, Alexander J: Different roles for interleukin-4 during the course of *Toxoplasma gondii* infection. Infect Immun 1996;64:897–904.

109 Gazzinelli RT, Wysocka M, Hieny S, Scharton-Kersten T, Cheever A, Kuhn R, Muller W, Trinchieri G, Sher A: In the absence of endogenous IL-10 mice acutely infected with *Toxoplasma gondii* succumb to a lethal immune response dependent on CD4+ T cells and accompanied by overproduction of IL-12, IFN-γ and TNF-α. Immunol 1996;157:798–805.

110 Suzuki Y, Yang Q, Yang S, Nguyen N, Lim S, Liesenfeld O, Kojima T, Remington JS: IL-4 is protective against development of toxoplasmic encephalitis. J Immunol 1996;157:2564–2569.

111 Kamogawa Y, Minasi LE, Carding SR, Bottomly K, Flavell RA: The relationship of IL-4 and IFNγ-producing T cells studied by lineage ablation of IL-4-producing cells. Cell 1993;75:985–995.

112 Ferguson DJP, Graham DI, Hutchison WM: Pathological changes in the brains of mice infected with *Toxoplasma gondii*: A histological, immunocytochemical, and ultrastructural study. Int J Exp Pathol 1991;72:463–474.

113 Chao CC, Hu S, Gekker G, Novick WJ, Remington JS, Peterson PK: Effects of cytokines on multiplication of *Toxoplasma gondii* in microglial cells. J Immunol 1993;150:3404–3410.

114 Peterson PK, Gekker G, Hu S, Chao C: Intracellular survival and multiplication of *Toxoplasma gondii* in astrocytes. J Infect Dis 1993;168:1472–1478.

115 Jun CD, Kim SH, Soh CT, Kang SS, Chung HT: Nitric oxide mediates the toxoplasmastatic activity of murine microglial cells in vitro. Immunol Invest 1993;22:487–501.

116 Peterson PK, Gekker G, Hu S, Chao CC: Human astrocytes inhibit intracellular multiplication of *Toxoplasma gondii* by a nitric oxide-mediated mechanism. J Infect Dis 1995;171:516–518.

117 Hunter CA, Suzuki Y, Subauste CS, Remington JS: Cells and cytokines in resistance to *Toxoplasma gondii*. Curr Top Microbiol Immunol 1996;219:113–125.

118 Black CM, Israelski DM, Suzuki Y, Remington J: Effect of recombinant tumour necrosis factor on acute infection in mice with *Toxoplasma gondii* or *Trypanosoma cruzi*. Immunology 1990;68:570–574.

119 Alexander J, Jebbari H, Bluethmann H, Satoskar A, Roberts CW: Immunological control of *Toxoplasma gondii* and appropriate vaccine design. Curr Top Microbiol Immunol 1996;219:183–195.

120 Clark IA, Rockett KA, Cowden WB: Proposed link between cytokines, nitric oxide and human cerebral malaria. Parasitol Today 1991;7:205–207.

121 Ellis Neyer L, Grunig G, Fort M, Remington JS, Rennick D, Hunter CA: Role of interleukin-10 in regulation of T cell-dependent and T cell-independent mechanisms of resistance to *Toxoplasma gondii*. Infect Immun 1997;65:1675–1682.

122 Candolfi E, Hunter CA, Remington JS: Mitogen- and antigen-specific proliferation of T cells in murine toxoplasmosis is inhibited by reactive nitrogen intermediates. Infect Immun 1994;62:1995–2001.

123 Haque S, Khan I, Hague A, Kasper LH: Impairment of the cellular immune response in acute murine toxoplasmosis: Regulation of interleukin-2 production and macrophage-mediated inhibitory effects. Infect Immun 1994;62:2908–2916.

124 Khan IA, Matsuura T, Kasper LH: IL-10 mediates immunosuppression following acute infection with *T. gondii* in mice. Parasite Immunol 1995;17:185–195.

125 Sharma SD, Hofflin JM, Remington JS: In vivo recombinant IL-2 enhances survival against a lethal challenge with *T. gondii*. J Immunol 1985;135:4160–4163.

126 Kasper LH, Matsuura T, Khan IA: IL-7 stimulates protective immunity in mice against the intracellular pathogen, *Toxoplasma gondii*. J Immunol 1995;155:4798–4804.

127 Roberts CW, Cruickshank SM, Alexander J: Sex-determined resistance to *Toxoplasma gondii* is associated with temporal differences in cytokine production. Infect Immun 1995;63:2549–2555.

128 Walker W, Roberts CW, Ferguson DJP, Jebbari H, Alexander J: Innate immunity to *Toxoplasma gondii* infection is gender-influenced and is associated with differences in interleukin-12 and interferon-γ production. Infect Immun 1997;65:1119–1121.

129 Buxton D: Toxoplasmosis: The first commercial vaccine. Parasitol Today 1993;9:335–337.

130 Dubey JP: Toxoplasmosis. J Am Vet Med Assoc 1994;205:1593–1598.

131 Dubey JP, Baker DG, Davis SW, Urban JD, Sken SK: Persistence of immunity to toxoplasmosis in pigs vaccinated with a nonpersistent strain of *Toxoplasma gondii*. Am J Vet Res 1994;55:982–987.

132 Buxton D, Thomson K, Maley S, Wright S, Bos HJ: Vaccination of sheep with a live incomplete strain (S48) of *Toxoplasma gondii* and their immunity to challenge when pregnant. Vet Rec 1991;129:89–93.

133 Gallicha WS, Rosenthal KL: Long-lived cytotoxic T lymphocyte memory in mucosal tissues after mucosal but not systemic immunity. J Exp Med 1996;184:1871–1879.

134 McLeod R, Skamene E, Brown CR, Eisenhauer PB, Gibori G: Subcutaneous and intestinal vaccination with tachyzoites of *Toxoplasma gondii* and acquisition of immunity to peroral and congenital *Toxoplasma* challenge. J Immunol 1988;140:1632–1637.

135 Debard N, Buzoni-Gatel D, Bout D: Intranasal immunization with SAG1 protein of *Toxoplasma gondii* in association with cholera toxin dramatically reduces development of cerebral cysts after oral infection. Infect Immun 1996;64:2158–2166.

136 Fischer HG, Reichmann G, Hadding U: Toxoplasma proteins recognized by protective T lymphocytes. Curr Top Microbiol Immunol 1996;219:175–182.

137 Roberts CW, Brewer JM, Alexander J: Congenital toxoplasmosis in the Balb/c mouse: Prevention of vertical disease transmission and fetal death by vaccination. Vaccine 1994;12:1389–1394.

138 Kasper LH: Identification of stage specific antigens of *Toxoplasma gondii*. Infect Immun 1989;57:668–672.

139 Zhang YW, Smith JE: *Toxoplasma gondii*: Reactivity of murine sera against tachyzoite and cyst antigens via FAST-ELISA. Int J Parasitol 1995;25:637–640.

140 Freyre A, Choromanski L, Fishback JL, Popiel I: Immunisation of cats with tissue cysts, bradyzoites, tachyzoites of the T-263 strain of *Toxoplasma gondii*. J Parasitol 1993;79:716–719.

141 Lunden A, Lovgren K, Uggla A, Araujo FG: Immune responses and resistance to *Toxoplasma gondii* in mice immunized with antigens of the parasite incorporated into immunostimulating complexes. Infect Immun 1993;61:2639–2643.

142 Bulow R, Boothroyd JC: Protection of mice from fatal *Toxoplasma gondii* infection by immunization with p30 antigen in liposomes. J Immunol 1991;147:3496–3500.

143 Kasper LH, Currie KM, Bradley MS: An unexpected response to vaccination with a purified membrane tachyzoite antigen (P30) to *Toxoplasma gondii*. J Immunol 1985;134:3426–3431.

144 Lopes LM, Chain BM: Liposome mediated delivery stimulates a class I restricted cytotoxic T cell response to soluble antigen. Eur J Immunol 1992;22:287–290.

145 Carson WE, Giri JG, Lindermann MJ, Linett ML, Ahdieh M, Paxton R, Anderson D, Eisenmann J, Grabstein K, Caligiuri C: Interleukin (IL-15) is a novel cytokine that activates human natural killer cells via components of the IL-2 receptor. J Exp Med 1994;180:1395.

J. Alexander, Department of Immunology, University of Strathclyde,
31 Taylor Street, Glasgow G4 0NR (UK)
Fax +44 141 552 6674

Liew FY, Cox FEG (eds): Immunology of Intracellular Parasitism.
Chem Immunol. Basel, Karger, 1998, vol 70, pp 103–123

..........................

# Immunological Control of *Cryptosporidium* Infection

*Vincent McDonald, Gregory J. Bancroft*

Department of Clinical Sciences, London School of Hygiene and Tropical Hygiene, London, UK

Cryptosporidiosis, an important infectious disease affecting mucosal surfaces, is commonly found in snakes, lizards, birds and mammals. The infectious agent is the coccidian parasite *Cryptosporidium* which develops in mucosal epithelial cells and is transmitted in a faecal-oral manner through oocysts. Ingested oocysts contain four sporozoites which, after release in the digestive tract, invade host cells and initiate cycles of asexual reproduction by merogony to produce merozoites (fig. 1). Further merogony occurs in other cells and future generations of merozoites either continue to reproduce themselves or undergo sexual development leading to oocyst formation. Infection with different species may cause serious respiratory illness in domestic fowl or gastrointestinal disease in humans, domestic mammals and birds. One parasite species, *C. parvum,* which is found worldwide, causes debilitating gastrointestinal illness in humans and other mammals and is an important opportunistic pathogen in AIDS patients. Previous reviews have described in detail the biology of the parasite, clinical features of the disease and epidemiology of the infection [1, 2].

*C. parvum* infects the gastrointestinal tract, producing a cholera-like diarrhoea, vomiting, abdominal pain and weight loss. The mechanisms of pathogenesis are unclear at present but malabsorption has been demonstrated and parasite toxins may be involved. In immunocompetent hosts the symptoms may last for only a few days or up to 2–3 weeks. Cryptosporidiosis contributes to the economically important neonatal scour of farmed sheep and cattle and in some instances, particularly in sheep, overwhelming infections may lead to death. The human disease, which occurs in all age groups, accounts for 1–4% of reported cases of diarrhoea in western countries and is rarely fatal in otherwise healthy persons. Waterborne outbreaks of cryptosporidiosis have been reported in recent years involving hundreds or thousands of cases and examinations of rivers and reservoirs have shown that they are commonly contaminated with oocysts, often presumed to originate from agricultural waste. The incidence of the human disease is higher in the tropics where infants are particularly vulnerable to cryptosporidial infection. The symptoms in these young children may be quite severe or persistent, particularly when associated with malnourishment, and in some cases death may ensue. There is a high frequency of cryptosporidiosis in immunocompromised hosts, including individuals with AIDS, and the symptoms are often severe, chronic and life-threatening. In these cases, very large volumes of diarrhoea can be produced daily and widespread intestinal pathology with villous atrophy, crypt hyperplasia and erosion of the epithelium has been reported. Spread of infections to other mucosal sites including the gall bladder, biliary tract, pancreas, lungs and trachea has also been found. Chemotherapeutic agents, even those which are effective against other coccidial parasites, usually have little value in the treatment of cryptosporidiosis.

As an alternative approach to treatment, different forms of immunotherapy have been actively investigated and some have been significantly beneficial. Dissection of the host immune responses leading to elimination of infection should improve the prospects for development of more effective and refined immunological treatments. Detailed immunological studies with *Cryptosporidium* began only a few years ago, however, and compared with the quantities of information available on host responses to many other protozoa, relatively little is currently known about the immunology of cryptosporidiosis.

Elucidation of immune responses against *Cryptosporidium* will ultimately involve a focus on mucosal immunology. As the endogenous development of the parasite is confined to the mucosal surface, studies in this area should also help to increase the general understanding of local immune functions during infection with an intracellular parasite – particularly within the epithelium. Interest in the nature of these host responses is heightened by a unique feature of the parasite's development: the intracellular stages remain anchored at the lumenal surface and segregated from the host cell cytoplasm (fig. 1).

Cryptosporidiosis of animals is generally found in neonates (whereas all human age groups are susceptible) and, indeed, animals develop a refractoriness to *C. parvum* infection, which is partly immunologically mediated, 2–3 weeks after birth [2, 3]. This feature has undoubtedly hampered experimental investigation of cryptosporidiosis. Investigators, therefore, have commonly used as hosts suckling mice or, alternatively, immunocompromised mice which are highly susceptible to infection (see below). As an alternative to using *C. parvum*, some investigations have employed *C. muris*, a gastric parasite of rodents and cattle. The advantages of using *C. muris* are that adult immuno-

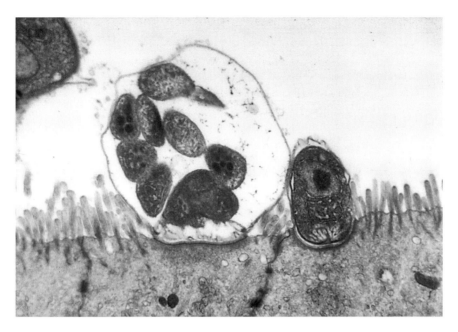

*Fig. 1.* Electron micrograph showing intracellular asexual developmental stages of *C. parvum* in intestinal epithelial cells. The organism on the right, with a single nucleus, has recently invaded the host cell, the one on the left is a mature meront with numerous merozoites present. Notable features include the extracytoplasmic location of the parasites at the lumenal surface, the electron-dense band which separates the parasite from the host cell cytoplasm and the absence of microvilli on the host cell membrane surrounding the parasite.

competent mice are susceptible to infection and adequate amounts of lymphoid tissues or serum may be recovered for analyses during infection [4].

This chapter will review recent advances in research on the mechanisms of immunity to *Cryptosporidium*, describe attempts to treat the disease by immunotherapy and examine possible areas of future research with this clinically important parasite.

### Innate Immune Responses to *Cryptosporidium*

A number of intracellular pathogens, including another coccidian, *Toxoplasma gondii*, have been shown to activate a T-cell-independent innate immune response leading to IFN-γ production which mediates macrophage activation and partial control of microbial reproduction [5]. In the activation pathway, TNF-α and IL-12 produced by macrophages trigger NK cells to produce

IFN-γ and the process is modulated by IL-10 [5–8]. This nonspecific immunity may be important in the early stages of infection before the onset of sterilizing T-cell responses or in providing a degree of immunological control of infection in immunocompromised hosts.

Cryptosporidiosis in T-cell-deficient individuals, such as those with AIDS, is often chronic and may be characterized by continuous diarrhoea, gradual expansion of foci of infection throughout the intestine and parasitization of extraintestinal mucosal tissues [1, 2]. The nature of *C. parvum* infection and also innate immune responses to the parasite have been examined in T-cell-deficient nude or SCID mice. These animals develop chronic infections which remain mild for several weeks but eventually increase in intensity and cause morbidity and death [9–13]. Several studies, however, have shown that there is an IFN-γ-dependent partially protective innate immune response since treatment with anti-IFN-γ-neutralizing antibodies exacerbated infections and shortened the time to death [9, 13–15]. We observed that weekly administration of anti-IFN-γ antibodies reduced the prepatent period from 2–4 weeks to less than 1 week and the time to death was reduced from > 12 weeks to 5–6 weeks [15]. Urban et al. [14] reported that treatment of neonatal SCID mice with anti-IL-12 also increased the susceptibility to infection, indicating that IL-12 was important in the innate response.

The involvement of both IFN-γ and IL-12 is consistent with the activation by *C. parvum* of the innate mechanism described above, but further in vivo experiments have failed to confirm NK cells as the source of IFN-γ. Administration to mice of anti-ASGM-1, which efficiently depletes NK cell numbers in vivo, had no effect on susceptibility to infection [15, 16]. It is possible that (a) this antibody had less activity in the gut than in other organs; (b) NK cells in the gut were not responsible for IFN-γ production in response to infection or (c) NK cells involved in the response expressed little ASGM-1. Similarly, attempts to demonstrate a role for TNF were also unsuccessful as injections with anti-TNF-neutralizing antibodies failed to affect the course of infection [13, 15]. In other experiments we performed, *C. parvum* infection of SCID mice was not influenced by regular injections with recombinant IL-2 which activates NK cells [15]. Thus, the in vivo data conflict with results of similar experiments obtained in studies of innate responses to nonmucosal intracellular infections, although it cannot be discounted that the T-cell-independent IFN-γ response against *Cryptosporidium* occurs by a different mechanism.

Studies of innate immunity in vitro have suggested, however, that *Cryptosporidium* is able to trigger an IFN-γ response by splenic NK cells. Chen et al. [13] demonstrated that SCID mouse splenocytes, which are rich in NK cells and macrophages, released IFN-γ when cultured in the presence of a *C. parvum* oocyst antigen preparation. Recently, R. Smith, G.J. Bancroft and V. McDon-

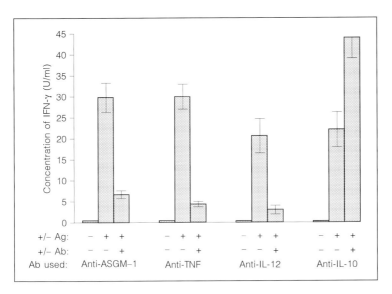

*Fig. 2.* ELISA measurement of production of IFN-γ by SCID mouse splenocytes in the presence of sporozoites of *C. muris*. 5 × 10⁵ cells were added with 2 × 10⁵ oocysts to wells in 96-well plates and cultured for 48 h at 37 °C (sporozoites are released from oocysts within 60 min). Supernatants were then examined for concentrations of IFN-γ present. Studies were made of the effect on amounts of IFN-γ produced following depletion of NK cells with rabbit antiserum against ASGM-1 (1:50 dilution) and complement, or neutralization of cytokine activity by addition of monoclonal antibodies against either murine TNF (10 μg/ml), IL-12 (2 μg/ml) or IL-10 (3 μg/ml).

ald [submitted for publication] showed that SCID mouse splenocytes also produced IFN-γ in the presence of sporozoites of *C. muris*. NK cells appeared to be the predominant source of the cytokine as depletion of these cells with anti-ASGM-1 antibodies almost abolished IFN-γ production (fig. 2). IL-12 and TNF-α were necessary for stimulation of this IFN-γ production and the response was negatively regulated by IL-10.

*Cryptosporidium*, therefore, can trigger splenic NK cells to produce IFN-γ by a similar mechanism to that found in other infection systems, but the cell type in the mucosa which produces this cytokine remains to be identified. Our studies have indicated that intraepithelial lymphocytes (IELs) may play a major part in T-cell-mediated immune responses to cryptosporidia (see later) and it is possible that NK cells present in this cell population [17] are important in the innate immune response. The accessory cells involved in this local T-cell-independent response have also to be identified since gut epithelium contains few macrophages [17]. Epithelial cells might replace macrophages for this function, however, as they are able to produce inflammatory cytokines.

## The Role of T Cells in Response to Cryptosporidial Infection

*C. parvum* induces an intestinal inflammatory response in different host species, with increased numbers of lymphocytes, plasma cells and macrophages being found in the lamina propria [2]. Increased numbers of both CD4[+] and CD8[+] cells have been observed in the Peyer's patches of mice during infection with *C. parvum* [18] and purified splenic T cells from previously infected hosts proliferated in vitro in the presence of parasite antigen [19]. Rats recovered from *C. parvum* infection demonstrated parasite-specific delayed-type hypersensitivity reactions following injection of oocyst antigen [20]. These observations suggested that T cells were involved in the immune response to cryptosporidial infection and Heine et al. [21] demonstrated that these cells were necessary for elimination of *C. parvum* infestation. These workers observed that, whereas immunocompetent suckling mice had a transient patent infection with little associated intestinal pathology, athymic nude mice had intense chronic infections with severe pathology and mortality. Similar observations were made in studies with other T-cell-deficient hosts, including newborn nude rats, adult nude mice, SCID mice or immunocompetent mice depleted of T cells by administration of anti-T-cell antibodies [9–13, 22, 23] and the histopathological pattern observed in the intestine – crypt hyperplasia, villous atrophy, erosion of epithelium and extraintestinal infection – was similar to that sometimes found in immunocompromised patients with cryptosporidiosis [2]. In studies with *C. muris*, adult nude or SCID mice developed chronic infections which could not be eliminated and the susceptibility of immunocompetent mice to infection was increased following treatment with anti-Thy.1 + anti-Lyt.1 antibodies [4, 10]. Chronic infections in nude or SCID mice may be overcome by injection of immunocompetent lymphocytes contained in bone marrow, thymus, mesenteric lymph node (MLN) or spleen cells, but depletion of T cells from the donor population was found to abolish the protective effect of donor cells [4, 10, 22–25]. T cells defined by either αβ or γδ T-cell receptors were both involved in immunity against *C. parvum* infection since neonatal mice deficient in either type of receptor were more susceptible to infection than control animals [26]. The αβ T cells appeared to be more crucial than γδ T cells, however, as in experiments with adult mice, those deficient in αβ T cells developed infections as before but those deficient in γδ T cells and control animals were refractory to infection.

Clinical studies of human cryptosporidiosis and investigations with murine infection models have indicated that CD4[+] cells played a major protective role in immunity. Susceptibility to *C. parvum* infection in HIV patients appears to increase with the progression to AIDS and the most severe symptoms have been observed in patients with the lowest CD4[+] cell counts [27]. However, in one study, no reduction in the ratio of $CD4^+:CD8^+$ cells was found in infants with chronic cryptosporidiosis in West Africa [28]. In murine studies, continuous administration of anti-CD4 antibodies to suckling or adult mice allowed chronic *C. parvum* infections to develop [9, 22] and treatment of mice with similar antibodies increased susceptibility to *C. muris* [4]. Conversely, SCID mice reconstituted with functional lymphocytes from immunocompetent mice developed immunity to cryptosporidial infection but depletion of $CD4^+$ cells from the donor population abrogated the protective effect [15, 22, 24, 25]. McDonald et al. [4] reported that MLN or spleen cells from immunocompetent donor mice recovered from *C. muris* infection could be used to transfer immunity adoptively to SCID mice, but depletion of T cells or $CD4^+$ cells from donor cells abolished this immunity. In another approach, Aguirre et al. [29] observed that mice with MHC class II deficiency (therefore lacking functional $CD4^+$ cells) were as susceptible to *C. parvum* as SCID mice.

In contrast with the dominant role of $CD4^+$ cells described above, $CD8^+$ cells appear to have either a minor role in host protection against *Cryptosporidium* or are not relevant. Some investigators have observed no effect on cryptosporidial infection when $CD8^+$ cells in the host were depleted using antibodies [24, 25]. In one investigation, splenic cells from mice repeatedly challenged with *C. parvum* demonstrated parasite antigen-specific proliferative responses but when the cells were enriched for $CD4^+$ or $CD8^+$ cells, only the subset of enriched $CD4^+$ cells could be stimulated by antigen [19]. Further evidence of a lack of $CD8^+$ cell involvement in immunity came from a study showing that mice lacking $CD8^+$ cell function as a result of MHC class I deficiency were no more susceptible to cryptosporidial infection than control mice [29]. In studies with both *C. parvum* and *C. muris*, however, we reported that depletion of $CD8^+$ cells, either in immunocompetent mice or in SCID mice injected with functional T cells from naive or infection-primed animal donors, consistently produced a small increase in oocyst production and/or prolonged the duration of patent infection [4, 10, 15]. In a study with *C. parvum*, Ungar et al. [9] found that adult immunocompetent mice, which are normally refractory to infection, developed chronic infections when administered anti-CD4 antibodies and that the susceptibility increased further by simultaneous administration of anti-CD8 antibodies. The contradictory observations made by different investigators in experiments of this type might be explained by differences in the potency or amounts of the anti-CD8 antibodies used or variation in the sensitivity of methods for measurement of infection levels. So far, few studies have been made to characterize the protective T cells in the mucosa or the migration pattern and location of these cells at the site of infection. We have obtained results, however, which suggest that IELs, which are predominately T cells, may play an important part in the establishment of host resistance.

*Table 1.* Effect of anti-IFN-γ-neutralizing antibody on the adoptive transfer of immunity against *C. muris* to CB.17 SCID mice obtained using IELs from previously infected BALB/c mice

| Treatment given to SCID mice[a] | Mean number of oocysts produced ($\times 10^6$)[b] | Number of days taken for recovery |
|---|---|---|
| None | 82 ± 9* | > 36[c] |
| Naive IELs | 72 ± 8* | > 36[c] |
| Immune IELs | 6 ± 3** | 21–24 |
| Immune IELs + anti-IFN-γ | 48 ± 6*** | 30–35 |

[a] Prior to infection with *C. muris*, SCID mice were injected intravenously with medium or $1 \times 10^6$ intestinal IELs from BALB/c mice which were naive or had recovered from *C. muris* infection. Mice also received intraperitoneally 250 μg H22 hamster anti-mouse IFN-γ IgG monoclonal antibody in saline or saline alone on days 0, 7, 14 and 21. Infection data are derived from the study of Culshaw et al. [34].

[b] The values in this column represent the mean of the total numbers of oocysts produced by each group up to day 36 of infection. Values with different numbers of asterisks are significantly different (p < 0.0001).

[c] SCID control mice given no IELs or IELs from naive BALB/c did not recover from infection.

Immunity to *C. muris* infection was obtained in SCID mice injected with as few as $1 \times 10^6$ intestinal IELs isolated from previously infected immunocompetent donor mice [30] (table 1). Interestingly, SCID mice given IELs from naive immunocompetent donors were as susceptible to infection as control SCID mice, whereas injection with MLN or spleen cells from naive immunocompetent animals allowed SCID mice to recover [4, 30]. T cells were found in the IEL population of SCID mice given naive IELs, so failure of these cells to provide any protection was not associated with an inability to migrate to the gut [unpubl. data]. There is evidence to suggest that most T cells present in the gut epithelium have previously been activated [17] and it is possible that in our study the IEL population contained many cells which were effete or lacked the pluripotential of lymphocytes from other tissues. The adoptive transfer of immunity obtained using immune IELs required the presence of CD4[+] cells in the immune donor cell population since immunity was abrogated by depletion of CD4[+] cells with anti-CD4 antibodies. Furthermore, CD4[+] cells were located in the gut IEL population of the recipient SCID mice which had recovered from infection. In comparison, depletion of CD8[+] cells produced only a small decrease in the protective effect of immune IELs although they formed about 90% of the donor cell population [30]. These observations are consistent with earlier observations on the relative importance of CD4[+] and CD8[+] cells in resistance against *Cryptosporidium* and indicate that CD4[+] IELs play a major part in the induction of immunity. Future studies in this area need to characterize further the phenotype of the protective mucosal T cells and determine the source(s) of these cells and their eventual location in the mucosa during the recovery phase of infection.

### Involvement of IFN-γ in T-Cell-Mediated Immunity

Host production of IFN-γ has been shown to be pivotal in T-cell-mediated effector mechanisms against cryptosporidial infection. Susceptibility of immunocompetent mice to either *C. parvum* or *C. muris* infection is increased following treatment with IFN-γ-neutralizing antibodies [9, 10] and in one study a similar treatment abolished the protection conferred on SCID mice against *C. parvum* infection by injected spleen cells obtained from immuno-competent animals [24]. However, IFN-γ-independent mechanisms of immunity may also operate as it has been observed that mice continuously treated with anti-IFN-γ antibodies eventually overcome *C. parvum* or *C. muris* infection [9, 10].

In studies to examine *C. parvum*-induced T-cell cytokine production, Harp et al. [19] reported that splenic T cells from immunized mice produced IFN-γ in the presence of oocyst antigen and that this production was associated with CD4[+] cells but not CD8[+] cells. Similarly, Tilley et al. [31] measured IFN-γ released by spleen cells at different times during *C. muris* infection of mice and observed increasing amounts of the cytokine starting from the early stages of recovery; once again, production of IFN-γ appeared to be predominantly (but not entirely) associated with CD4[+] T cells. Recently, increased levels of IFN-γ production or mRNA expression during either *C. parvum* or *C. muris* infection were observed in MLN cells [14, 32]. In an investigation of variation between MHC congenic strains of mice in susceptibility to *C. muris* infection, Davami et al. [32] observed that BALB/c mice were more resistant than BALB/b mice, but the strains demonstrated similar patterns of IFN-γ production by splenocytes during infection. This indicated that the difference in susceptibility between these strains was not related to the ability to mount an IFN-γ response.

Recently, attempts have been made to measure IFN-γ responses in the mucosa during or after cryptosporidial infection. Kapel et al. [33], examining IFN-γ concentrations in ileal homogenates of *C. parvum*-infected suckling immunocompetent mice, demonstrated an increase during the acute phase of infection and then a decrease to control levels as the mice recovered. Using the same model, Urban et al. [14] showed an increase in IFN-γ mRNA expression in intestinal homogenates during infection. In the above studies, no attempts were made to identify the cells producing IFN-γ but, as we had previously shown that IELs were sensitized to mobilize mechanisms for elimination of C. muris [30], we have now examined the possible requirement for IFN-γ production in the protective role of IELs. Thus, Culshaw et al. [34] (table 1) compared C. muris infections in SCID mice reconstituted with IELs from immunocompetent mice recovered from infection and similar reconstituted mice which also received anti-IFN-γ antibodies during infection. As in previous studies [30], control SCID mice and those given naive IELs failed to control infections and produced large numbers of oocysts. The mice given immune IELs, in contrast, had mild infections and recovered by day 24 postinfection. Mice given immune IELs and also treated with anti-IFN-γ antibodies (on days 0, 7, 14 and 21), however, produced a number of oocysts 8-fold greater than that obtained for animals given immune IELs only. These mice failed to begin recovery until at least 9 days after the final injection of anti-IFN-γ and patent infections were observed until day 35. These observations demonstrated that the resistance against infection conferred on SCID mice by immune IELs was IFN-γ-dependent.

Further experiments by Culshaw et al. [34] compared production of IFN-γ by IELs from C. muris-immune and naive mice, using an enzyme-linked immunospot assay (ELISPOT) for detection of individual cells producing IFN-γ. It was found that the IELs from immune mice stimulated with concanavalin A or rat anti-mouse CD3 monoclonal antibodies contained up to 9-fold more IFN-γ-producing cells compared with IELs from naive mice. This bias towards production of IFN-γ shown by activated immune IELs was compatible with the finding that animals recovered from infection were completely resistant to reinfection [10]. Culshaw et al. [34] also examined parasite antigen-specific stimulation of IELs and observed that, in the presence of oocyst antigen, IFN-γ-producing cells developed in the immune IEL population but not in the corresponding naive population. Our findings, therefore, suggest that infection-primed IELs, which promote development of immunity, are an important mucosal source of IFN-γ required for the elimination of the parasite.

The mechanism by which IFN-γ exerts its protective effect against Cryptosporidium remains to be determined, however. Intestinal epithelial cells express IFN-γ receptors [35] and IFN-γ increases MHC class I and II expression in epithelial cells [36, 37]. IFN-γ has been found to increase production of the secretory component for transportation of IgA across the mucosal epithelium to the lumen [37] and parasite-specific secretory antibody might play some part in immunity to infection (see below). IFN-γ is also important in T-cell-mediated clearance of two other coccidian parasites, *Eimeria* and *Toxoplasma* [38, 39] and, in vitro, has been observed to inhibit intracellular reproduction of these parasites in epithelial cell lines [40, 41]. IFN-γ may kill intracellular organisms in nonepithelial cells by activation of reactive oxygen intermediates or arginine-derived nitric oxide and, in fibroblasts infected with *Toxoplasma*, may alter the host cell metabolism to starve the parasite of tryptophan [41–43]. It is not known whether intestinal epithelial cells can effect nitric oxide-mediated parasite killing but Kuhls et al. [44] reported that treatment of mice with an inhibitor of nitric oxide production, aminoguanidine, previously shown to exacerbate *Listeria* development, had no effect on the reproduction of *C. parvum*. Finally, IFN-γ may increase epithelial cell turnover and in cryptosporidial infection this would serve to accelerate the sloughing of parasitized cells from the villi [45].

In summary, sterilizing immunity to cryptosporidial infection is associated with the production of IFN-γ by protective T cells. Further studies are needed to characterize factors which regulate IFN-γ production by mucosal T cells. In addition, in vitro culture systems of *C. parvum* are available [46] and it should be possible to use these to determine whether IFN-γ directly induces intracellular killing of *Cryptosporidium* and, if so, establish the mechanisms for parasite inactivation.

## Production of Other T Cell Cytokines during Infection

The finding that IFN-γ, a key Th1 type cytokine, plays a highly influential role in the development of immunity to *Cryptosporidium* suggests that infection may activate a Th1 inflammatory response more effectively than a Th2 antibody-dominating response [47]. In support of this view, Urban et al. [14] demonstrated that treatment of newborn mice with neutralizing antibody against IL–12, a cytokine which strongly induces Th1 T-cell development, increased the intensity of *C. parvum* infection. Furthermore, treatment of mice with exogenous IL-12 conferred complete resistance against infection induced by oocysts administered a day later. The efficacy of the exogenous IL-12 appeared to be related to IFN-γ production, since administration of anti-IFN-γ antibodies abolished the protective effect conferred by the cytokine. If administration of IL-12 was delayed until 2 days after infection, however, the exogenous cytokine had no effect on parasite reproduction.

Splenic and/or MLN cells from mice recovering from *C. muris* infection or immunized against *C. parvum* infection have been shown to produce increased amounts of IL-2, another Th1 cytokine [19, 32] but, in another murine study with *C. parvum*, no increase in IL-2 mRNA expression by MLN cells was obtained during infection [14]. In the first two of these studies [19, 32], however, the isolated lymphoid cells were stimulated in vitro with parasite antigen first before cytokine measurements whereas no stimulation was done in the latter study [14]. Administration of anti-IL-2-neutralizing antibodies to mice infected with *C. parvum* increased oocyst production [48] and in a human study IL-2 therapy was found to reduce the levels of diarrhoea and oocyst shedding in AIDS patients with cryptosporidiosis [49]. These results suggest, therefore, that IL-2 is important in the development of immunity to cryptosporidiosis. In our studies, TNF has not been implicated in the immune response to *C. muris* as it was not produced by spleen cells or MLN cells from animals recovering from infection [32] and treatment with anti-TNF-neutralizing antibodies during infection had no effect on parasite development [10].

Th2 cytokines have been examined in only a small number of studies of cryptosporidial infections. In mice repeatedly challenged with oocysts of *C. parvum*, no splenic IL-4 production was detected by ELISA [19] and during infection with the same parasite no change in IL-4 or IL-10 mRNA expression was found in the intestine or MLN cells [14]. However, treatment of mice during infection with *C. parvum* with anti-IL-4 or anti-IL-5 antibodies increased oocyst shedding compared with control animals while administration of both antibodies together was more effective than either alone in increasing susceptibility to infection [48]. During *C. muris* infection of BALB/c mice, a low level of IL-4 was released by spleen cells stimulated by parasite antigen around the time of elimination of infection [31, 32]. IL-5 and IL-4, therefore, may contribute to the development of immunity against cryptosporidial infection. These cytokines are particularly important in proliferation of eosinophils and mast cells, respectively, but, histopathological observations do not show a large infiltration of eosinophils during infection and mast cell-deficient mice were not significantly more susceptible to infection than control mice [2, 50]. In another study, we examined the immunological basis of variation in susceptibility to *C. muris* infection between BALB/b mice and BALB/c mice. Davami et al. [32] observed that BALB/c was significantly more resistant to infection than BALB/b and, in examining Th1 (IFN-$\gamma$, IL-2) and Th2 (IL-4, IL-10) cytokine production by spleen cells during infection, the only cytokine which had a different pattern of release in each strain was IL-4: BALB/c produced none until towards the end of the patent infection when small amounts were measured but BALB/b produced high concentrations starting a few days after infection and the onset of recovery in this strain coincided with a reduction in the amount of IL-4 produced. This suggested that overproduction of IL-4 correlated with increased susceptibility to infection.

Th1 cytokines are important, therefore, in generating host resistance to *Cryptosporidium* infection. The role of Th2 cytokines in immunity is less clear, however, although some evidence has suggested that a Th2 response contributes to the control of infection. It is possible that in the early stages of the development of the host response, Th1 cytokines have a predominant protective role but become less important in the later stages of recovery. Indirect evidence for this comes from two studies which showed that although continual treatment with IFN-γ-neutralizing antibodies at first significantly exacerbated *C. parvum* or *C. muris* infection in mice, the animals eventually recovered [9, 10]. Determining the relative importance of Th1 and Th2 responses and characterizing the cytokine profile produced by protective CD4$^+$ mucosal T cells will help in elucidating the nature of parasite killing mechanisms and could lead to the development of valuable immunotherapies for use with immunocompromised hosts.

## Antibody Response to Infection

Titres of parasite-specific antibodies of different classes increase in the serum and mucosal secretions during *C. parvum* infections of humans, cattle and sheep and may persist for months or years postinfection [2, 51–54]. Serum IgM antibodies develop before IgG antibodies but IgM titres decline rapidly after recovery whereas IgG could persist for several months [51, 52]. Titres of IgM and IgA coproantibodies increase during infection and then decrease after recovery, although the rate of decrease for IgM is greater [52, 53].

Antibodies from convalescent hosts of different species have been shown to recognize a number of immunodominant sporozoite antigens, including polypeptides of approximately 11, 15, 20/23, 44, 100, 180 and > 200 kD [1, 52, 53, 55] and at least some of these antigens may be protective (see below). Anti-*C. parvum* murine monoclonal antibodies have been generated against sporozoites and may recognize one of the above antigens or any of many other parasite antigens which have been identified [56]. Following intramammary immunization of cattle with oocyst antigen and Freund's complete adjuvant, 'hyperimmune' bovine colostrum (HBC) has been obtained which contained high titres of anti-*C. parvum* sporozoite antibodies [57–60]. Monoclonal or HBC antibodies which recognize the sporozoite have been shown to inhibit significantly *C. parvum* development either in vitro or in suckling mice when administered orally [61–64]. In addition, treatment of immunocompromised patients with HBC has often proved to be highly effective in attenuating the clinical effects of cryptosporidial infection [57–59]. Therapeutic antibodies were found to produce a circumsporozoite precipitation effect similar to that observed with anti-*Plasmodium* sporozoite-neutralizing antibodies which may help to inactivate the extracellular parasite [65].

Protective antibodies reactive with sporozoites may recognize the whole organism, the pellicle or the anterior end which attaches to the host cell prior to invasion and contains the apical complex organelles involved in invasion. A number of sporozoite antigens recognized by protective antibodies have been cloned and/or partially characterized and these clones will be valuable in future studies in immunology and immunotherapy [60, 66–68]. Clearly, immunodominant protective antigens shared by sporozoites and merozoites would be attractive candidates for development of immunotherapy and, indeed, epitopes common to the respective invasive stages have been demonstrated using inhibitory monoclonal antibodies [67–69]. In addition to the extracellular invasive stages, the host cell membrane at the lumenal surface surrounding the intracellular parasite might be a target for immunological attack by antibody as it has been demonstrated in this laboratory that two antigens found in sporozoites were also expressed on this membrane in all infected cells [70].

Although antibodies developed by immunization with antigens could inhibit parasite development, there is considerable doubt about the protective role played by antibodies developed during infection. In human studies, AIDS patients with severe chronic cryptosporidiosis have had high titres of anti-*C. parvum* secretory IgA, perhaps suggesting that the antibody was not protective [71]. Although passive immunity has been demonstrated with HBC (see above), no protective activity has been found in colostrum from animals previously exposed to cryptosporidial infection or repeatedly infected with *C. parvum* [72, 73]. More evidence that antibody was not required for the development of immunity was obtained in studies which examined the effect of B-cell depletion on cryptosporidial infection in mice. Taghi-Kilani et al. [74] observed that neonatal mice depleted of B cells by anti-μ chain treatment, and lacking the ability to produce immunoglobulin, were able to control *C. parvum* infection as efficiently as controls with normal B-cell function. Using a similar approach, M.H. Davami and V. McDonald [unpubl. data] found that SCID mice injected with immunocompetent spleen cells depleted of 99% of B cells were able to control *C. muris* infection as effectively as those given the whole spleen population containing approximately 40% B cells: parasite-specific antibody was detectable in the serum of the latter group only.

There is some evidence, however, supporting a protective role for antibody produced during infection. For example, there have been a number of reports of chronic infections in patients with congenital hypogammaglobulinaemia

[1, 2]. In addition, some epidemiological studies [1, 2] have indicated that breast-fed babies were less likely to experience cryptosporidiosis, suggesting protection could be provided by lactogenic immunity. Finally, in an experimental investigation, there was reduced C. parvum development and pathology in nude mice if treated with bile from previously infected immunocompetent rats which contained parasite-specific secretory IgA [75].

Overall, infection antibodies appear to have a minor role in protection but there is sufficient evidence to the contrary to support a closer examination of this area. In the future, continuing work on identification and cloning of protective antigens should be followed by investigation of T-cell responses against these antigens. These studies may provide valuable information on immune mechanisms and in the long term provide effective forms of immunotherapy.

## Immunotherapy against Cryptosporidiosis

The lack of an effective drug for chemotherapy against cryptosporidiosis has encouraged the investigation of development of immunotherapy. Most immunocompetent individuals infected with C. parvum feel extremely unwell for several days but recover fully with no after-effects. The most worthwhile use for therapy, therefore, would probably be for newborn livestock (which are highly susceptible for only 2–3 weeks after birth) or immunocompromised patients. Different forms of immunotherapy against cryptosporidiosis in experimental animal infection models or patients have met with varying degrees of success.

The most consistently fruitful results have been obtained with HBC treatment which produced alleviation of symptoms and significant reduction or elimination of the parasite burden in mice, calves or humans [57–59, 64]. Parasite-specific antibodies of different classes have been demonstrated to be important protective components of this colostrum [63, 64]. Similarly, hens immunized against C. parvum by subcutaneous injection of antigen and adjuvant produced eggs containing yolks with high anti-C. parvum antibody titres and oral administration of the yolk to infected mice reduced parasite development by 85% [76]. One problem with this approach may be that patients with severe symptoms of cryptosporidiosis (e.g. anorexia or vomiting) may be unable to ingest these products but this could probably be overcome by administering purified antibodies in a small protective capsule. Another difficulty with this form of treatment may be that extraintestinal sites of infection (e.g. respiratory and biliary tracts) commonly reported in immunocompromised patients [1, 2] may be inaccessible to orally administered reagents. Other potential problems with these products may be variability in potency of batches, limitations in the amounts that can be obtained and a possible lack of commercial viability. Large-scale production of protective monoclonal antibodies may circumvent some of these obstacles, but a cocktail of antibodies recognizing different epitopes may be required for effectiveness [62].

Experimental studies have also been carried out on the treatment of cryptosporidial infection with soluble T-cell products. One of the earliest investigations employed a bovine dialysable leucocyte (DLE) extract, or transfer factor, prepared from lymph node lymphocytes from calves immunized by *C. parvum* infection [77]. Six out of 7 AIDS patients with cryptosporidiosis given 'immune' DLE orally had improved symptoms and eradicated oocysts from stools. No attempt was made to identify the protective component, however, and, in another report, this product failed to provide any efficacy in infected calves [78].

In the investigation of the efficacy of cytokines there have been reports of both success and failure in treatment. One of the most promising results has been obtained in an experimental study to examine the effect of IL-12 on *C. parvum* infection in suckling mice [14]. A single injection of either immunocompetent or SCID mice with IL-12 a day before oocyst inoculation provided complete immunity against infection. Unfortunately, no protection was observed when the treatment was given 1–2 days postinfection. Although IFN-γ has been shown to play a prominent part in both innate and acquired immunity against *Cryptosporidium*, treatment of mice with IFN-γ was found in separate studies to be ineffective [15, 44], but one report has suggested that remission of chronic cryptosporidiosis in a child was obtained as a result of treatment with IFN-γ [79]. In studies of *C. parvum*-infected SCID mice given IL-2, McDonald and Bancroft [15] failed to observe any reduction in parasite reproduction. In contrast, Connolly et al. [49] reported that oocyst shedding decreased and symptoms were significantly reduced in AIDS patients treated with IL-2.

The principle of immunological therapy against cryptosporidial infection, therefore, has been demonstrated experimentally and in patients using either antibodies or cytokines. Future considerations for therapy should arise from elucidation of local immune effector mechanisms, including examination of the role of products from T cells or epithelial cells. The development of means to stimulate mucosal B-cell function or IgA production may increase the titres of local antibody and prove beneficial. The design of procedures to deliver increased concentrations of exogenous cytokines to the site of infection may also be valuable.

## Conclusions

T-cell-independent and T-cell-dependent mechanisms of immunity have been identified in rodent models of cryptosporidial infection. In each case, IFN-γ was involved in the development of effector mechanisms leading to parasite killing but the parasite life-cycle stages affected by immunity and the means of killing have not been elucidated. T-cell immunity via CD4$^+$ cells was necessary for elimination of infection and immunity correlated with the ability of CD4$^+$ cells to proliferate in response to parasite antigens and produce IFN-γ. In contrast, the involvement of CD8$^+$ cells in immunity has been determined to be relatively minor. In the gut, immunity was associated with the presence of protective CD4$^+$ IELs and local production of IFN-γ, but the role of mucosal T cells in elimination of infection is otherwise poorly understood.

Many studies have shown that cryptosporidial infection stimulated an antibody response, including secretory IgA. Examination of the protective role of antibody has generally suggested that it is not significant but some evidence to the contrary has been provided. In contrast, monoclonal or poly-clonal antibodies developed by immunization with parasite antigens have been shown to confer passive immunity against infection when administered orally. At least partial protection and relief of symptoms of cryptosporidiosis have been obtained with antibody or cytokine therapies. Investigations to clone and characterize immunodominant antigens have been initiated in recent years and examination of the host response to these antigens should lead to the development of more refined immunotherapies.

## References

1     Current WL, Garcia LS: Cryptosporidiosis. Microbiol Rev 1991;4:325–358.
2     Tzipori S: Cryptosporidiosis in perspective. Adv Parasitol 1988;27:63–129.
3     Sherwood DK, Angus KW, Snodgrass DR, Tzipori S: Experimental cryptosporidiosis in laboratory mice. Infect Immun 1982;38:471–475.
4     McDonald V, Robinson HA, Kelly JP, Bancroft GJ: *Cryptosporidium muris* in adult mice: Adoptive transfer of immunity and roles of CD4 versus CD8 cells. Infect Immun 1994;62:2289–2294.
5     Bancroft GJ, Schreiber RD, Unanue ER: Natural immunity: A T-cell-independent pathway of macrophage activation, defined in the SCID mouse. Immunol Rev 1991;124:5–24.
6     Tripp CS, Wolf SF, Unanue ER: Interleukin-12 and tumor necrosis factor alpha are costimulators of interferon gamma production by natural killer cells in severe combined immunodeficiency mice with listeriosis, and interleukin-10 is a physiologic antagonist. Proc Natl Acad Sci USA 1993;90: 3725–3729.
7     Gazzinelli RT, Hieny S, Wynn TA, Wolf S, Sher A: Interleukin-12 is required for the T-lymphocyte-independent induction of interferon-γ by an intracellular parasite and induces resistance in T-cell-deficient hosts. Proc Natl Acad Sci USA 1993;90:6115–6119.

8    Hunter CA, Subauste CS, Van Cleave VH, Remington JS: Production of gamma interferon by natural killer cells from *Toxoplasma gondii*-infected SCID mice: Regulation by interleukin-10, interleukin-12, and tumor necrosis factor alpha. Infect Immun 1994;62:2818–2824.

9    Ungar BLP, Kao T-C, Burris JA, Finkelman FD: *Cryptosporidium* infection in an adult mouse model. Independent roles for IFN-γ and CD4+ T lymphocytes in protective immunity. J Immunol 1991;147:1014–1022.

10   McDonald V, Deer R, Uni S, Iseki S, Bancroft GJ: Immune responses to *Cryptosporidium muris* and *Cryptosporidium parvum* in adult immunocompetent or immunocompromised (nude and SCID mice). Infect Immun 1992;60:3325–3331.

11   Kuhls S, Greenfield RA, Mosier DA, Crawford DL, Joyce WA: Cryptosporidiosis in adult and neonatal mice with severe combined immunodeficiency. J Comp Pathol 1992;106:399–410.

12   Mead JR, Arrowood MJ, Sidwell RW, Healey MC: Chronic *Cryptosporidium parvum* infections in congenitally immunodeficient SCID and nude mice. J Infect Dis 1991;163:1297–1304.

13   Chen W, Harp JA, Harmsen AG, Havell EA: Gamma interferon functions in resistance to *Cryptosporidium parvum* infection in severe combined immunodeficient mice. Infect Immun 1993;61:3548–3551.

14   Urban JF Jr, Fayer R, Chen S-J, Gause WC, Gately MK, Finkelman FD: IL-12 protects immunocompetent and immunodeficient neonatal mice against infection with *Cryptosporidium parvum*. J Immunol 1996;156:263–268.

15   McDonald V, Bancroft GJ: Mechanisms of innate and acquired immunity in SCID mice infected with *Cryptosporidium parvum*. Parasite Immunol 1994;16:315–320.

16   Rohlman V, Kuhls T, Mosier D, Crawford D, Greenfield R: *Cryptosporidium parvum* infection after abrogation of natural killer cell activity in normal and severe combined immunodeficiency mice. J Parasitol 1993;79:295–297.

17   Sim G-K: Intraepithelial lymphocytes and the immune system. Adv Immunol 1995;58:297–343.

18   Boher Y, Perez-Schael I, Caceres-Dittmar G, Urbina G, Gonzalez R, Kraal G, Tapia FJ: Enumeration of selected leukocytes in the small intestine of BALB/c mice infected with *Cryptosporidium parvum*. Am J Trop Med Hyg 1994;50:145–151.

19   Harp JA, Whitmire WM, Sacco R: In vitro proliferation and production of gamma interferon by murine CD4+ cells in response to *Cryptosporidium parvum* antigen. J Parasitol 1994;80:67–72.

20   Gardner AL, Roche JK, Weikel CS, Guerrant RL: Intestinal cryptosporidiosis: Pathophysiologic alterations and specific cellular and humoral immune responses in RNU/+ and RNU/RNU (athymic) rats. Am J Trop Med Hyg 1991;44:49–62.

21   Heine J, Moon HW, Woodmansee DB: Persistent *Cryptosporidium* infection in congenitally athymic (nude) mice. Infect Immun 1984;43:856–859.

22   Ungar BLP, Burris JA, Quinn CA, Finkelman FD: New mouse models for chronic *Cryptosporidium* infection in immunodeficient hosts. Infect Immun 1990;58:961–969.

23   Mead JR, Arrowood MJ, Healey MC, Sidwell RS: Cryptosporidial infections in SCID mice reconstituted with human or murine lymphocytes. J Protozool 1991;38:59S–61S.

24   Chen W, Harp JA, Harmsen AG: Requirements for CD4+ cells and gamma interferon in resolution of established *Cryptosporidium parvum* infection in mice. Infect Immun 1993;61:3928–3932.

25   Perryman LA, Mason PH, Chrisp CE: Effect of spleen cell populations in resolution of *Cryptosporidium parvum* infection in SCID mice. Infect Immun 1994;62:1474–1477.

26   Waters WR, Harp JA: *Cryptosporidium parvum* infection in T-cell receptor (TCR)-α- and TCR-δ-deficient mice. Infect Immun 1996;64:1854–1857.

27   Flanigan T, Whalen C, Turner J, Soave S, Toerner J, Havlir D, Kotler D: *Cryptosporidium* infection and CD4 counts. Ann Intern Med 1992;116:840–842.

28   Molbak K, Lisse IM, Hojling N, Aaby P: Severe cryptosporidiosis in children with normal T-cell subsets. Parasite Immunol 1994;16:275–277.

29   Aguirre SA, Mason PH, Perryman LE: Susceptibility of major histocompatibility class I- and class II-deficient mice to *Cryptosporidium parvum* infection. Infect Immun 1994;62:697–699.

30   McDonald V, Robinson HA, Kelly JP, Bancroft GJ: Immunity to *Cryptosporidium muris* in mice is expressed through gut CD4+ intraepithelial lymphocytes. Infect Immun 1996;64:2556–2662.

31  Tilley M, McDonald V, Bancroft GJ: Resolution of cryptosporidial infection in mice correlates with parasite-specific lymphocyte proliferation associated with Th1 and Th2 cytokine secretion. Parasite Immunol 1995;17:459–464.

32  Davami MH, Bancroft GJ, McDonald V: *Cryptosporidium* infection in MHC congenic strains of mice: Variation in susceptibility and the role of T-cell cytokine responses. Parasitol Res 1997;83:257–263.

33  Kapel N, Benhamou Y, Buraud M, Magne D, Opolon P, Gobert J-G: Kinetics of mucosal ileal gamma-interferon response during cryptosporidiosis in immunocompetent neonatal mice. Parasitol Res 1996;82:664–667.

34  Culshaw RJ, Bancroft GJ, McDonald V: Gut intraepithelial lymphocytes induce immunity against *Cryptosporidium* infection through a mechanism involving interferon gamma production. Infect Immun 1997;65:3074–3079.

35  Valente GL, Ozmen L, Novelli F, Geuna M, Palestro G, Forni G, Garotta G: Distribution of IFN-$\gamma$ receptor in human tissues. Eur J Immunol 1992;22:2403–2412.

36  Colgan SP, Parkos CA, Mathhews JB, D'Anrea L, Awtrey CS, Lichtman AH, Delp-Archer C, Madara JL: Interferon-gamma induces a cell surface phenotype switch on T84 intestinal epithelial cells. Am J Physiol 1994;267:C402–C410.

37  Kvale D, Brandtzaeg P, Lovhaug D: Up-regulation of the secretory component and HLA molecules in human colonic cell line by tumor necrosis factor-$\alpha$ and gamma interferon. Scand J Immunol 1988;28:351–357.

38  Rose ME, Wakelin D, Hesketh P: Interferon-gamma-mediated effects upon immunity to coccidial infections in the mouse. Parasite Immunol 1991;13:63–74.

39  Suzuki Y, Conley FK, Remington JS: Treatment of toxoplasmic encephalitis in mice with recombinant gamma interferon. Infect Immun 1990;58:3050–3055.

40  Rose ME, Smith AL, Wakelin D: Gamma interferon-mediated inhibition of *Eimeria vermiformis* growth in cultured fibroblasts and epithelial cells. Infect Immun 1991;59:59–65.

41  Dimier IH, Bout DT: Rat intestinal epithelial cell line IEC-6 is activated by recombinant interferon-$\gamma$ to inhibit replication of the coccidian *Toxoplasma gondii.* Eur J Immunol 1993;23:981–983.

42  Cox FEG, Liew FY: T cell subsets and cytokines in parasitic infections. Immunol Today 1992;13:445–448.

43  Pfefferkorn ER: Interferon-$\gamma$ blocks the growth of *Toxoplasma gondii* in human fibroblasts by inducing the host cell to degrade tryptophan. Proc Natl Acad Sci USA 1984;81:908–912.

44  Kuhls TL, Mosier DA, Abrams VL, Crawford DL, Greenfield RA: Inability of interferon-gamma and aminoguanidine to alter *Cryptosporidium parvum* infection in mice with severe combined immunodeficiency. J Parasitol 1994;80:480–485.

45  MacDonald TT, Spencer J: Cell-mediated immune injury in the intestine. Gastroenterol Clin North Am 1992;21:367–386.

46  Griffiths JK, Moore R, Dooley S, Keusch GT, Tzipori S: *Cryptosporidium parvum* infection of Caco-2 cell monolayers induces an apical monolayer defect, selectively increases transmonolayer permeability and causes epithelial cell death. Infect Immun 1994;62:4506–4514.

47  Abbas AK, Murphy KM, Sher A: Functional diversity of helper T lymphocytes. Nature 1996;383:787–793.

48  Enriquez FJ, Sterling CR: Role of CD4+ TH1- and TH2-cell-secreted cytokines in cryptosporidiosis. Folia Parasitol 1993;40:307–311.

49  Connolly GM, Owen SL, Hawkins DA, Gazzard BG: Treatment of cryptosporidial infection with recombinant interleukin-2. 5th Int Congr AIDS, Montreal 1989, WBP47, p 359.

50  Harp JA, Moon HW: Susceptibility of mast cell-deficient W/Wv mice to *Cryptosporidium parvum.* Infect Immun 1991;59:718–720.

51  Ungar BLP, Soave R, Fayer R, Nash TE: Enzyme immunoassay detection of immunoglobulin M and G antibodies to *Cryptosporidium* in immunocompetent and immunocompromised persons. J Infect Dis 1986;153:570–578.

52  Peeters JE, Villacorta I, Vanopdenbosch E, Vandergheynst D, Naciri M, Ares-Maras E, Yvorre P: *Cryptosporidium parvum* in calves: Kinetics and immunoblot analysis of specific serum and local antibody responses (immunoglobulin A [IgA], IgG, and IgM) after natural and experimental infections. Infect Immun 1992;60:2309–2316.

53   Hill BD, Blewett DA, Dawson AM, Wright S: Analysis of the kinetics, isotype and specificity of serum and coproantibody in lambs infected with *Cryptosporidium parvum.* Res Vet Sci 1990;48: 76–81.

54   Williams RO, Burden DJ: Measurement of class specific antibody against *Cryptosporidium* in serum and faeces from experimentally infected calves. Res Vet Sci 1987;43:264–265.

55   Mead JR, Arrowood MJ, Sterling CR: Antigens of *Cryptosporidium* sporozoites recognized by immune sera of infected animals and humans. J Parasitol 1988;74:135–143.

56   McDonald V, Deer RMA, Nina JMS, Wright S, Chiodini PL, McAdam KPWJ: Characteristics and specificity of hybridoma antibodies against oocyst antigens of *Cryptosporidium parvum* from man. Parasite Immunol 1991;13:251–259.

57   Tzipori S, Roberton D, Chapman C: Remission of diarrhoea due to cryptosporidiosis in an immuno-deficient child treated with hyperimmune bovine colostrum. Br Med J 1986;293:1276–1277.

58   Ungar BLP, Ward DJ, Fayer R, Quinn CA: Cessation of *Cryptosporidium*-associated diarrhea in an acquired immunodeficiency syndrome patient after treatment with hyperimmune bovine colostrum. Gastroenterology 1990;98:486–489.

59   Fayer R, Andrews C, Ungar BLP, Blagburn B: Efficacy of hyperimmune bovine colostrum for prophylaxis of cryptosporidiosis in neonatal calves. J Parasitol 1989;75:393–397.

60   Tilley M, Fayer R, Guidry A, Upton SJ, Blagburn BL: *Cryptosporidium parvum* (Apicomplexa: Cryptosporidiidae) oocysts and sporozoite antigens recognized by bovine colostral antibodies. Infect Immun 1990;58:2966–2971.

61   Perryman LE, Riggs MW, Mason PH, Fayer R: Kinetics of *Cryptosporidium parvum* sporozoite neutralization by monoclonal antibodies, immune bovine serum, and immune bovine colstrum. Infect Immun 1990;58:257–259.

62   Arrowood MJ, Mead JR, Mahrt JL, Sterling CR: Effects of immune colostrum and orally adminis-tered antisporozoite monoclonal antibodies on the outcome of the *Cryptosporidium parvum* infections in neonatal mice. Infect Immun 1989;57:2283–2288.

63   Doyle PS, Crabb J, Petersen C: Anti-*Cryptosporidium parvum* antibodies inhibit infectivity in vitro and in vivo. Infect Immun 1993;61:4079–4084.

64   Fayer R, Guidry A, Blagburn BL: Immunotherapeutic efficacy of bovine colostral immunoglobulins from a hyperimmunized cow against cryptosporidiosis in neonatal mice. Infect Immun 1990;58: 2962–2965.

65   Riggs MW, Cama VA, Leary HL Jr, Sterling CR: Bovine antibody against *Cryptosporidium parvum* elicits a circumsporozoite precipitate-like reaction and has immunotherapeutic effect against persist-ent cryptosporidiosis in SCID mice. Infect Immun 1994;62:1927–1939.

66   Petersen C, Gut J, Leech JH, Nelso RG: Identification and initial characterization of five *Cryptospori-dium parvum* antigen genes. Infect Immun 1992;60:2343–2348.

67   Petersen C, Gut J, Doyle PS, Crabb JH, Nelson RG, Leech JH: Characterization of a >900,000-$M_r$ *Cryptosporidium parvum* sporozoite glycoprotein recognized by protective hyperimmune bovine colostral immunoglobulin. Infect Immun 1992;60:5132–5138.

68   Bjorneby JM, Riggs MW, Perryman LE: *Cryptosporidium parvum* merozoites share neutralization-sensitive epitopes with sporozoites. J Immunol 1990;145:298–304.

69   Tilley M, Upton SJ, Fayer R, Barta JR, Chrisp CE, Freed PS, Blagburn BL, Anderson BC, Barnard SM: Identification of a 15-kilodalton surface glycoprotein on sporozoites of *Cryptosporidium parvum.* Infect Immun 1991;59:1002–1007.

70   McDonald V, McCrossan MV, Petry F: Localization of parasite antigens in *Cryptosporidium parvum*-infected epithelial cells using monoclonal antibodies. Parasitology 1995;110:259–268.

71   Cozon G, Biron F, Jeannin M, Cannella D, Revillard J-P: Secretory IgA antibodies to *Cryptosporid-ium parvum* in AIDS patients with chronic cryptosporidiosis. J Infect Dis 1994;169:696–699.

72   Saxon A, Weinstein W: Oral administration of bovine colostrum anti-cryptosporidia antibody fails to alter the course of human cryptosporidiosis. J Parasitol 1987;73:413–415.

73   Moon HW, Woodmansee HW, Harp JA, Abel S, Ungar BLP: Lacteal immunity to enteric crypto-sporidiosis in mice: Immune dams do not protect their suckling pups. Infect Immun 1988;56:649–653.

74   Taghi-Kilani R, Sekla L, Hayglass KT: The role of humoral immunity in *Cryptosporidium* spp. infection studies with B-cell-depleted mice. J Immunol 1990;145:1571–1576.

75    Albert MM, Rusnak J, Luther MF, Graybill JR: Treatment of murine cryptosporidiosis with anticryptosporidial immune rat bile. Am J Trop Med Hyg 1994;50:112–119.

76    Cama VA, Sterling CR: Hyperimmune hens as a novel source of anti-*Cryptosporidium* antibodies suitable for passive immune transfer. J Protozool 1991;38:42S–43S.

77    McMeeking A, Borkowsky W, Klesius PH, Bonk S, Holzman RS, Lawrence HS: A controlled trial of bovine dialyzable leukocyte extract for cryptosporidiosis in patients with AIDS. J Infect Dis 1990;161:108–112.

78    Fayer R, Klesius PH, Andrews C: Efficacy of bovine transfer to protect neonatal calves against experimentally induced clinical cryptosporidiosis. J Parasitol 1987;73:1061–1062.

79    Gooi HC: Gastrointestinal and liver involvement in primary immunodeficiency; in Heatley RV (ed): Gastrointestinal and Hepatic Immunology. Cambridge Rev Clin Immunol. Cambridge, Cambridge University Press, 1994, pp 169–177.

Vincent McDonald, Department of Clinical Sciences,
London School of Hygiene and Tropical Medicine,
Keppel Street, London WC1E 7HT (UK)

Liew FY, Cox FEG (eds): Immunology of Intracellular Parasitism.
Chem Immunol. Basel, Karger, 1998, vol 70, pp 124–143

..........................
# Immunology of *Trypanosoma cruzi* Infections

*Steven G. Reed*

Infectious Disease Research Institute, Seattle, Wash., USA

## Introduction

*Trypanosoma cruzi* is an intracellular protozoan parasite infecting humans
as well as a wide variety of other mammals. Among the trypanosomes, it is
by far the most important human pathogen, with an estimated 18 million
infected individuals in which it is most often associated with chronic, disabling
heart disease. The parasite is restricted to the Americas, following the distribution of its vector insects, and is found from Argentina to California. *T. cruzi*
has been widely studied in animal models for its ability to induce potent
immune depression in susceptible rodents. The effects of the parasite on the
immune system have been studied at the cellular and molecular levels and will
be the subject of discussion in this chapter. These immune alterations are
relevant to human infections which are characterized in the acute phase by
immune depression and in the chronic phase by autoimmune pathology.

## The Parasite

Few if any of the protozoan pathogens of humans compare with *T. cruzi*
in terms of virulence and ability to infect such a broad range of cell types. It
is believed that this parasite can infect virtually any nucleated cell. There are
three main forms of the parasite: the epimastigote, found in the insect vector
and readily cultured in a variety of media; the trypomastigote, the flagellated
form found in infected mammals, and the amastigote, which has no free
flagellum and which replicates inside cells. *T. cruzi* has the ability to escape
the phagocytic vacuole, so amastigotes may be detected both within such

vacuoles as well as free in the cytoplasm. Amastigotes may be released from ruptured cells, transform into trypomastigotes, and exit from the cell in the flagellate form. Trypomastigotes are the most infective forms, but amastigotes are also capable of initiating infection in macrophages.

*T. cruzi* is among the most successful of the intracellular parasites. Its principal means of escaping destruction by the immune system is by limiting its extracellular exposure and performing its replication inside cells, many of which have little in the way of internal defense mechanisms. This intracellular habit means that *T. cruzi* has not found it necessary to evolve elaborate means of adaptive genetic variation, such as occurs in African trypanosomes which can alter expression of surface proteins in response to the presence of lytic antibodies. However, the ability of *T. cruzi* to invade, survive, and replicate within host cells, particularly within macrophages with their potent armament of chemical warfare, demonstrates an equally admirable evolutionary achievement. The lack of antigenic variation has proven to be of crucial importance for the development of *T. cruzi*-specific diagnostic reagents, and also has implications for vaccine development.

*T. cruzi* is transmitted to humans by bloodsucking insects of the reduviid group. The insects are nocturnal, and deposit hindgut contents containing infective trypomastigotes while feeding. These are rubbed into the eye (the insects often bite the soft tissue under the eye) or bite wound by the victim and intracellular infection begins. This form of 'posterior station' transmission is an aspect separating *T. cruzi* from the trypanosomes that cause African sleeping sickness which are transmitted from the salivary gland ('anterior station') of a biting fly. Because of the domestic nature of the reduviid bugs, they often live in cracks in the walls and roofs of poorly constructed houses, eradication efforts have focused on the application of insecticides with prolonged residual activity. This, along with improving the quality of construction, has proven to be an effective way to decrease human infection.

*Infection and Disease*

Although *T. cruzi* is classified as a single species, there is a great deal of diversity between strains. This is manifested in both biochemical and genetic variations. A fascinating but not elucidated characteristic is the tremendous difference between different strains or isolates in terms of virulence and types of pathology induced. Thus laboratory isolates have been classified as having increased propensity for either muscle cells or macrophages and as inducing characteristic pathologies in rodents. Some laboratory strains produce rapidly fatal infections in mice, while others produce mild infections and no disease. In nature, this type of strain diversity seems to be an important determinant of clinical outcome. In laboratory studies, differences in *T. cruzi* strains can greatly influence the immunological characteristics and disease outcome. Similarly, inbred mouse strains have been classified as being susceptible or resistant to *T. cruzi* infection, but this pattern depends on the parasite strain as well. Thus the C57Bl mouse is resistant to the Y strain of *T. cruzi*, but highly susceptible to the Tulahuen strain.

Human infections with *T. cruzi* are classified as acute, chronic, and indeterminate. Acute and chronic refer to disease, while indeterminate refers to infection without disease symptoms. Early infections may produce acute, even fatal disease, characterized by circulating parasites, fever, splenomegaly, and a variety of other symptoms which may include myocarditis and CNS involvement. Chronic disease is characterized by few circulating parasites, no fever or splenomegaly, but by progressive deterioration of cardiac or intestinal function. Collectively, these different stages are referred to as Chagas disease, after Carlos Chagas who meticulously described the parasite and characterized the symptoms [1]. The underlying mechanisms of these pathologies appear to be mediated, at least in part, by tissue-reactive T cells rather than by excessive numbers of parasites. Typical of chronic Chagas pathology is an enlarged heart with thin ventricular walls and apical thinning of the myocardium. This results in a flaccid organ incapable of efficiently pumping blood. Lymphocytic infiltrates, rather than high numbers of amastigotes, characterize histological sections of the chagasic heart. Pathology may also occur in the form of enlarged esophagus or colon, resulting in a debilitating condition which may progress to death.

The majority of human infections are thought to be asymptomatic, or indeterminate. These individuals have antibody against *T. cruzi*, which indicates active infection, but no disease or detectable pathology. In many cases, circulating parasites can be demonstrated by culturing a blood sample in laboratory culture medium. Another method of parasite detection using the insect vector is called xenodiagnosis and consists of allowing uninfected bugs to feed on the suspect, waiting for 30 days, and examining the bugs' gut for parasites. This is still used as a diagnostic tool, incredible as it may seem. The indeterminate infections illustrate an important aspect of the natural history of *T. cruzi* in mammals. A large reservoir of infected, but not diseased, hosts presents continuing opportunities for generations of insects to acquire the parasite and thus ensure its survival. Thus it appears that at least some strains of *T. cruzi* have evolved into highly successful parasites, while others, because of their high degree of virulence, are less efficient at inducing asymptomatic infections and end up killing their hosts.

## Immunobiology of *T. cruzi* Infection

*Experimental Models*

Mouse models of *T. cruzi* infection have been used by many investigators to study vaccines, therapeutics, and immune regulation. This latter area has received the most attention, and is most pertinent to the subject of this text. Many of us started working in this area before the era of cytokines and recombinant proteins, interested in how an intracellular parasite, particularly one that infects macrophages, can subvert the host immune system to its own advantage. Although perhaps more of a laboratory biohazard than most other protozoan parasites, *T. cruzi* is relatively easy to maintain and passage, and mice can be infected with the same parasites that cause human disease. Infections can be monitored by sampling a drop of blood, and a rapid onset of disease and death make it possible to perform experiments on acute infections in a matter of days. Another attractive aspect of *T. cruzi* infection in mice is the ability to study both acute and chronic infections with ease. Aside from the use of an infection model to elucidate molecular immunological pathways, and in this regard protozoan parasites have provided excellent models as illustrated in this text, understanding how *T. cruzi* alters host immune function may also elucidate mechanisms of autoimmune pathology.

Studies by Kuhn and colleagues [2] on the suppression of heterologous humoral immune responses, as well as other studies on depressed cellular immune responses [3, 4], began two decades of work to understand immune dysfunction in *T. cruzi*-infected mice. It was observed early on that acute infections produced profound suppression in multiple components of the immune system, and that control of *T. cruzi* infection and disease involved virtually all of the host defenses. Reviews have been written on these earlier studies [5].

Several studies have described the effects of *T. cruzi* infection on both T-cell and Th-dependent antibody responses. The most profound suppression occurs during acute disease, but also extends into the chronic phase. One of the first attempts to define mechanisms of immune suppression focused on the failure of infected mice to mount a cellular response to oxazalone, a contact-sensitizing agent used to study delayed-type hypersensitivity (DTH) responses. Even though infected mice could not manifest a DTH response, they had, upon sensitization with oxazalone, activated T cells in their draining lymph nodes that were as effective in transferring contact sensitivity to uninfected syngeneic recipients as were cells from sensitized normal mice [4]. This indicated that the initial phases of the immune response, such as antigen processing and presentation, were not blocked during *T. cruzi* infection. This proved to be an important aspect of distinguishing between deficiencies in afferent versus efferent arms of the immune response during infection with intracellular pathogens. Understanding of a molecular basis for decreased effector function awaited elucidation of cytokine pathways.

The first cytokine shown to be able to reconstitute immune responsiveness in infected mice was IL-2, which restored Th function both in vitro and in vivo [6–8]. These studies were performed not only in mice with acute infections, but also in those allowed to enter into a stage of prolonged chronicity following chemotherapy. These mice present a more interesting system in which to evaluate immune deregulation in that they remain selectively immunocompromised in the absence of any overt disease, and do not have increased susceptibility to secondary infections. By 2–3 months after the acute phase, their spleens have returned to near normal size, although low numbers of intracellular parasites can be detected indefinitely. In these experiments the immunological lesion in chronically infected animals was characterized as an inability to mount an antibody response to a previously unencountered T-dependent antigen. With the development of recombinant mouse and human cytokines, tools became available to allow molecular dissection of specific and nonspecific immune responses during infection. In addition to IL-2, both GM-CSF [9] and IL-1 [10] were also effective in restoring immune competence to spleen cells from chronically infected mice, both in vitro and in vivo. It has never been fully understood how these individual cytokines mediated restoration of Th function in infected mice, but it is likely that much of the effect is ultimately mediated by IL-2, again suggesting that the processing of heterologous antigen was not impaired in infected mice, but that effector cytokines, including those involved in T-cell stimulation via IL-2 production, were not functional in the spleen of infected animals. While the above studies did not directly address the role of soluble mediators in resistance or susceptibility to *T. cruzi* infection, they did point to the fact that both acute and chronic infections with this parasite led to immunological abnormalities that could be corrected by the addition of exogenous cytokine.

## The Role of T Cells in *T. cruzi* Infections

A key role for T cells in mediating resistance to *T. cruzi* was established with the observation that purified T cells, but not B cells, from immunized animals could passively confer protection to susceptible hosts [11, 12]. Understanding the nature of the anti-parasite T-cell response came largely from work by Tarleton [13, 14], who demonstrated a role for both CD4+ and CD8+ T cells in experimental infections; ablation of either component led to enhanced susceptibility. These studies, along with the observation that $\beta_2$-

microglobulin knockout mice, which lack clas I-mediated defense mechanisms, had increased susceptibility to *T. cruzi* infection [15], demonstrate the complexity of trying to define a central mechanism that is the key to resistance to this (or any other) intracellular pathogen. However, all these observations are consistent with a crucial role for IFN-γ, produced by both CD4+ and CD8+ T cells, in mediating resistance to *T. cruzi* infection. The intracellular replication of *T. cruzi* in macrophages is readily inhibited in vitro by the early addition of IFN-γ [16], not unlike the situation with most other intracellular microbes. In a relatively homogenous population of macrophages, such as those obtained from the peritoneal cavities of mice, in vitro activation by IFN-γ results in a near complete elimination of intracellular amastigotes. With human PBMC-derived macrophages, the intracellular killing is less complete, but IFN-γ is still highly effective. In vivo, the importance of an intact IFN-γ response, in both afferent and efferent aspects, has been demonstrated in several studies, including the therapeutic efficacy of recombinant IFN-γ [16, 17]. It appears clear that the early production of IFN-γ is important in controlling disease [18, 19]; however, fatal infections may also develop in the presence of vigorous IFN-γ production because of the inability of macrophages to become activated.

Human *T. cruzi* infections are often dormant for decades. Such infections may be activated to produce acute, even fatal, infections upon immunosuppresive conditions. This has been observed, for example, during intentional immunosuppression for organ transplants, including heart transplants as a therapeutic approach for chronic Chagas disease [20]. Thus, it has been recognized that *T. cruzi* may be an opportunistic protozoal infection as, for example *Toxoplasma gondii*. More recently, several examples of *T. cruzi* as an opportunist in AIDS patients have been reported [21]. As may be expected, these patients have extraordinary parasite levels in the blood, as well as in cerebrospinal fluid.

Experimental studies have also demonstrated the effect of an immunosuppressive viral co-infection on the exacerbation of *T. cruzi* infections [22]. MuLv is a murine leukemia virus with immunosuppressive effects. However, as with *T. cruzi* infections, inbred mouse strains vary in their susceptibility to this virus. Therefore, models can be developed to study the effects of each of these infections on one another. Not suprisingly, MuLv was found to reactivate latent *T. cruzi* infections in mice. More interesting, however, was the observation that chronic *T. cruzi* infection also exacerbated viral disease in an MuLv-resistant mouse strain. This demonstrates the potentially severe immunosuppressive effects of *T. cruzi* infection. Although not well studied it is likely that chronic *T. cruzi* infections also predispose humans to other infections.

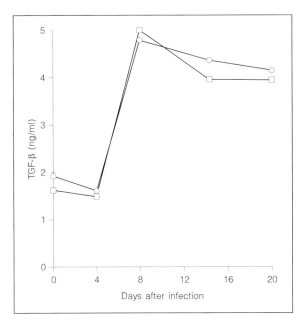

*Fig. 1.* Production of active TGF-β by spleen cells from mice infected with *T. cruzi.* Spleen cells from B6 mice obtained at different days after infection with $10^3$ trypomastigotes of *T. cruzi* were incubated for 48 h in the presence (□) or absence (○) of trypomastigote lysate, and supernatants were tested for biologically active TGF-β. The first points (day 0) indicate uninfected control mice.

## TGF-β

The observations that effector mechanisms were impaired in mice infected with *T. cruzi* led to the search for soluble mediators of this deficiency. It appears intuitive that a macrophage pathogen would induce the production of mediators to prevent macrophage activation, and, with the key observations that transforming growth factor beta (TGF-β) could impair macrophage-killing mechanisms, a candidate for such a mediator was found [23, 24]. TGF-β is actually a family of peptides found in vertebrates that stimulate cell growth and differentiation and play a critical role in embryological development and wound healing. TGF-β is tightly regulated and secreted as an inactive precursor molecule which is cleaved enzymatically (or in the laboratory by low pH) into an active homodimer capable of binding to receptors. Latent (or precursor) TGF-β is produced by a number of cell types, including macrophages. A role for TGF-β in mediating pathology of *T. cruzi* infection became apparent when it was observed that cultured spleen cells from mice with acute infections released active TGF-β [25] (fig. 1). This led to a number of observations on

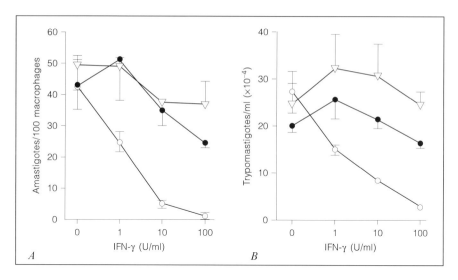

*Fig. 2.* TGF-β inhibits cytokine activation of macrophages to kill *T. cruzi* in vitro. The cells were plated on 13-mm² round glass coverslips (*A*) or 48-well plates (*B*) and incubated for 24 h with the indicated concentration of rMuIFN-γ without (○), or with 1 ng/ml rMuTGF-β before (●), or before and after (▽) infection with *T. cruzi*. *A* Coverslips were fixed 48 h after infection, and numbers of amastigotes per 100 macrophages determined. *B* Extracellular trypomastigotes were counted 5 days after infection. Points represent mean ± SD.

the role of TGF-β in mediating susceptibility to disease from *T. cruzi* infections. It was demonstrated that macrophages treated with TGF-β could not become activated upon treatment with IFN-γ. Furthermore, TGF-β could have potent immunosuppressive effects on T-cell effector functions, including proliferation and cytokine production. The observations that the sensitization of T cells and the production of activating cytokines such as IFN-γ did not appear to be impaired in infected mice fit with the hypothesis that *T. cruzi* infection, rather than producing a general T-cell deficiency, may lead to the production of negative response mediators. Such mediators could prevent T-cell cytokines from effectively inhibiting parasite replication and from mediating heterologous immune responses (fig. 2).

These in vitro observations demonstrated that *T. cruzi* infection can lead to the production of a cytokine capable of preventing parasite killing by macrophages. Determination of a role for TGF-β in vivo next required developing a model of resistance to infection with this highly virulent organism. This was accomplished by testing a variety of parental and F₁ hybrids for susceptibility to infection and disease by determining parasite numbers, mor-

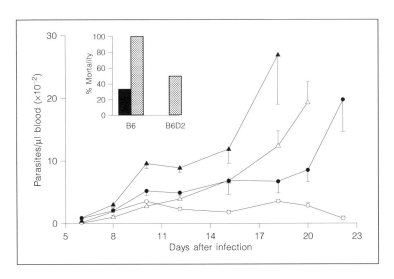

*Fig. 3.* Treatment of resistant mice with TGF-β increases susceptibility to *T. cruzi* infection. Effects of TGF-β on the course of *T. cruzi* infection in resistant (B6D2) (○) or B6 mice (△) treated i.p. with PBS (open symbols) or 10 μg of rMuTGF-β (solid symbols) on −1, 0, 2, 5 and 9 days after i.p. injection with $10^3$ trypomastigotes. Points represent the mean ± SEM of 6 mice. At 10, 12, 15, 18, 20 and 22 days TGF-β treated vs. control, $p < 0.05$ for both mouse strains. Inset shows cumulative mortality on day 20 after infection in PBS (black bar) or TGF-β (gray bar) treated mice.

bidity, and mortality following infection. This led to a serendipitous finding that an $F_1$ hybrid mouse from the cross of C57Bl/6 and DBA.2, both highly susceptible strains, was resistant to acute *T. cruzi* infection. This hybrid, B6D2, could resist infection with up to $10^6$ parasites, whereas the parental strains developed fatal infections with $10^2$ or fewer organisms. It was found that in B6D2 mice the administration of recombinant TGF-β could significantly increase both morbidity and mortality in these animals, pointing to a role for TGF-β in mediating disease susceptibility (fig. 3).

More recent studies have focused on the activation of TGF-β by *T. cruzi* based on the observations that both spleen cells from infected mice, as well as macrophages infected in vitro, elaborated already activated TGF-β. In most cases, TGF-β is produced in the latent form. Treatment with acid can reduce the disulfide bond to produce active TGF-β capable of binding to its receptors. However, in *T. cruzi* infections, all of the TGF-β produced appeared to be activated; treatment with acid did not further increase its biological activity. This led to the search for a mechanism by which activation occurred, and suggested two possibilities. One is that infection increased the enzyme activity

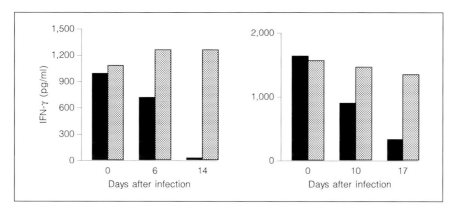

*Fig. 4.* Production of IL-10 by spleens of mice with acute *T. cruzi* infections. IL-10 activity in spleen cell supernatants from B6 (solid bar) and B6D2 (stippled bar) mice infected with *T. cruzi*. 48-Hour supernatants of $5 \times 10^6$ unstimulated spleen cells from uninfected and from mice infected for 6–17 days with *T. cruzi* were assayed for CSIF activity. Representative data from two experiments are shown. Each point represents pooled spleen cells from 3 mice.

of macrophages, or possibly other cells. Another is that the parasite itself could directly activate TGF-β. Several observations suggested the latter to be the case. Recombinant latent TGF-β incubated with live, but not heat-inactivated, *T. cruzi* trypomastigotes was reduced to its active form. The conclusions of these studies [submitted for publication] were that the parasite itself has potent enzyme activity capable of activating TGF-β. This observation demonstrates a novel mechanism for pathogenesis, and suggests an intricate communication between a pathogen and the immune system.

*IL-10*

Another candidate for a mediator of macrophage inhibition which could play a role in *T. cruzi* virulence is IL-10. The importance of this cytokine in *T. cruzi* infections was suggested by demonstrating the production of a soluble mediator that blocked the production of IFN-γ and which was inhibited by anti-IL-10 mAb [26]. Paradoxically, however, in spite of the in vitro demonstration of anti-IFN-γ producing activity, there was no in vivo evidence for a lack of IFN-γ production in highly susceptible mice. In fact, susceptible mice had higher levels of IFN-γ message and of circulating IFN-γ than did resistant mice with comparatively mild infections. Studies performed in the SCID mouse confirmed that IL-10 is produced by macrophages during experimental *T. cruzi* infections, as well as by B and T cells (fig. 4). IL-10 is clearly a potent inhibitor

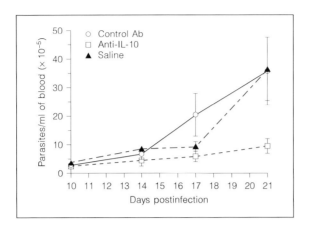

*Fig. 5.* Anti-IL-10 mAb inhibits mortality in susceptible mice infected with *T. cruzi.* B6 mice (5 per group) were injected i.p. with 200 μg of anti-IL-10 or control rat IgG 4 h before infection with $10^3$ trypomastigotes of *T. cruzi.* Data from one of three experiments are shown, represented as mean ± SD.

of the production of INF-γ and of the IFN-γ-mediated killing of the parasite through T cells as well as NK cells [27, 28].

A definitive role for IL-10 in mediating susceptibility to acute disease was established with the observation that administration of neutralizing anti-IL-10 mAb could block the development of acute disease in susceptible B6 mice. In this study, it was found that an intermediate dose of anti-IL-10 mAb [29] blocked morbidity and mortality indicating that early production of IL-10 played an important role in the development of disease (fig. 5). However, another interesting observation was not pursued in this study, namely, that higher doses of anti-IL-10 had lesser therapeutic effects. It was thought that perhaps the higher doses of mAb may actually have a stabilizing effect on circulating IL-10, potentially prolonging or exacerbating its activity.

Although these experiments fit the hypothesis that infection of macrophages by *T. cruzi* led to the production of a macrophage-inactivating cytokine, IL-10, and that this excessive production of IL-10 eventually resulted in the development of disease, the situation proved not to be so simple. Although a dual role for IL-10 in mediating both resistance and susceptibility was indicated by the dose dependency of the anti-IL-10 effects, it was only recently, with the studies of Hunter et al. [30], that the complexities of the situation became known when it was found that IL-10 was actually needed to prevent the development of pathology in mice infected with the Tulahuen strain of *T. cruzi.* IL-10 knockout mice infected with the virulent Tulahuen strain had fewer

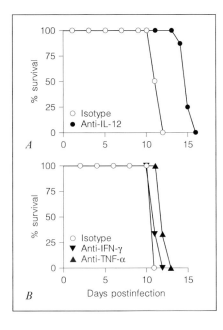

*Fig. 6.* Effect of anticytokine Abs on time to death of IL-10 –/– mice infected with *T. cruzi.* Mice were infected with *T. cruzi* and treated i.p. with 1 mg/mouse of an isotype control or anti-IL-12 (*A*), anti-TNF-α, or anti-IFN-γ (*B*) on days 5, 7 and 9 postinfection. The results presented are the pooled data from two separate experiments with 8 mice per experimental group. Administration of anti-TNF-α or anti-IL-12, but not anti-IFN-γ, resulted in a statistically significant delay in time to death.

parasites than the IL-10 competent mice, an observation apparently consistent with studies demonstrating decreased parasitemias in mice treated with neutralizing anti-IL-10 mAb. In contrast to the IL-10 neutralization studies, however, knockout mice had accelerated mortality, as compared to wild-type mice, and this manifestation of increased susceptibility was effectively reversed by administering rIL-10. A similar 'protective' effect could also be achieved using anti-IL-12 mAb to treat the knockout mice. The authors postulate a role for IL-10 in preventing a toxic immune response characterized by overproduction of IL-12 and IFN-γ associated with acute *T. cruzi* infections. Such a mechanism could explain why low doses of anti-IL-10 protected against acute disease, whereas higher doses did not, as well as the observation that susceptible mice made more IFN-γ than did resistant mice during acute infection [29]. The production of IL-10 is not sufficient to protect mice; both knockout and wild-type mice died of acute infection. Rather, either an excess or complete absence of IL-10 production appears to adversely affect the course of infection. These studies demonstrate the importance of a balance between key macrophage and T cell cytokines in regulating disease from an intracellular infection (fig. 6, 7).

Another example of the importance of maintaining a proper cytokine balance for controlling intracellular pathogens comes from studies on IL-12. This pivotal cytokine is, as are others, a double-edged sword. Small amounts of IL-12 are needed for the development of a protective Th1 response, with

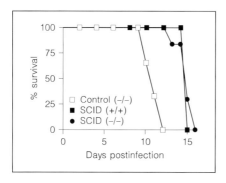

Fig. 7. T. cruzi infection in IL-10 knockout mice. Time to death of IL-10 –/– (n = 12), SCID IL-10 –/– (n = 13), and SCID IL-10 +/+ (n = 8) mice infected with T. cruzi. Results presented are the pooled data from three separate experiments.

corresponding IFN-γ production. However, excess IL-12 is associated with increased IL-10, excess IFN-γ, and the development of shock symptoms. Thus, while Hunter et al. demonstrated that neutralizing excessive IL-12 in the IL-10 knockout mice reversed the accelerated mortality observed in these animals, they also showed, in a different study, that administration of rIL-12 at low doses ($< 100$ ng/day) during the first week of infection had significant protective effects in terms of parasitemia, pathology, and mortality [31]. The protective effects were dependent on the production of IFN-γ, and, perhaps to a lesser extent, TNF. In contrast, administration of higher doses of IL-12 increased pathology and accelerated mortality. Taken together, these studies on IL-10 and IL-12 demonstrate the importance of an intact Th1 response for a favorable outcome of T. cruzi infections in mice, as well as the importance of preventing an overexuberant Th1 response from developing, resulting in a detrimental outcome. Indeed, it is likely that an excessive Th1 response pattern could contribute to the development of autoimmune pathology, which is characteristic of chronic Chagas disease (fig. 8, table 1).

### Cytokine Responses in Human T. cruzi Infections

Limited studies have been performed on the immunoregulation of human T. cruzi infections. The complexity of disease states, determination of infection status, documentation of time of infection, etc. make these analyses difficult to perform. Howevera, we analyzed the molecular immune response occurring in humans with different stages of T. cruzi infection, by examining cytokine RNAs in PBMC from patients with chronic disease or with indeterminate infections. Diagnosis of infection was based upon positive serological tests for T. cruzi, while diagnosis of chronic disease status was based on clinical findings of either chagasic cardiac or digestive tract disease symptoms. Cells were

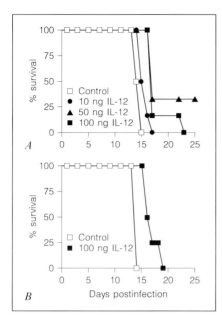

A

B

*Fig. 8.* Administration of IL-12 to BALB/c mice infected with *T. cruzi* delays time to death. *A* Groups of 4–6 BALB/c mice were treated i.p. with IL-12 (10, 50 or 100 ng/mouse) at 24 h prior to infection and every day thereafter for 6 days. All three treatments resulted in a significant delay in the time to death (p=0.02, 0.002, and 0.0002, respectively). *B* Mice were treated with IL-12 (100 ng/mouse) beginning 3 days after infection and for a further 6 days. This treatment resulted in a significant delay in the time to death (p=0.008).

*Table 1.* rIL-10 blocks the IFN-γ-mediated inhibition of *T. cruzi* in mouse peritoneal macrophages[1]

| | IFN-γ | Experiment 1 | | Experiment 2 | |
|---|---|---|---|---|---|
| | | amastigotes/100 macrophages ($\bar{X} \pm$ SD)) | percent inhibition | amastigotes/100 macrophages ($\bar{X} \pm$ SD) | percent inhibition |
| Medium | − | 33.1 ± 3.9 | | 137.9 ± 13.5 | |
| | + | 5.6 ± 0.6 | 83.1 | 41.1 ± 8.7 | 70.2 |
| COS-control | − | 36.6 ± 6.3 | | 130.0 ± 2.8 | |
| | + | 3.5 ± 1.6 | 90.4 | 32.6 ± 6.9 | 74.9 |
| rIL-10 | − | 30.5 ± 1.7 | | 166.8 ± 20.6 | |
| | + | 14.6 ± 2.6 | 52.1 | 120.9 ± 2.1 | 27.5 |

[1] BALB/c peritoneal macrophages were treated with rMu-IFN-γ and rIL-10 or COS-supernatant control for 48 h, washed, and infected with *T. cruzi* trypomastigotes. The cells were washed thoroughly 2 h later and incubated for 48 h (Exp. 1) or 72 h (Exp. 2) and intracellular amastigotes enumerated. IFN-γ and COS-control + IFN-γ groups vs. rIL-10 + IFN-γ, p < 0.05.

stimulated in vitro with mitogen or with *T. cruzi* antigens, and mRNA profiles between patient and uninfected control groups were compared.

We found that stimulated PBMC from both patient groups produced a range of cytokines, including IL-2, IL-4, IL-10, and IFN-$\gamma$, in response to *T. cruzi* antigens. Indeed, even PBMC from uninfected individuals responded to *T. cruzi* antigens with IL-2 production, as we and others have previously reported [32, 33]. Of interest, however, were the differences observed in cytokine profiles in unstimulated or 'resting' PBMC from the two patient groups. While IL-2 mRNA was seen in most individuals with either chronic disease or indeterminate infections, IL-4 and IL-10 mRNA were detected only in PBMC from individuals with indeterminate infections, and not in those obtained from chronic disease patients or from uninfected individuals. This surprising finding of cytokine message in PBMC from infected but not diseased individuals may indicate a variable state of immune activation which influences the transition from indeterminate infection to chronic disease.

Other studies have examined the responses of normal human PBMC to *T. cruzi* antigens. Homogenates of both epimastigotes and trypomastigotes have potent stimulatory effects on PBMC, as manifested by intense proliferation and IL-2 production. IFN-$\gamma$ and IL-10 are not produced by normal PBMC in response to trypanosome antigens. *T. cruzi*-induced normal PBMC proliferation resembles mitogen-induced proliferation in magnitude, but not in other aspects such as kinetics and cytokine profiles. As mentioned above, the cytokine profile induced by parasites is more limited than a mitogen-induced response and the proliferation peaks at 5–6 days, versus 3–4 days for mitogens. These in vitro proliferative responses are not similar to those obtained with superantigens; responses to *T. cruzi* are processing dependent, and T cells with a wide range of V$\beta$ receptor types are involved in the response [32]. The stimulation appears to be in response to protein (proliferation does not occur when the lysate is treated with protease) and in fact at least one potent immunostimulatory protein of *T. cruzi*, a ribosomal P protein, has been cloned and characterized [34]. The significance of these observations relative to infection and pathology are not known. As acute infections are characterized by intense immunoproliferative responses with accompanying splenomegaly and lymphadenopathy, nonspecific proliferation to parasite proteins may play an important role in the disease process, including the subsequent development of autoimmune responses. In contrast, the presence of *T. cruzi* in an in vitro culture of human PBMC may also decrease mitogen-induced responses. This has been studied in detail by Kierszenbaum and colleagues [35], who have demonstrated in a co-culture system that the parasite decreases both IL-2 production and IL-2 R expression in normal human PBMC.

*Autoimmune Responses in Human* T. cruzi *Infection*

There is strong evidence that much of the pathology of chronic Chagas disease is autoimmune in nature. Understanding the pathological immune response occurring during *T. cruzi* infection has progressed with the discovery of parasite molecules that induce responses to host tissue. Chronic immune stimulation with these 'antigenic mimicry' antigens have been hypothesized to lead to a destructive autoimmune response in *T. cruzi* infection. One antigen, FL-160, has been implicated in molecular mimicry of nervous tissues. Nervous tissues are important targets of chronic Chagas disease, in that the myenteric plexus of the gut is destroyed leading to megaesophagus and megacolon. Destruction of the autonomic innervation of cardiac tissues may exacerbate cardiac manifestations [36], and destruction of nervous tissues leads to peripheral neuropathy [37]. FL-160 is a 160-kD surface protein of *T. cruzi* associated with the flagellar pocket [38]. FL-160 has two epitopes that mimic nervous tissues. One (12X), near the carboxy terminus of FL-160, shares an epitope with myenteric plexus and peripheral axons [39]. Affinity selected anti-12X antibodies from persons infected with *T. cruzi* cross-react with human sciatic nerve. The second molecular mimicry epitope of FL-160, near the amino terminus, shares epitopes with epineurium, nerve cell connective tissue. The second epitope has been limited to 240 amino acids by recombinant expression and a competitive staining assay with mammalian nerve [A. Centurion-Lara, M.C. Cetron, W.C. Van Voorhis, unpubl. data]. Antibodies to both of these epitopes have been shown to bind human sciatic nerve [39]. About 40% of persons with chronic *T. cruzi* infection in northeastern Brazil have antibodies to the FL-160 antigen, but uninfected persons do not have demonstrable titers.

Ribosomal P proteins are also potential mediators of autoimmunity in human *T. cruzi* infections. We have cloned and characterized members of the *T. cruzi* ribosomal P protein family. In the first study, *T. cruzi* P0 and other P protein family members were cloned and expressed [34, 40]; the first definitive report of the cloning of a full-length *T. cruzi* antigen gene that mimics a characterized host homologue in structure, function, and shared antigenicity. Of particular interest, the P proteins have also been implicated as autoimmune targets in SLE patients [41–43] and we found that SLE patient sera reacted strongly to *T. cruzi* P0 [34]. P0 represents an interesting target for autoimmune pathology as it was also shown that anti-P0 antibodies react with cell membranes [44].

Although the P0 gene is phylogenetically conserved, the majority of humans infected with *T. cruzi* have antibodies to both *T. cruzi* P0 and human P0. The mechanisms responsible for the induction of anti-human P0 antibody following *T. cruzi* infection are under investigation. The *T. cruzi* antigenic epitope was mapped to six amino acids at the C terminus of P0; thus we have begun to define epitopes which may be involved in autoimmune responses in human *T. cruzi* infection. We have recently expressed human P0, and have verified the autoreactivity in patient sera using recombinant HuP0. The reactivity of Chagas patient sera against HuP0 is also directed against the C terminus. Other P proteins, including TcP1, TcP2a, and TcP2b homologous with the human ribosomal phosphoproteins HuP0, HuP1, and HuP2 respectively, have also been cloned and characterized [4].

Further evidence of the potential role of *T. cruzi* P0 in pathological responses was obtained from animal studies. BALB/c mice immunized subcutaneously with 100 µg of purified P0, developed strong T-cell proliferative responses to P0 upon subsequent in vitro stimulation of draining lymph node cells. When the P0-immunized mice were infected with *T. cruzi*, they developed significantly higher parasitemias and increased myositis and cardiac inflammation, and increased mortality compared to control infected mice. These observations in experimental infections support the concept that P0 may be implicated in pathology resulting from *T. cruzi* infection.

Clinically, there are few studies to directly support the role of specific molecules in Chagas pathology. However, a recent study has identified an epitope of myosin that is cross-reactive with a *T. cruzi* antigen [45, 46]. Patients with Chagas cardiomyopathy have antibodies that react with both the myosin and parasite epitope. Heart-infiltrating T-cell clones isolated from a patient with chronic Cagas cardiomyopathy were found to react to cardiac myosin, but not to skeletal muscle myosin, as well as to the cross-reactive *T. cruzi* protein. This provides another example of the ability of *T. cruzi* to induce anti-self responses, and defines a clinically relevant epitope as well.

### Practical Considerations

*T. cruzi* has provided an interesting and important model system for the study of molecular and cellular immunoregulation for the past two decades. Unfortunately, little of the research in this area has led to tools or even the promise of tools for disease prevention or disease management. One exception is in the area of diagnosis, where peptides representing dominant B-cell epitopes have been identified, synthesized, and developed into diagnostic assays. The use of synthetic peptides means that assays can now be standardized and produced in a variety of ways, from rapid single test formats to automated systems amenable for blood bank use. We have recently described a multiepitope peptide reagent that combines several immunodominant epitopes to allow development of a diagnostic test capable of detecting > 99.9% of *T. cruzi*-infected individuals [47]. Thus, a new generation of synthetic reagents is now available for more effective management of disease and prevention of infection.

The cloning of *T. cruzi* antigens as well as the identification of important cross-reactive epitopes also means that vaccine development is a realistic goal. The idea that vaccination should not be attempted because of the risk of autoimmunity is probably not valid, particularly now that a subunit vaccine can be developed consisting of recombinant proteins selected on the basis of both immunogenicity and lack of host tissue cross-reactivity. Although prophylactic vaccination may not prevent infection by the parasite, an effective vaccine could prevent the development of acute disease, lead to reduced parasite burden, and decrease or eliminate the generation of autoreactive T cells and antibodies. The technology to produce such a vaccine is now in hand. However, the impetus to do so is lacking, largely because of the success of vector control programs [48] and advances in diagnostic and blood screen development in reducing the incidence of *T. cruzi* transmission. Thus, on several fronts, there is optimism that Chagas disease can and should be brought under control in the near future.

### References

1    Chagas C: American trypanosomiasis; in Kean BH, Mott KE, Russel AJ (eds): Tropical Medicine and Parasitology, Classic Investigations. London, Cornell University Press, 1978, vol 1, pp 214–220.
2    Cunningham DS, Kuhn RE, Rowland EC: Suppression of humoral responses during *Trypanosoma cruzi* infections in mice. Infect Immun 1978;22:155–160.
3    Reed SG, Larson CL, Speer CA: Suppression of cell-mediated immunity in experimental Chagas disease. Z Parasitenkd 1977;52:11–17.
4    Reed SG, Larson CL, Speer CA: Contact sensitivity responses in mice infected with *Trypanosoma cruzi*. Infect Immun 1978;22:548–554.
5    Kuhn RE: Immunology of *Trypanosoma cruzi* infections; in Mansfield JM (ed): Parasitic Diseases: The Immunology. New York, Decker, 1981, pp 137–166.
6    Harel-Bellan A, Joskowicz M, Fradelizi D, Eisen H: Modification of T cell proliferation and interleukin-2 production in mice infected with *Trypanosoma cruzi*. Proc Natl Acad Sci USA 1983; 80:3466–3469.
7    Reed SG, Inverso JA, Roters SB: Suppressed antibody responses to sheep erythrocytes in mice with chronic *Trypanosoma cruzi* infection are restored with interleukin-2. J Immunol 1984;133:3333–3337.
8    Tarleton RL, Kuhn RE: Restoration of in vitro immune responses of spleen cells from mice infected with *Trypanosoma cruzi* by supernatants containing interleukin-2. J Immunol 1984;133:1570–1577.
9    Reed SG, Grabstein KH, Pihl DL, Morrissey PJ: Recombinant GM-CSF restores depressed immune responses in mice with chronic *Trypanosoma cruzi* infections. J Immunol 1990;145:1564–1570.
10   Reed SG, Pihl DL, Conlon PJ, Grabstein KH: Interleukin-1 as adjuvant: Role of T cells in the augmentation of specific antibody production by recombinant human IL-1-α. J Immunol 1989;142: 3132–3133.
11   Reed SG: Adoptive transfer of resistance to *Trypanosoma cruzi* infection with T lymphocyte-enriched spleen cells. Infect Immun 1980;28:404–410.
12   Araujo FG: Development of resistance to *Trypanosoma cruzi* in mice depends on a viable population of L3T4+ (CD4+) T lymphocytes. Infect Immun 1989;57:2246–2248.

13   Tarleton RL: Depletion of CD8+ T cells increases susceptibility and reverses vaccine-induced immunity in mice infected with *Trypanosoma cruzi*. J Immunol 1990;144:717–724.

14   Tarleton RL: The role of T cells in *Trypanosoma cruzi* infections. Parasitol Today 1995;11:7–9.

15   Tarleton RL, Koller BH, Latour A, Postan M: Susceptibility of $\beta_2$-microglobulin deficient mice to *Trypanosoma cruzi* infection. Nature 1992;356:338–340.

16   Reed SG: In vivo administration of recombinant interferon-gamma induces macrophage activation, and prevents acute disease, immune suppression, and death in experimental *Trypanosoma cruzi* infection. J Immunol 1988;140:4342–4347.

17   Plata F, Wietzerbin F, Pons FG, Falcoff E, Eisen H: Synergistic protection by specific antibodies and interferon against infection by *Trypanosoma cruzi* in vitro. Eur J Immunol 1984;14:930–936.

18   Minoprio P, Cury-El-Cheikh M, Murphy E, Hontebeyrie-Joskowicz M, Coffman R, Coutinho A, O'Garra A: Xid-associated resistance to experimental Chagas disease is IFN-$\gamma$ dependent. J Immunol 1993;151:4200–4208.

19   Gazzinelli RT, Oswald IP, Hieny S, James SL, Sher A: The microbicidal activity of interferon-$\gamma$-treated macrophages against *Trypanosoma cruzi* involves an *L*-arginine-dependent, nitrogen oxide-mediated mechanism inhibitable by interleukin-10 and transforming growth factor-$\beta$. Eur J Immunol 1992;22:2501–2506.

20   de Carvalho VB, Sousa FL, Vila JHA: Heart transplantation in Chagas disease. 10 years after the initial experience. Circulation 1996;94:1815–1819.

21   Ferreira MS, Nishioka SDA, Rocha A, Silva AM, Ferreira RG, Olivier W, Tostes S Jr: Acute fatal *Trypanosoma cruzi* meningoencephalitis in a human immunodeficiency virus-positive hemophiliac patient. Am J Trop Med Hyg 1991;45:723–727.

22   Silva JS, Barral-Netto M, Reed SG: Aggravation of both *Trypanosoma cruzi* and murine leukemia virus by concomitant infections. Am J Trop Med Hyg 1993;49:589–597.

23   Tsunawaki S, Sporn M, Ding A, Nathan CF: Deactivation of macrophages by transforming growth factor-$\beta$. Nature 1988;334:260–262.

24   Ding A, Nathan CF, Graycar J, Derynck R, Stuehr DJ, Srimal S: Macrophage deactivating factor and transforming growth factor-$\beta_1$, -$\beta_2$, and -$\beta_3$ inhibit induction of macrophage nitrogen oxide synthesis by IFN-$\gamma$. J Immunol 1990;145:940–944.

25   Silva JS, Twardzik DR, Reed SG: Regulation of *Trypanosoma cruzi* infection in vitro and in vivo by transforming growth factor-beta. J Exp Med 1991;174:539–545.

26   Silva JS, Morrissey PJ, Grabstein KH, Mohler KM, Anderson D, Reed SG: IL-10 and IFN-$\gamma$ regulation of experimental *Trypanosoma cruzi* infection. J Exp Med 1992;175:169–174.

27   Gazzinelli RT, Oswald IP, James SL, Sher A: IL-10 inhibits parasite killing and nitrogen oxide production by IFN-$\gamma$-activated macrophages. J Immunol 1992;148:1792–1796.

28   Cardillo F, Voltarelli JC, Reed SG, Silva JS: Regulation of *Trypanosoma cruzi* infection in mice by gamma interferon and interleukin-10: Role of NK cells. Infect Immun 1996;64:128–134.

29   Reed SG, Brownell CE, Russo DM, Silva JS, Grabstein KH, Morrissey PJ: Interleukin-10 mediates susceptibility to *Trypanosoma cruzi* infection. J Immunol 1994;153:3135–3140.

30   Hunter CA, Ellis L, Slifer T, Kanaly S, Grunig G, Rennick D, Araujo F: IL-10 is required to prevent immune hyperactivity during infection with *Trypanosoma cruzi*. J Immunol 1997;158:3311–3316.

31   Hunter CA, Slifer T, Araujo F: Interleukin-12-mediated resistance to *Trypanosoma cruzi* in dependent on tumor necrosis factor-alpha and gamma interferon. Infect Immun 1996;64:2381–2386.

32   Piuvezam MR, Russo DM, Burns JM Jr, Grabstein KH, Reed SG: Characterization of responses of normal human T cells to *Trypanosoma cruzi* antigens. J Immunol 1993;150:916–924.

33   van Voorhis WC: Co-culture of human peripheral blood mononuclear cells with *Trypanosoma cruzi* leads to proliferation of lymphocytes and cytokine production. J Immunol 1992;148:239–248.

34   Skeiky YAW, Benson DR, Parsons M, Elkon K, Reed SG: Cloning and expression of *Trypanosoma cruzi* ribosomal protein P0 and epitope analysis of anti-P0 autoantibodies in Chagas disease patients. J Exp Med 1992;176:201–211.

35   Sztein MB, Cuna WR, Kierszenbaum F: *Trypanosoma cruzi* inhibits the expression of CD3, CD4, CD8, and IL-2R by mitogen-activated helper and cytotoxic human lymphocytes. J Immunol 1990;144:3558–3562.

36  Wendel SL, Brenner Z, Camargo ME, Rassi A: Chagas Disease (American Trypanosomiasis): Its Impact on Transfusion and Clinical Medicine. ISBT Brazil '92 – Sociedade Brasileira de Hematologia e Hemoterapia, São Paulo, Brazil 1992, pp 1–271.

37  Sica REP, Filipini D, Panizza M, Fumo T, Basso S, Lazzari J, Molina H: Involvement of the peripheral nervous system in human chronic Chagas disease. Medicina 1986;46:662–670.

38  van Voorhis WC, Eisen H: Fl-160: A surface antigen of *Trypanosoma cruzi* that mimics mammalian nervous tissue. J Exp Med 1989;169:641–652.

39  van Voorhis WC, Schlekewy L, Trong HL: Molecular mimicry by *Trypanosoma cruzi*: The Fl-160 epitope that mimics mammalian nerve can be mapped to a 12-amino acid peptide. Proc Natl Acad Sci USA 1991;88:5993–5997.

40  Skeiky YAW, Benson DR, Guderian J, Sleath PR, Parsons M, Reed SG: *Trypanosoma cruzi* acidic ribosomal P protein gene family. Novel P proteins encoding unusual cross-reactive epitopes. J Immunol 1993;151:5504–5515.

41  Elkon K, Skelly S, Parnassa A, Moller W, Danho W, Weissbach H, Brot N: Identification and chemical synthesis of a ribosomal protein antigenic determinant in systemic lupus erythematosus. Proc Natl Acad Sci USA 1986;83:7419–7423.

42  Elkon K, Parnassa AP, Foster CL: Lupus autoantibodies target ribosomal P proteins. J Exp Med 1985;162:459–470.

43  Mesri EA, Levitus G, Hontebeyrie-Joskowicz M, Dighiero G, van Regenmortel MHV, Levin MJ: Major *Trypanosoma cruzi* antigenic determinant in Chagas heart disease shares homology with the systemic lupus erythematosus ribosomal P protein epitope. J Clin Microbiol 1990;28:1219–1224.

44  Koren E, Reichlin MW, Koscec M, Fugate RD, Reichlin M: Autoantibodies to the ribosomal P proteins react with a plasma membrane-related target on human cells. J Clin Invest 1992;89:1236–1241.

45  Cunha-Neto E, Duranti M, Gruber A, Zingales B, de Messias I, Stolf N, Bellotti G, Pilleggi F, Patarroyo ME, Kalil J: Autoimmunity in Chagas disease cardiopathy: Biological relevance of a cardiac myosin-specific epitope cross-reactive to an immunodominant *Trypanosoma cruzi* antigen. Proc Natl Acad Sci USA 1995;92:3541–3545.

46  Cunha-Neto E, Coelho V, Guilherme L, Fiorelli A, Stolf N, Kalil J: Autoimmunity in Chagas disease. Identification of cardiac myosin-B13 *Trypanosoma cruzi* protein cross-reactive T cell clones in heart lesions of a chronic Chagas cardiomyopathy patient. J Clin Invest 1996;98:1709–1712.

47  Burns JM, Shreffler WG, Rosman DR, Sleath PR, March CJ, Reed SG: Identification and synthesis of a major conserved antigenic epitope of *Trypanosoma cruzi*. Proc Natl Acad Sci USA 1992;89:1239–1243.

48  World Health Organization: The World Health Report 1996. Geneva, WHO, 1996, p 56.

Steven G. Reed, Infectious Disease Research Institute, 1124 Columbia St., Suite 464,
Seattle, WA 98104 (USA)

Liew FY, Cox FEG (eds): Immunology of Intracellular Parasitism.
Chem Immunol. Basel, Karger, 1998, vol 70, pp 144–162

..........................

# The Immune Response to Asexual Blood Stages of Malaria Parasites

*Nick C. Smith, Andrew Fell, Michael F. Good*

Queensland Institute of Medical Research, The Bancroft Centre,
PO Royal Brisbane Hospital, Brisbane, Qld, Australia

## Introduction

Malaria is by far the most serious parasitic disease of humans, with up
to 300 million people currently infected. According to the World Health
Organisation, 40% of the world's population is at risk from malaria and about
3 million people die from the disease every year – most of them children under
5 years old.

Malaria is caused by infection with Apicomplexan protozoa of the genus,
*Plasmodium, P. falciparum* being the most serious form. Infection begins when
the female *Anopheles* mosquito takes a blood meal. Part of this process involves
the mosquito injecting an anticoagulant from her salivary glands into the
bloodstream and accompanying the anticoagulant are the sporozoite stages
of the malaria parasite. Usually fewer than 100 sporozoites enter the bloodstream and within 45 min they have invaded the liver cells (hepatocytes) and
initiated what is called the pre- or exo-erythrocytic stage. This stage is not
pathogenic and lasts about 6 days for *P. falciparum.* During this time the
parasite grows and multiplies – a single sporozoite can give rise to 30,000
merozoites, the next stage in development. Eventually, the infected hepatocytes
burst and the ovoid merozoites enter the bloodstream. Within 20–30 s each
has attached to and entered a red blood cell.

Inside the red blood cell (erythrocyte) the merozoite becomes an erythrocytic trophozoite. The trophozoite ingests and digests haemoglobin and multiplies asexually to produce schizonts. It takes only 2–3 days from entry into a
red blood cell before up to 24 new merozoites rupture the cell and rapidly
invade new red blood cells. This asexual reproductive cycle is repeated several
times and up to 40% of red blood cells may become infected. Furthermore,

these cycles of multiplication cause all the symptoms of malaria including the periodic fever which is initiated by the release of pyrogens when the schizonts burst.

In the final third of the asexual cycle of *P. falciparum* the infected red blood cells stop circulating and instead adhere to endothelial cells of the capillaries. This is known as 'sequestration' and is probably a parasite adaptation to keep it away from the spleen which is a crucial organ for killing malaria parasites, possibly by providing an architecture and environment where the necessary combination of parasite and a variety of effector mechanisms are brought together. Sequestration of infected erythrocytes in capillaries of the brain would also appear to play a role in causing the comas associated with cerebral malaria, one of the most severe and dangerous manifestations of the disease, with a 20% mortality rate.

Eventually, some merozoites differentiate into the sexual forms, gametocytes, which mature to extracellular gametes only in the blood meal in the midgut of another female mosquito. Fertilization of macrogametes by microgametes soon follows, producing a zygote which becomes a motile ookinete. The ookinete burrows through the midgut wall, encysts on the outer surface and becomes an oocyst. Sporozoites develop within the oocyst and are ultimately shed into the insect's haemocoel and migrate to the salivary glands, ready to start the cycle again.

Thus, only two stages of the malaria parasite are truly intracellular; that which infects the liver and the asexual stage which resides within red blood cells. Intracellular parasitism is widely assumed to be a strategy for evading antibody-dependent immune responses. Camouflaged by a host cell, the parasite makes minimal necessary contact with the surrounding tissues, hiding from the patrols of the immune system. T cells can trump this strategy by recognizing antigens from intracellular parasites presented by lysosomal (class II) or, for parasites lying in the cytoplasm, endogenous (class I) pathways. For instance, protective immunity to intracellular protozoan parasites like *Toxoplasma gondii* and *Leishmania major* depends on responses mediated by T cells involving the activation of macrophages whilst cytotoxic CD8 or 'killer' T cells mediate killing of the liver stage of *Plasmodium*, possibly by secretion of cytokines such as IFN-γ and tumour necrosis factor (TNF) leading to activation of nitric oxide synthase (NOS) and production of the highly reactive and toxic nitric oxide (NO) (and metabolites thereof) by the infected hepatocyte [1]. The liver stage of *Plasmodium* will not be discussed any further in this chapter. The asexual blood stage of malaria, however, presents the immune system with a rather more intriguing problem because the parasite is carried within an erythrocyte, a cell that can neither process antigen nor present peptides to T cells.

## T Cells in Resistance to Asexual Blood Stage Malaria

Studies on T-cell responses in *Plasmodium* blood stage infections in humans present several difficulties: (1) the only tissue easily available for sampling is peripheral blood, which contains a fraction of the lymphocyte pool at any time and peripheral blood mononuclear cells (PBMC) probably do not accurately reflect the composition, specificity or activation state of cells in other tissues of the body – venous blood samples do not even contain all the cells present in the bloodstream, as cells in the marginal pool adjacent to the endothelium will not be sampled [2]; (2) unlike mouse models of malaria, immunity to human malaria does not develop after one or two infections but requires repeated exposure [3] – such immunity is age-related and may be strain-specific; (3) natural infections are initiated by sporozoite exposure and it is therefore difficult to separate liver stage from blood stage immunity in resistant populations, and (4) experimental manipulations which are technically feasible in mice are ethically impossible in humans. As a result, a great deal of experimental work on malaria has been done in murine systems, and then extended to human malaria by analogy.

Indeed, much of the evidence for a role for antibody-independent T-cell-mediated responses in malaria has been derived from studies on malaria infections in rodents. These species of malaria were mostly isolated from African thicket rats [4], and laboratory mice are therefore not their natural hosts. However, some of these parasites can be maintained in mice and rats. Different species display differing characteristics in pathology and immunology; additionally, inbred mouse strains vary in susceptibility and resistance to a particular strain of the parasite. It is therefore possible to select a combination of parasite species and strain, and inbred mouse strain, which shows particular characteristics. For example, the AS strain of *P. chabaudi* causes a self-limiting infection in C57Bl/6 mice, but a lethal infection in A/J mice [5].

In a nonimmune mouse, infection with any of the rodent malarias leads to a high parasitaemia. For some parasite species, parasitaemia progressively increases until the mice die (e.g. *P. berghei, P. yoelii* 17XL), whereas for others, the infection will eventually resolve (e.g. *P. yoelii* 17XNL). Evidence that T cells play an important role in this innate resistance came from studies showing that athymic (nude) mice are unable to resolve infections [6].

T cells are also critical for development of acquired immunity to *Plasmodium.* Mice can be successfully immunized against the rodent malarias by infection, followed by drug cure if necessary. Following challenge of immunized mice, parasites typically cannot be detected in peripheral blood. Immunity induced in this manner can persist for several months at least [7]. B cells do not appear to be essential for the induction of immunity; mice treated from birth with antibodies to IgM ('μ-suppressed'), and which have neither antibodies nor B cells can be immunized, although such mice are unable to completely resolve their infection [8]. More recently, experiments have been performed with B-cell and antibody-deficient μMT mice and $J_H D$ mice [9, 10]. B-cell-deficient mice can greatly reduce, but not eliminate infections with *P. chabaudi*, *P. chabaudi chabaudi* or *P. vinckei petteri*. Treatment of B-cell-deficient infected mice with antibodies to CD4 T cells results in high parasitaemia. Furthermore, nude mice do not develop immunity following infection and cure [11], implicating T cells as being critical to the development and/or effector phase of immunity.

Further evidence for the importance of T cells in resistance to malaria comes from studies in mice deleted of specific genes ('knockout' mice). For instance, mice lacking the TCR-α chain and, therefore of, TCR-αβ T cells, are unable to control *P. chabaudi* infection [12]. However, mice do not usually die during the first 60 days after infection. These results are similar to those obtained by in vivo treatment of mice with anti-T-cell antibodies [13], although this study reported a significantly increased mortality amongst T-cell-depleted mice. In *P. vinckei*, immunodepletion of CD4 T cells from immune mice with antibodies leads to a complete loss of immunity and death [14]. These studies all implicate CD4 TCR-αβ T cells in immunity. In contrast, mice with a disrupted TCR-γ chain, and therefore no TCR-γδ T cells[1], are able to control *P. chabaudi* parasitaemia, albeit with a slightly longer period of patent parasitaemia than heterozygous controls [12].

Collectively, these studies suggest that T cells are essential for the induction of immunity. Furthermore, the studies in which immunodepletion occurred after immunization showed that, at least in some models [14], CD4 T cells operate as effectors of immunity. However, B cells appear to be essential for the complete clearance of parasites. Human CD4 T cells can inhibit growth of *P. falciparum* parasites in vitro [16, 17] and it is tempting to consider that, based on this and the animal model data, they could function as effectors in vivo.

Adoptive transfer experiments also indicate the importance of CD4 T cells in immunity to malaria. In 1982, it was demonstrated that transfer of spleen cells

[1] γδ T cells build a TCR complex similar to that of αβ T cells, but from a different set of germline genes. The repertoire of γ and δ V chains is more limited than that of α and β chains, suggesting a more limited repertoire of antigens can be recognized [15]. The method of antigen recognition by γδ T cells is obscure; they are not directly restricted by MHC class I or II molecules, so they may recognize antigen directly. It has been suggested that they recognize stress proteins such as heat-shock proteins. The function of these cells is unclear; they do not appear to be essential for resistance to any particular type of pathogen but they may have an immunoregulatory role.

from immune mice to naive recipients confers immunity to *P. yoelii* 17X strain in CBA mice [18]. Fractionation experiments showed that the cells responsible are CD4 T cells. Similar results have since been obtained using other models; in most cases, CD4 T cells are required for transfer of immunity, although in some studies a role for CD8 T cells has been claimed [19]. The first study to use clones [20] demonstrated that specific T-cell lines and clones derived from immune mice could transfer protection of nude mice against challenge with *P. chabaudi adami*. The protective clone secreted IFN-γ and interleukin (IL)-2 and may have been a Th1-like clone, although the secretion of other cytokines was not monitored. More recently in *P. yoelii*, it has been demonstrated that Th1-like lines and clones can adoptively transfer immunity [21]. Such T cells can also reduce parasitaemia in SCID mice, but the animals die early at low parasitaemia, indicating T-cell-mediated immunopathology (see below).

The mechanism of protection mediated by adoptively transferred T cells has been investigated using *P. c. chabaudi* infections in mice. *P. c. chabaudi* parasitaemia peaks on day 10 after infection and then falls to a low level. A recrudescence of parasites occurs 2–3 weeks later. Characterization of CD4 T-cell clones shows that those derived from mice early in infection have a Th1-type cytokine profile (secreting IFN-γ and IL-2 in vitro), while clones derived after clearance of the infection have a Th2-type profile (secreting IL-4, providing B-cell help in vitro) [22, 23]. When transferred into mice depleted of CD4 T cells, both Th1 and Th2 clones confer resistance to challenge with *P. chabaudi*. Treatment of adoptively transferred mice with an inhibitor of NO metabolism, *L*-NMMA, ablates protection afforded by Th1 but not Th2 T-cell clones [24]. NO and related compounds can inhibit *P. falciparum* in vitro [25]; hence, NO, which readily diffuses across cell membranes, may be an effector molecule against the parasite. However, data show that immunity mediated by *P. yoelii*-specific CD4 Th1-like cells is not dependent on NO [21] and similar results have been found for *P. berghei* [C. Hirunpetcharat et al., unpubl. data]. Furthermore, serum nitrite and nitrate levels and levels of expression of inducible NOS (iNOS) are correlated with parasitaemia in populations from malaria hyperendemic areas [26]. Thus, whether NO plays an anti-parasitic role is not yet resolved. In contrast to immunity mediated by Th1-like cells, Th2-mediated immunity depends on the presence of B cells and immunity is associated with the rapid production of IgG1 antibodies [24, 27].

The observation that both Th1- and Th2-like clones could adoptively transfer protection was highly relevant to an earlier observation [28] that Th1- and Th2-like T cells appear in successive waves during infection with *P. chabaudi* and it has been suggested that this switch is driven by the density of parasite antigens and differential presentation of antigen by B cells and dendritic cells [27, 29]. There is good reason to believe that a similar switch occurs in human malaria: levels of the soluble IL-2 receptor (sIL-2R), a useful in vivo marker of T-cell activation, decline with age and, therefore, malaria exposure and immunity in endemic populations [30, 31]; levels of neopterin, indicative of macrophage activation and correlated with IFN-$\gamma$ production, decline in clinical *P. falciparum* cases after chemotherapy, and also decrease with the number of previous bouts of malaria the patient has suffered and the decreasing severity of the disease [32, 33]; and studies on heavily malaria-exposed populations in endemic areas such as sub-Saharan Africa and Papua New Guinea show a lack of in vitro T-cell responsiveness in adults who are presumably immune [34, 35], while levels of specific antibody increase with age.

A difficulty in accepting that effector CD4 T cells can control malaria is that the HIV pandemic has not had a major effect on the incidence of malaria or disease severity, especially in sub-Saharan Africa where HIV infection rates approach 25% in some areas. HIV has been associated with an increase in tuberculosis cases worldwide, with a predicted 1.4 million HIV-associated cases by 2000 [36]. Control of tuberculosis is classically associated with Th1-type T-cell-mediated responses. Other intracellular protozoan parasites, such as *T. gondii*, are controlled by Th1-type responses and are exacerbated by HIV and progression to AIDS [37]. However, no increase in cases of malaria, nor in their severity, has been found associated with HIV infection [38], apart from a few individual case reports of patients with unusually high parasitaemias. On face value, it is difficult to see how this fact can be reconciled with a major role for Th1 T-cell-mediated responses in infection with malaria. However, these observations may simply reflect the possibility that immunity to malaria involves a switch from a Th1-type T-cell-mediated response to a Th2-type response. In highly endemic areas such as sub-Saharan Africa, resistance to malaria (at least in adults) may be a function of antibody-mediated immunity and HIV would not be expected to have a substantial effect in this scenario if progression to AIDS involves a preferential depletion of Th1-type CD4 T cells and not Th2-type CD4 T cells [39]. It will be necessary to assess the effect of HIV and AIDS on malaria in areas of less intense transmission, where Th1-type cell-mediated mechanisms may be more important for resistance to malaria, before drawing firm conclusions. Certain analogies may be drawn here with the effect of pregnancy on susceptibility to malaria; increased susceptibility to malaria as a result of pregnancy is usually only noted in areas of relatively low malaria endemicity and not in areas of high transmission [40, 41]. This may reflect the possibility that, in areas of low endemicity, control of malaria relies on effective cell-mediated responses, which are down-regulated during pregnancy to protect the foetus [42], whereas in areas of intense transmission women have switched to antibody-dependent means of parasite control prior to becoming pregnant and these are unaffected by pregnancy [43].

A second difficulty in accepting that effector CD4 T cells can control a malaria infection is that the parasites are carried in red cells – cells that can neither process antigen nor present peptide epitopes to T cells. The prevalent model to explain the activation of T cells is that cross-presentation of parasite antigens occurs by professional antigen-presenting cells (such as macrophages) that take up either infected cells or antigen liberated from infected cells. However, there is still no clear answer as to how the activated T cells then mediate parasite death. It is widely believed that the effector T-cell response is nonspecific and mediated by cytokines such as IL-12 [44], TNF [45, 46], and IFN-γ [45, 47, 48] either directly or through the action of inflammatory molecules such as NO (see above) or oxygen radicals [49, 50]. These small molecules can permeate red cells and possibly kill the parasites inside leading to 'crisis' forms of parasites [51]. This process is thought to be facilitated by the spleen since splenectomy can completely abrogate immunity in models for which CD4 T cells are critical [14, 52].

The cellular immune response to malaria is also involved in the pathogenesis of the disease. Although CD4 T cells are known to be directly involved in the causation of cerebral malaria in a mouse model [53], there is debate about their role in human cerebral malaria [54–57]. However, there is evidence that the systemic pathology associated with malaria may be due to an exuberant inflammatory response to the parasite resulting in such diverse manifestations of disease as hypoglycaemia, hypertriglyceridaemia, nausea, diarrhoea, fever, anaemia and cerebral malaria [reviewed in 58–61]. The central molecule in this scenario is TNF, high serum levels of which are associated with a poor outcome of cerebral malaria [62, 63]. Furthermore, homozygosity of the TNF2 allele (which is in the TNF promoter region and increases TNF transcription) predisposes children to cerebral malaria [64].

TNF could originate directly from macrophages but it could also come from malaria parasite-activated T cells. A more critical question is what drives TNF production. Most interest has focussed on a malaria 'toxin'. Several proteins are known to induce TNF production including ring-infected erythrocyte surface antigen (RESA) [65], a soluble antigen complex known as AG7 [66, 67] and the merozoite surface proteins, MSP1 and MSP2 [68]. However, most attention has focussed on a (still incompletely characterized) lipid moiety as the major malaria toxin that induces TNF production: Bate et al. [see 58 for a review] demonstrated that the fraction of parasite lysate that induces TNF production is resistant to proteolysis and deglycosylation but susceptible to deacylation, dephosphorylation and phospholipase C; they also showed that the TNF-inducing activity of parasite lysates can be inhibited by antibodies to phosphatidylinositol (PI). Taken together, these data imply that the toxin is a glycosylphosphatidylinositol (GPI)-like structure and, indeed, Schofield and

Hackett [68] demonstrated that the TNF-inducing ability of MSP1 and MSP2 is likely to be due to their GPI moieties. These observations now enable testing of a proposal by Playfair et al. [69] that a malaria vaccine might be aimed at neutralizing a malaria toxin thereby preventing severe disease. This proposal was supported by the finding that antibodies to TNF-inducing PI can be induced in experimental rodent malaria [70] and can be found in the serum of malaria patients [71]. Unfortunately, however, these antibodies are almost invariably short-lived, low-affinity IgM isotypes.

The fact that T cells capable of reacting strongly to malaria parasites are detectable at high frequency in the periphery prior to malaria exposure raises another possible mechanism to drive production of TNF in response to *Plasmodium*. In 1975, Greenwood and Vick [72] presented evidence that malaria parasites are mitogenic for T cells, as parasite extracts could induce proliferation of T cells from nonmalaria exposed humans. Since then, it has been shown that this effect is more likely to be due to recognition of specific epitopes by cross-reactive T cells. The response is dependent on antigen processing, requires CD45RO (previously activated) T cells, has the kinetics of a conventional antigenic response [73, 74], and T-cell clones reactive to blood stage antigens can be generated readily in vitro [75]. Such T-cell clones can be shown to react to nonmalaria antigens from a panel of common organisms [74, 76]. They are heterogeneous in usage of V segment families of the TCR-β chain, indicating that the effect is not due to a 'malaria superantigen', and that it is probably driven by a large number of epitopes [77]. These responses are low or absent in cord blood but increase with age such that T cells from about half of the children and all adults in one study were capable of responding [76]. It therefore seems that humans acquire these cross-reactive T cells by exposure to environmental antigens. Infected blood taken directly from donors can trigger T-cell clones generated from nonexposed donors. Release of parasite antigens during infection would certainly be expected to activate such T cells. Furthermore, most clones generated from nonexposed donors to parasitized red blood cells secrete IFN-γ, and TNF can be detected in the supernatants of most activated clones. Thus, T cells, generated as a result of cross-reactive stimulation, must be considered as a source of potentially harmful TNF during malaria infection.


### Evidence for Involvement of Antibodies in Resistance to Asexual Blood Stage Malaria

The evidence that humoral immune mechanisms play a major role in immunity to malaria is not just derived from the observation of an apparent switch in reliance from Th1-type responses to Th2-type responses; the evidence that antibodies can protect against the asexual blood stages of the malaria parasite is simple and direct. In both humans [78–80] and mice [81, 82], passive transfer of antibodies from immune individuals to those suffering acute malaria reduces parasitaemia dramatically and rapidly. This passive immunity is dependent on the IgG subset transferred; it appears that in most cases IgG2a is critical in the mouse models [81, 82] and IgG1 and IgG3 in humans [83, 84]. Several recent epidemiological studies [35, 85–88] have confirmed the strong association of IgG1 and IgG3 antibodies with immunity to *P. falciparum* and it is also possibly significant that the predominant isotypes transferred from mother to foetus in malaria endemic areas are IgG1 and IgG3, which presumably accounts for the apparent resistance of newborns to malaria [89]; it is interesting to note that immunoglobulin derived from cord blood in hyperendemic areas can be used to transfer passive immunity to *P. falciparum* [79]. The ability to produce IgG1 and IgG3 antibodies to asexual blood stages of *P. falciparum* appears to be age-dependent [86, 88] and, combined with the demonstration [80] that immune IgG could protect people in a geographically disparate area, this observation supports Baird's contention [3] that the delayed development of immunity to malaria is as much to do with an intrinsic inability of children to develop an appropriate immune response as a necessity for several years of exposure to the parasite in order to encounter a broad spectrum of antigenic varieties.

IgG2a in mice and IgG1 and IgG3 in humans are cytophilic isotypes; they promote activation of phagocytes and monocytes via Fc receptors. Thus, it is significant that, in the murine model, the antibody-dependent parasite killing is mediated by neutrophils [90] and, in an in vitro assay system that predicted the in vivo efficacy of human IgG, parasite growth is only inhibited when both monocytes and IgG1 or IgG3 antibodies are present [84]. These results are in accord with earlier observations demonstrating the opsonic activity of human sera for *P. falciparum*-infected red blood cells [91, 92]; IgG antibodies opsonize only schizonts and trophozoites but not ring forms of the parasite and implicate antigens expressed on the surface of infected red blood cells as important factors in immunity to the malaria parasite. Cross-sectional and longitudinal studies performed in The Gambia [93] also indicate the importance of such parasite-derived erythrocyte surface antigens in immunity to malaria; these studies tested for correlations between several immunoassays (indirect immunofluorescence for blood stage antigens including RESA, inhibition of cell invasion, enzyme-linked immunosorbent assays to detect schizont antigens, schizont-infected red blood cell opsonization and infected red blood cell agglutination) and parasitaemia but found that only agglutination of infected erythrocytes is significantly and consistently associated with reduced parasite density. Agglutination is, however, also significantly associated with opsonization ability [93] so that this result may reflect the importance of antibody recognition of antigens expressed on the surface of infected red blood cells rather than agglutination per se.

It now seems likely that opsonizing antibodies [91, 92] and agglutinating antibodies [93, 94] recognize PfEMP1 (for *P. falciparum*-infected erythrocyte memebrane protein 1), a collection of antigenically diverse, large (200–350 kD) proteins inserted into the red cell membrane by mature asexual blood stage parasites [see 95 for a review]. PfEMP1 allows the *P. falciparum*-infected red blood cell to adhere to a variety of endothelial receptors, including vascular cell adhesion molecule 1, intercellular adhesion molecule 1, CD36, E-selectin and the extracellular matrix protein, thrombospondin, resulting in the retention of the parasite in vascular beds and, thus, the parasite avoids circulating through the spleen. An intriguing possibility is that the recently demonstrated adherence of parasitized red blood cells to chondroitin sulphate A, allowing preferential sequestration in the placenta [96], is due to yet another variant of PfEMP1. PfEMP1 represents an extraordinary effort by *P. falciparum* to avoid the spleen; several reports from human, monkey and rodent systems have demonstrated the crucial role played by the spleen in immunity to malaria (as discussed below).

Clearly, antibodies to PfEMP1 could inhibit the binding of parasitized erythrocytes to endothelia and thus make it inevitable that these infected red blood cells will pass through the spleen. Indeed, Quinn and Wyler [97] showed that while transfused *P. berghei* hyperimmune sera can clear parasites from eusplenic rats, this does not occur in splenectomized rats. If these antibodies were cytophilic, this would facilitate interaction of infected red blood cells with the phagocytic cells within the framework of the splenic architecture (see section on 'Spleen' below), resulting in their endocytosis and removal from the circulation. Indeed, it has been shown that the spleen plays a key role in the effective IgG2a antibody-dependent clearance of two rodent malarias, *P. berghei* [90] and *P. yoelii* [98]. Thus, the importance of particular specific antibody isotypes for effective immunity to the asexual blood stage of the malaria parasite can be rationalized with the central role of the spleen in immunity to malaria. There is also evidence that the spleen is crucial in regulating which type of IgG antibody is produced in response to *Plasmodium*. In rodents the presence of a spleen appears to down-regulate IgG1 (noncytophilic) responses and favour IgG2a responses [99, 100]; it may be that the cytokine milieu generated as a result of antigen presentation within the spleen is an important factor [101].

Bouharoun-Tayoun et al. [102] have suggested another model for the mechanism underlying the monocyte-mediated, antibody-dependent killing of *P. falciparum* asexual blood stages. These authors believe that the cytophilic antibodies actually recognize a surface antigen of the extracellular merozoite and the Fc receptor interactions of these antibodies with monocytes stimulates release of TNF. TNF then blocks the division of nearby intracellular parasites – a 'bystander' effect; the fact that neutralization of TNF prevents asexual parasite growth inhibition by the combination of cytophilic antibodies and monocytes and the fact that cell-free supernatants, presumably containing TNF, can mediate growth inhibition supports this contention [102]. At the same time, however, the inability of exogenous TNF to mediate these effects in the absence of immune IgG [102] is extremely puzzling, more so when one considers that red blood cells are not known to bear any receptors for TNF. Nevertheless, the striking association of IgG1 and IgG3 antibodies to MSP1 and MSP2 and immunity to malaria in endemic populations [85, 88] suggests that this idea deserves further investigation.

It must be pointed out, however, that the antibody isotype (cytophilic versus noncytophilic) is apparently a less critical factor in the induction of immunity by vaccination as opposed to natural immunity; this is demonstrated by vaccine studies with MSP1. MSP1 is a very large protein of molecular mass 190–230 kD found in most if not all species of malaria parasites. Early studies using native protein purified from *P. yoelii* showed that immunity could be induced by vaccination [103], and suggested that, on the basis of passive transfer studies, antibody-dependent mechanisms of immunity were not operative [104]. MSP1 is a highly polymorphic protein which undergoes processing during the time of merozoite invasion of erythrocytes. The carboxylterminal 19-kD domain, which is comparatively highly conserved, as well as the larger 42-kD domain, have now been shown to be targets on the protein for protective antibodies. Studies have been undertaken in mice (in *P. yoelii*) [105–108] and in monkeys (*P. falciparum*) [109, 110] using recombinant fragments and showed very solid protection following challenge. In some of the murine studies, sera from immunized animals was able to adoptively transfer protection. However, not all strains of mice could be immunized with recombinant $MSP1_{19}$, even though protected and not-protected strains showed similar levels of serum antibodies binding $MSP1_{19}$ in enzyme-linked immunosorbent assay. These results may indicate a difference in the fine specificity of the protective and nonprotective antibodies since it has been shown that in a protected strain (BALB/c), there is a very strong correlation between the titre and the degree of protection. Interestingly in this system, the isotype of antibodies was not IgG2a (shown to be critical in the development of natural immunity, above), but IgG2b and IgG1 [108]. Similarly, an $MSP1_{19}$-specific monoclonal antibody that can transfer protection to *P. yoelii* is an IgG3 [111]. For protection in this system, however, the titre of antibodies must be very high ($> 10^6$) and protective antibodies may therefore function simply by neutralizing merozoites [108].

## The Role of the Spleen in Resistance to Malaria

The prevalence of an enlarged spleen (commonly referred to as 'spleen rate') is a reliable indicator to the degree of endemicity of malaria in a population, and it has therefore been widely assumed that the spleen does play an important role in immunity to malaria. Supporting this are various case report studies of the effect on parasitaemia of splenectomy. One such example is that of a patient who had asymptomatic *Plasmodium malariae* for 53 years but then, following an incidental splenectomy, developed acute malaria [112]. Evidence supporting a role for the spleen in innate resistance comes from a case in which a splenectomized man developed a very high falciparum parasitaemia following initial infection. Interestingly, his peripheral blood contained all the developmental stages of the parasite, indicating that the spleen is involved in sequestration [113]. This is in keeping with previous demonstrations that the spleen is required for the expression on parasitized red blood cells of ligands for cytoadherence [114]. Other reports, however, question the role of the spleen in human immunity. A man who was previously immune to malaria and, while developing a high parasitaemia with *P. malariae* after splenectomy, subsequently during long-term follow-up was able to maintain parasite densities at levels similar to other villagers with intact spleens [115]. These data suggest that while the spleen can control parasitaemia, and may be the principal organ involved in this control, other tissues in the body also have the capacity to do so.

Data from mice also give conflicting views on the role of the spleen in immunity. An intact spleen has been shown to be critical to maintaining immunity in mice previously exposed to *P. vinckei* [14]; this immunity is CD4 T-cell-dependent. The absence of a spleen has also been shown to significantly delay (by >40 days) the clearance of *P. c. adami* parasites in mice not previously exposed to the parasite [52]. However, the importance of the spleen to innate resistance varies with the strain of mouse and the strain of parasite [116] and splenectomized C57 mice experienced significantly lower parasitaemias following infection with *P. yoelii* 17X than did eusplenic mice.

Recently, spleen transplantation between immune and nonimmune rats has been used to study the role of this organ in innate resistance and immunity to *P. berghei* [117]. In this model, innate resistance is dependent on the presence of an intact spleen, and immune rats lose the ability to clear parasites after splenectomy, although parasitaemia is maintained between 0.1 and 1%. Parasites are undetectable in the periphery of immune eusplenic rats. In this system it was shown that nonimmune rats became immune following transplantation with an immune spleen (fig. 1). However, dispersed immune spleen cells were not able to adoptively transfer immunity to a normal rat. On the other hand,

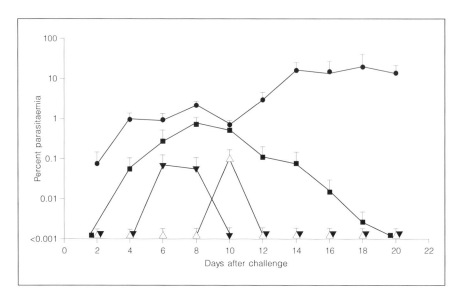

*Fig. 1.* Parasitaemias postchallenge in spleen-chimeric rats. Combined pancreas-spleen transplants were performed between normal and immune rats. Three normal DA rats were transplanted with a normal spleen (●, NL→NL), 4 immune rats were transplanted with a normal spleen (■, NL→IMM), 2 normal rats were transplanted with an immune spleen (△, IMM→NL) and 2 immune rats were transplanted with an immune spleen (▼, IMM→IMM). Between 5 and 21 days after transplantation, rats were challenged with $10^6$ *P. berghei*-parasitized erythrocytes intraperitoneally. Data points are mean parasitaemias and error bars represent SEM. [From 117 with permission].

immune rats whose spleens were swapped for those of nonimmune rats displayed significantly higher parastemias following challenge. The inability of the dispersed cells to transfer resistance indicates that the architecture of the organ is critical for immunity, and indeed architectural changes in the spleen as a result of malaria have been noted [118].

## Conclusions

The asexual blood stage of the malaria parasite presents the immune system with a unique challenge; how to control a parasite that resides within a cell incapable of processing and presenting antigens. The two factors of most importance to the immune system's success in dealing with malaria appear to be (1) the spleen and (2) the presence of parasite antigens on the surface of infected erythrocytes (although other factors such as merozoite surface antigen-specific antibodies can also play a vital role). The spleen plays important roles in clearing infected red cells from the circulation and in regulating parasite sequestration during infection. It appears to play a critical role in many, but not necessarily all types of innate resistance to malaria, as well as in the maintenance of acquired immunity, although other organs or tissues may be able to adapt to play this role in the absence of the spleen. It has been shown to be involved in both antibody-dependent as well as antibody-independent immunity. A possible model to explain these various observations is that exposure to the malaria parasite modifies the spleen in such a way that inter-action between T cells, macrophages, neutrophils and parasitized red blood cells is optimized, leading to parasite death via release of mediators such as free oxygen radicals and NO derivatives produced by phagocytic cells. This process would also be facilitated by cytophilic antibodies to antigens on the infected red blood cell's surface. The key to rational and effective development of a vaccine against malaria may well lie in better understanding precisely why the spleen is such a vital element in immunity to *Plasmodium*.

## Acknowledgements

The research of the authors is supported by the UNDP/World Bank/WHO Special Programme for Research and Training in Tropical Diseases; the National Health and Medical Research Council (Australia); The Cooperative Research Centre for Vaccine Technology; and the Australian Centre for International and Tropical Health and Nutrition.

## References

1   Hoffman SL, Franke ED, Hollingdale MR, Druihle P: Attacking the infected hepatocyte; in Hoffman SL (ed): Malaria Vaccine Development: A Multi-Immune Response Approach. Washington, ASM Press, 1996, pp 105–143.
2   Jandl JH: Blood: Textbook of Haematology, ed 2. Boston, Little, Brown, 1996.
3   Baird JK: Host age as a determinant of naturally acquired immunity to *Plasmodium falciparum.* Parasitol Today 1995;11:105–111.
4   Carter R, Walliker D: New observations on the malaria parasites of rodents of the Central African Republic – *Plasmodium vinckei petteri* subsp. nov. and *Plasmodium chabaudi* Landau, 1965. Ann Trop Med Parasitol 1975;69:187–196.
5   Stevenson MM, Lyanga JJ, Skamene E: Murine malaria: Genetic control of resistance to *Plasmodium chabaudi.* Infect Immun 1982;38:80–88.
6   Weinbaum FI, Evans CB, Tigelaar RE: Immunity to *Plasmodium berghei yoelii* in mice. I. The course of infection in T cell and B cell deficient mice. J Immunol 1976;117:1999–2005.
7   Winkel KD, Good MF: Inability of *Plasmodium vinckei*-immune spleen cells to transfer protection to recipient mice exposed to vaccine vectors or heterologous plasmodia. Parasite Immunol 1991; 13:517–530.
8   Grun JL, Weidanz WP: Immunity to *Plasmodium chabaudi adami* in the B-cell-deficient mouse. Nature 1981;290:143–145.

9    van der Heyde HC, Huszar D, Woodhouse C, Manning DD, Weidanz WP: The resolution of acute malaria in a definitive model of B cell deficiency, the J$_H$D mouse. J Immunol 1994;152:4557–4562.

10   von der Weid T, Honarvaar N, Langhorne J: Gene-targeted mice lacking B cells are unable to eliminate a blood stage malaria infection. J Immunol 1996;156:2510–2516.

11   Roberts DW, Rank RG, Weidanz WP, Finerty JF: Prevention of recrudescent malaria in nude mice by thymic grafting or by treatment with hyperimmune serum. Infect Immun 1977;16:821–826.

12   Langhorne J, Mombaerts P, Tonegawa S: αβ and γδ T cells in the immune response to the erythrocytic stages of malaria in mice. Int Immunol 1995;7:1005–1011.

13   Sayles PC, Rakhmilevich L: Exacerbation of Plasmodium chabaudi malaria in mice by depletion of TCRαβ+ T cells, but not TCRγδ+ T cells. Immunology 1996;87:29–33.

14   Kumar S, Good MF, Dontfraid F, Vinetz JM, Miller LH: Interdependence of CD4+ T cells and malarial spleen in immunity to Plasmodium vinckei: Relevance to vaccine development. J Immunol 1989;143:2017–2023.

15   Haas W, Pereira P, Tonegawa S: Gamma/delta cells. Annu Rev Immunol 1993;11:637–685.

16   Brown J, Greenwood BM, Terry RJ: Cellular mechanisms involved in recovery from acute malaria in Gambian children. Parasite Immunol 1986;8:551–564.

17   Fell AH, Currier J, Good MF: Inhibition of Plasmodium falciparum growth in vitro by CD4+ and CD8+ T cells from non-exposed donors. Parasite Immunol 1994;16:579–586.

18   Jayawardena AN, Murphy DB, Janeway CA, Gershon RK: T cell mediated immunity in malaria. I. The Ly phenotype of T cells mediating resistance to Plasmodium yoelii. J Immunol 1982;129: 337–381.

19   Mogil RJ, Patton CL, Green DR: Cellular subsets involved in cell-mediated immunity to murine Plasmodium yoelii 17X malaria. J Immunol 1987;138:1933–1939.

20   Brake DA, Long CA, Weidanz WP: Adoptive protection against Plasmodium chabaudi adami malaria in athymic nude mice by a cloned T cell line. J Immunol 1988;140:1989–1993.

21   Amante F, Good MF: Prolonged Th1-like response generated by a Plasmodium yoelii-specific T cell clone allows complete clearance of infection in reconstituted nude mice. Parasite Immunol. 1997; 19:111–126.

22   Taylor-Robinson AW, Phillips RS: Functional characterization of protective CD4+ T cell clones reactive to the murine malaria parasite Plasmodium chabaudi. Immunology 1992;77:99–105.

23   Stevenson MM, Tam MF: Differential induction of helper T cell subsets during blood stage Plasmodium chabaudi AS infection in resistant and susceptible mice. Clin Exp Immunol 1993;92:77–83.

24   Taylor-Robinson AW, Phillips RS, Severn A, Moncada S, Liew FY: The role of Th1 and Th2 cells in a rodent malaria infection. Science 1993;260:1931–1934.

25   Rockett KA, Awburn MM, Cowden WB, Clark IA: Killing of Plasmodium falciparum in vitro by nitric oxide derivatives. Infect Immun 1991;59:3280–3283.

26   Anstey NM, Weinberg JB, Hassanali MY, Mwaikambo ED, Manyenga D, Misukonis MA, Arnelle DR, Hollis D, McDonald MI, Granger DL: Nitric oxide in Tanzanian children with malaria: Inverse relationship between malaria severity and nitric oxide production/nitric oxide synthase type 2 expression. J Exp Med 1996;184:557–567.

27   von der Weid T, Langhorne J: Altered response of CD4+ T cell subsets to Plasmodium chabaudi chabaudi in B-cell-deficient mice. Int Immmunol 1993;5:1343–1348.

28   Langhorne J, Gillard S, Simon B, Slade S, Eichmann K: Frequencies of CD4+ T cells reactive with Plasmodium chabaudi chabaudi: Distinct response kinetics for cells with Th1 and Th2 characteristics during infection. Int Immunol 1989;1:416–424.

29   Taylor-Robinson AW: Regulation of immunity to malaria: Valuable lessons learned from murine models. Parasitol Today 1995;11:334–342.

30   Riley EM, Rowe P, Allen SJ, Greenwood BM: Soluble plasma IL-2 receptors and malaria. Clin Exp Immunol 1993;91:495–499.

31   Jakobsen PH, Morris-Jones S, Theander TG, Hviid L, Hansen MB, Bendtzen K, Ridley RG, Greenwood BM: Increased plasma levels of soluble IL-2R are associated with severe Plasmodium falciparum malaria. Clin Exp Immunol 1994;96:98–103.

32   Brown AE, Webster HK, Teja-Isavadharm P, Keeratithakul D: Macrophage activation in falciparum malaria as measured by neopterin and interferon-gamma. Clin Exp Immunol 1990;82:97–101.

33    Brown AE, Teja-Isavadharm P, Webster HK: Macrophage activation in vivax malaria: Fever is associated with increased levels of neopterin and interferon-gamma. Parasite Immunol 1991;13:673–679.

34    Doolan DL, Beck H-P, Good MF: Evidence for limited activation of distinct CD4+ T cell subsets in response to the *Plasmodium falciparum* circumsporozoite protein in Papua New Guinea. Parasite Immunol 1994;16:129–136.

35    Beck H-P, Felger I, Genton B, Alexander N, Al-Yaman F, Anders RF, Alpers M: Humoral and cell-mediated immunity to the *Plasmodium falciparum* ring-infected erythrocyte surface antigen in an adult population exposed to highly endemic malaria. Infect Immun 1995;63:596–600.

36    World Health Organization: The World Health Report 1996. Geneva, WHO, 1996, p 31.

37    Lockwood DNJ, Weber JN: Parasite infections in AIDS. Parasitol Today 1989;5:310–316.

38    Butcher GA: HIV and malaria: A lesson in immunology? Parasitol Today 1992;8:307–311.

39    Clerici M, Shearer GM: The Th1-Th2 hypothesis of HIV infection: New insights. Immunol Today 1994;15:575–581.

40    McGregor IA: Epidemiology, malaria and pregnancy. Am J Trop Med Hyg 1984;33:517–525.

41    Menendez C: Malaria during pregnancy: A priority area of malaria research and control. Parasitol Today 1995;11:178–183.

42    Wegmann TG, Lin H, Guilbert L, Mosmann TR: Bidirectional cytokine interactions in the maternal-fetal relationship: Is successful pregnancy a Th2 phenomenon? Immunol Today 1993;14:353–356.

43    Smith NC: An immunological hypothesis to explain the enhanced susceptibility to malaria during pregnancy. Parasitol Today 1996;12:4–6.

44    Stevenson MM, Tam MF, Wolf SF, Sher A: IL-12-induced protection against blood-stage *Plasmodium chabaudi AS* requires IFNγ and TNFα and occurs via a nitric oxide dependent mechanism. J Immunol 1995;155:2545–2556.

45    Clark IA, Hunt NH, Butcher GA, Cowden WB: Inhibition of murine malaria (*Plasmodium chabaudi*) in vivo by recombinant interferon-γ or tumor necrosis factor, and its enhancement by butylated hydroxyanisole. J Immunol 1987;139:3493–3496.

46    Stevenson MM, Ghadirian E: Human recombinant tumour necrosis factor alpha protects susceptible A/J mice against lethal *Plasmodium chabaudi AS* infection. Infect Immun 1989;57:3936–3939.

47    Stevenson MM, Tam MF, Belosevic M, van der Meide PH, Podoba JE: Role of endogenous gamma interferon in host response to infection with blood-stage *Plasmodium chabaudi AS*. Infect Immun 1990;58:3225–3232.

48    Meding SJ, Cheng SC, Simon-Haarhaus B, Langhorne J: Role of gamma interferon during infection with *Plasmodium chabaudi chabaudi*. Infect Immun 1990;58:3671–3678.

49    Clark IA, Hunt NH: Evidence for reactive oxygen intermediates causing hemolysis and parasite death in malaria. Infect Immun 1983;39:1–6.

50    Wozencraft AO, Dockrell HM, Taverne J, Targett GAT, Playfair JHL: Killing of human malaria parasites by macrophage secretory products. Infect Immun 1984;43:664–669.

51    Ockenhouse CF, Schulman S, Shear HL: Induction of crisis forms in the human malaria parasite *Plasmodium falciparum* by γ-interferon activated, monocyte-derived macrophages. J Immunol 1984; 133:1601–1608.

52    Grun JL, Weidanz WP: Effects of splenectomy on antibody-independent immunity to *Plasmodium chabaudi adami* malaria. Infect Immun 1985;48:853–858.

53    Grau GE, Piguet P-F, Engers HD, Louis JA, Vassalli P, Lambert P-H: L3T4+ T lymphocytes play a major role in the pathogenesis of murine cerebral malaria. J Immunol 1986;137:2348–2354.

54    Grau GE, de Kossodo S: Cerebral malaria: Mediators, mechanical obstruction or more? Parasitol Today 1994;10:408–409.

55    Clark IA, Rockett KA: The cytokine theory of human cerebral malaria. Parasitol Today 1994;10: 410–412.

56    Berendt AR, Turner GDH, Newbold CI: Cerebral malaria: The sequestration hypothesis. Parasitol Today 1994;10:412–414.

57    Clark IA, Cowden WB, Rockett KA: The pathogenesis of human cerebral malaria. Parasitol Today 1994;10:417–418.

58    Jakobsen PH, Bate CAW, Taverne J, Playfair JHL: Malaria: Toxins, cytokines and disease. Parasite Immunol 1995;17:223–231.

---

59    Kwiatkowski D: Malarial toxins and the regulation of parasite density. Parasitol Today 1995;11: 206–212.

60    Mendis KN, Carter R: Clinical disease and pathogenesis in malaria. Parasitol Today 1995;11:2–16.

61    Clark IA, Rockett KA: Nitric oxide and parasitic disease. Adv Parasitol 1996;37:1–56.

62    Grau GE, Taylor TE, Molyneux ME, Wirima MB, Vassalli P, Hommel M, Lambert P-H: Tumor necrosis factor and disease severity in children with falciparum malaria. N Engl J Med 1989;320: 1586–1591.

63    Kwiatkowski D, Hill AVS, Sambou I, Twumasi P, Castracane J, Manogue KR, Cerami A, Brewster DR, Greenwood BM: TNF concentration in fatal cerebral, non-fatal cerebral, and uncomplicated *Plasmodium falciparum* malaria. Lancet 1990;336:1201–1204.

64    McGuire W, Hill AVS, Allsopp CEM, Greenwood BM, Kwiatkowski D: Variation in the TNF promotor region is associated with susceptibility to cerebral malaria. Nature 1994;371:508–511.

65    Picot S, Peyron F, Deloron P, Boudin C, Chumpitazi B, Barbe G, Vuillez JP, Donadille A, Ambroise-Thomas P: Ring-infected erythrocyte surface antigen (Pf/155RESA) induces tumour necrosis factor-alpha production. Clin Exp Immunol 1993;93:184–188.

66    Taverne J, Bate CAW, Kwiatkowski D, Jakobsen PH, Playfair JHL: Two soluble antigens of *P. falciparum* induce TNF release from macrophages. Infect Immun 1990;58:2923–2928.

67    Jakobsen PH, Moon R, Ridley RG, Bate CAW, Taverne J, Hansen MB, Tabacs B, Playfair JHL, McBride JS: Tumour necrosis factor and interleukin-6 production induced by components associated with merozoite proteins of *Plasmodium falciparum*. Parasite Immunol 1993;15:229–237.

68    Schofield L, Hackett F: Signal transduction in host cells by a glycosylphosphatidylinositol toxin of malaria parasites. J Exp Med 1993;177:145–153.

69    Playfair JHL, Taverne J, Bate CAW, de Souza JB: The malaria vaccine: Anti-parasite or anti-disease? Parasitol Today 1990;11:25–27.

70    Bate CAW, Taverne J, Bootsma HJ, Mason RCSt H, Skalko N, Gregoriadis G, Playfair JHL: Antibodies against phosphatidylinositol and inositol monophosphate specifically inhibit TNF induction by malaria exoantigens. Immunology 1992;76:35–41.

71    Bate CAW, Kwiatkowski D: Inhibitory immunoglobulin M antibodies to tumor necrosis factor-inducing toxins in patients with malaria. Infect Immun 1994;62:3086–3091.

72    Greenwood BM, Vick RM: Evidence for a malaria mitogen in human malaria. Nature 1975;257: 592–595.

73    Jones KR, Hickling JK, Targett GAT, Playfair JHL: Polyclonal in vitro proliferative responses from non-immune donors to *Plasmodium falciparum* malaria antigens require UCHL-1+ (memory) T cells. Eur J Immunol 1990;20:307–315.

74    Currier J, Sattabongkot J, Good MF: 'Natural' T cells responsive to malaria: Evidence implicating immunological cross-reactivity in the maintenance of TCRαβ+ malaria-specific responses from non-exposed donors. Int Immunol 1992;4:985–994.

75    Good MF, Quakyi IA, Saul A, Berzofsky JA, Carter R, Miller LH: Human T cell clones reactive to the sexual stages of *Plasmodium falciparum* malaria. J Immunol 1987;138:306–312.

76    Currier J, Beck H-P, Currie B, Good MF: Antigens released at schizont burst stimulate *Plasmodium falciparum*-specific CD4+ T cells from non-exposed donors: Potential for cross-reactive memory T cells to cause disease. Int Immunol 1995;7:821–833.

77    Fell AH, Silins SL, Baumgarth N, Good MF: *Plasmodium falciparum* specific T cell clones from non-exposed and exposed donors are highly diverse in TCR β chain V segment usage. Int Immunol 1996;8:1877–1887.

78    Cohen S, McGregor IA, Carrington S: Gamma-globulin and acquired immunity to human malaria. Nature 1961;192:733–737.

79    Edozien JC, Gilles HM, Udeozo IOK: Adult and cord blood gamma-globulin and immunity to malaria in Nigerians. Lancet 1962;ii:951–955.

80    Bouharoun-Tayoun H, Attanath P, Sabcharoen A, Chongsuphajaisiddhi T, Druilhe P: Antibodies that protect humans against *Plasmodium falciparum* blood stages do not on their own inhibit parasite growth and invasion in vitro, but act in cooperation with monocytes. J Exp Med 1990;172:1633–1641.

81    White WI, Evans CB, Taylor DW: Antimalarial antibodies of the immunoglobulin G2a isotype modulate parasitaemias in mice infected with *Plasmodium yoelii*. Infect Immun 1991;59:3547–3554.

82   Waki S, Uehara S, Kanbe K, Nariuch H, Suzuki M: Interferon-gamma and the induction of protective IgG2a antibodies in non-lethal *Plasmodium berghei* infections of mice. Parasite Immunol 1995;17:503–508.

83   Groux H, Gysin J: Opsonization as an effector mechanism in human protection against asexual blood stages of *P. falciparum*: Functional role of IgG subclasses. Res Immunol 1990;141:529–542.

84   Bouharoun-Tayoun H, Druilhe P: *Plasmodium falciparum* malaria: Evidence for an isotype imbalance which may be responsible for delayed acquisition of protective immunity. Infect Immun 1992;60: 1473–1481.

85   Taylor RR, Smith DB, Robinson VJ, McBride JS, Riley EM: Human antibody response to *Plasmodium falciparum* merozoite surface protein 2 is serogroup specific and predominantly of the immunoglobulin G3 subclass. Infect Immun 1995;63:4382–4388.

86   Aribot G, Rogier C, Sarthou J-F, Toure Balde A, Druilhe P, Roussilhon C: Pattern of immunoglobulin isotype response to *Plasmodium falciparum* blood-stage antigens in individuals in a holoendemic area of Senegal (Dielmo, West Africa). Am J Trop Med Hyg 1996;54:449–457.

87   Ferreira MU, Kimura EAS, de Souza JM, Katzin AM: The isotype composition and avidity of naturally acquired anti-*Plasmodium falciparum* antibodies: Differential patterns in clinically immune Africans and Amazonian patients. Am J Trop Med Hyg 1996;55:315–323.

88   Shi YP, Sayed U, Qari SH, Roberts JM, Udhayakumar V, Oloo AJ, Hawley WA, Kaslow DC, Nahlen BL, Lal AA: Natural immune response to the C-terminal 19-kilodalton domain of *Plasmodium falciparum* merozoite surface protein 1. Infect Immun 1996;64:2716–2723.

89   Chizzolini C, Trottein F, Bernard FX, Kaufmann M-H: Isotypic analysis, antigen specificity, and inhibitory function of maternally transmitted *Plasmodium falciparum*-specific antibodies in Gabonese newborns. Am J Trop Med Hyg 1991;45:57–64.

90   Waki S: Antibody-dependent neutrophil-mediated parasite killing in non-lethal rodent malaria. Parasite Immunol 1994;16:587–591.

91   Celada A, Cruchaud A, Perrin LH: Opsonic activity of human immune serum on in vitro phagocytosis of *Plasmodium falciparum* infected red blood cells by monocytes. Clin Exp Immunol 1982;47: 635–644.

92   Celada A, Cruchaud A, Perrin LH: Phagocytosis of *Plasmodium falciparum*-parasitized erythrocytes by human polymorphonuclear leukocytes. J Parasitol 1983;69:49–53.

93   Marsh K, Otoo L, Hayes RJ, Carson DC, Greenwood BM: Antibodies to blood stage antigens of *Plasmodium falciparum* in rural Gambians and their relation to protection against infection. Trans R Soc Trop Med Hyg 1989;83:293–303.

94   Newbold CI, Pinches R, Roberts DJ, Marsh K: *Plasmodium falciparum*: The human agglutinating antibody response to the infected red cell surface is predominantly variant specific. Exp Parasitol 1992;75:281–292.

95   Borst P, Bitter W, McCulloch R, van Leeuwen F, Rudenko G: Antigenic variation in malaria. Cell 1995;82:1–4.

96   Fried M, Duffy PE: Adherence of *Plasmodium falciparum* to chondroitin sulfate A in the human placenta. Science 1996;272:1502–1504.

97   Quinn TC, Wyler PJ: Mechanisms of action of hyperimmune serum in mediating protective immunity to rodent malaria (*Plasmodium berghei*). J Immunol 1979;123:2245–2249.

98   Hunter RL, Kidd MR, Olsen MR, Patterson PS, Lal AA: Induction of long-lasting immunity to *Plasmodium yoelii* malaria with whole blood-stage antigens and copolymer adjuvants. J Immunol 1995;154:1762–1769.

99   Sayles PC, Yanez DM, Wassom DL: *Plasmodium yoelii*: Splenectomy alters the antibody responses of infected mice. Exp Parasitol 1993;76:377–384.

100  Yap GS, Stevenson MM: Differential requirements for an intact spleen in induction and expression of B-cell-dependent immunity to *Plasmodium chabaudi AS*. Infect Immun 1994;62:4219–4225.

101  Smith NC, Favila-Castillo L, Monroy-Ostria A, Hirunpetharat C, Good MF: The spleen, IgG antibody subsets and immunity to *Plasmodium berghei* in rats. Immunol Cell Biol 1997;75:318–323.

102  Bouharoun-Tayoun H, Oeuvray C, Lunel F, Druilhe P: Mechanisms underlying the monocyte-mediated antibody-dependent killing of *Plasmodium falciparum* asexual blood stages. J Exp Med 1995;182:409–418.

103  Holder AA, Freeman RR: Immunization against blood-stage rodent malaria using purified parasite antigens. Nature 1981;294:361–364.

104  Freeman RR, Holder AA: Characteristics of the protective response of BALB/c mice immunized with a purified *Plasmodium yoelii* schizont antigen. Clin Exp Immunol 1983;54:609–616.

105  Ling IT, Ogun SA, Holder AA: Immunization against malaria with a recombinant protein. Parasite Immunol 1994;16:63–67.

106  Daly TM, Long CA: Humoral response to a carboxyl-terminal region of the merozoite surface protein-1 plays a predominant role in controlling blood-stage infection in rodent malaria. J Immunol 1995;155:236–243.

107  Tian J-H, Miller LH, Kaslow DC, Ahlers J, Good MF, Alling DW, Berzofsky JA, Kumar S: Genetic regulation of protective immune response in congenic strains of mice vaccinated with a subunit malaria vaccine. J Immunol 1996;157:1176–1183.

108  Hirunpetcharat C, Tian J-H, Kaslow DC, van Rooijen N, Kumar S, Berzofsky JA, Miller LH, Good MF: Complete protective immunity induced in mice by immunization with the 19-kilodalton carboxyl-terminal fragment of the merozoite surface protein-1 (MSP1 19) of *Plasmodium yoelii* expressed in *Saccharomyces cerevisiae*. J Immunol 1997;159:3400–3411.

109  Kumar S, Yadava A, Keister DB, Tian JH, Ohl M, Perdue-Greenfield KA, Miller LH, Kaslow DC: Immunogenicity and in vivo efficacy of recombinant *Plasmodium falciparum* merozoite surface protein-1 in *Aotus* monkeys. Mol Med 1995;1:325–332.

110  Chang SP, Case SE, Gosnell WL, Hashimoto A, Kramer KJ, Tam LQ, Hashiro CQ, Nikaido CM, Gibson HL, Lee-Ng CT, Barr PJ, Yokota BT, Hui GSN: A recombinant baculovirus 42-kilodalton C-terminal fragment of *Plasmodium falciparum* merozoite surface protein 1 protects *Aotus* monkeys against malaria. Infect Immun 1996;64:253–261.

111  Majarian WR, Daly TM, Weidanz WP, Long CA: Passive immunization against murine malaria with an IgG3 monoclonal antibody. J Immunol 1984;132:3131–3137.

112  Guazzi M, Grazi S: Considerazioni su un caso do malaria quartana recidivante dopo 53 ani di latenza. Rev Malariol 1963;42:55.

113  Israeli A, Shapiro M, Ephros MA: *Plasmodium falciparum* malaria in an asplenic man. Trans R Soc Trop Med Hyg 1987;81:233 234.

114  David PH, Hommel M, Miller LH, Udeinya IJ, Oligino LD: Parasite sequestration in *Plasmodium falciparum* malaria: Spleen and antibody modulation of cytoadherence of infected erythrocytes. Proc Natl Acad Sci USA 1983;80:5075–5079.

115  Petersen E, Hogh B, Marbiah NT, Hanson AP: The effect of splenectomy on immunity to *Plasmodium malariae* and *P. falciparum* in a malaria immune donor. Trop Med Parasitol 1992;43:68–69.

116  Sayles PC, Cooley AJ, Wassom DL: A spleen is not necessary to resolve infections with *Plasmodium yoelii*. Am J Trop Med Hyg 1991;44:42–48.

117  Favila-Castillo L, Monroy-Ostria A, Kobayashi E, Hirunpetcharat C, Kamada N, Good MF: Protection of rats against malaria by a transplanted immune spleen. Parasite Immunol 1996;18: 325–331.

118  Weiss L, Geduldig U, Weidanz WP: Mechanisms of splenic control of murine malaria: Reticular cell activation and the development of a blood-spleen barrier. Am J Anat 1986;176:251–258.

M.F. Good, The Queensland Institute of Medical Research,
PO Royal Brisbane Hospital, Brisbane 4029 (Australia)
Tel. +61 7 3362 0404, fax +61 7 3362 0104, e-mail michaelG@qimr.edu.au

Liew FY, Cox FEG (eds): Immunology of Intracellular Parasitism.
Chem Immunol. Basel, Karger, 1998, vol 70, pp 163–185

........................

# Immunology of Infections with *Theileria parva* in Cattle

*W. Ivan Morrison*[a], *Declan J. McKeever*[b]

[a] Institute for Animal Health, Compton, UK and
[b] International Livestock Research Institute, Nairobi, Kenya

## Introduction

*Theileria* are tick-borne protozoan parasites of ruminants, found predominantly in tropical and subtropical regions of the world. Two species, *T. parva* and *T. annulata,* are highly pathogenic for domestic cattle and cause economically important diseases. The distribution of these parasites mirrors that of the tick vector species: *T. parva,* transmitted by *Rhipicephalus appendiculatus,* occurs in Eastern, Central and Southern Africa where it causes a disease known as East Coast fever, while *T. annulata,* which is transmitted by *Hyalomma* species of ticks, is the causal agent of tropical theileriosis which occurs in North Africa, Southern Europe and Asia [reviewed in 1].

Infections with *Theileria* parasites in their mammalian hosts are characterized by successive developmental stages in leukocytes and erythrocytes. Unlike a number of other apicomplexan protozoa such as *Plasmodium* and *Babesia,* which cause disease by destruction or sequestration of erythrocytes, the diseases produced by *Theileria* are attributable mainly to the intraleukocyte stage of development. This is a consequence of the unique relationship that these parasites have evolved with host leukocytes, whereby development from the sporozoite to the schizont induces activation and proliferation of the host cell [2, 3]. In infections with pathogenic species, this process results in rapid clonal expansion of parasitized cells, thus allowing the parasite to remain in an intracellular location throughout this stage of development. As a consequence, immunological control of established infection relies largely on T-cell-mediated immune responses directed against parasitized leukocytes [4–7]. However, given that parasitized cells express receptors for cytokines that can act as growth factors, T-cell responses elicited by the parasite also have the potential to enhance the growth of parasitized cells [8]. Here, we will review current information on the immune responses that are implicated in the control of infections with *T. parva* and discuss the potential contribution of T-cell responses to enhancement of disease pathogenesis.

## Parasite-Host Cell Relationship

The natural reservoir host for *T. parva* is the African buffalo (*Syncerus caffer*), in which infection is essentially asymptomatic. By contrast, infection of cattle produces an acute lymphoproliferative disease resulting in the death of most animals within 3–4 weeks.

The development of methods for in vitro propagation of leukocytes infected with *T. parva* as continuously growing cell lines [9, 10], was a key factor not only in allowing analysis of T-cell-mediated immune responses to the parasite, but also in facilitating studies of the early events in host cell invasion and the cell tropism of the parasite. These studies have revealed a number of features that are relevant to considerations of immune recognition of the parasite and how it causes disease.

Parasitized cell lines can be established by isolation of cells from the lymphoid tissues of infected cattle or by infection of cells in vitro with sporozoites derived from infected ticks. Ultrastructural studies of cells incubated with sporozoites have shown that sporozoites enter host cells by receptor-mediated endocytosis, during which there is an intimate association of the host and parasite cell membranes [11, 12]. Unlike other apicomplexan parasites, there is no specific orientation of the apical complex organelles during the process of invasion. Following internalization of sporozoites, which takes only a few minutes, the surrounding host cell membrane is broken down so that within 15–30 min the parasite lies free within the cytoplasm. Disruption of the host cell membrane is associated with the release of rhoptry and microsphere contents. Over the next 24–48 h, development of the parasite to the multinuclear schizont stage occurs and results in activation of the host cell, which starts to divide. During mitosis, the parasite associates with the mitotic spindle and divides at the same time as the host cell, resulting in the schizont nuclei being distributed randomly to both daughter cells [2, 3]. In the case of *T. parva,* free schizonts do not readily infect other leukocytes. Moreover, merozoites produced by the eventual differentiation of schizonts also appear not to infect leukocytes. Hence, multiplication of *T. parva* in nucleated cells occurs largely by clonal expansion of the leukocytes initially infected by sporozoites.

The cell types that support infection with *T. parva* have been studied by examining the establishment of cell lines in limiting dilution cultures of purified populations of leukocytes to which sporozoites have been added. These studies have demonstrated that αβ T cells (both CD4+ and CD8+), γδ T cells and B cells can all be infected with similar frequencies and that the cells maintain distinct cell surface phenotypes following infection [13, 14]. However, the infection of unfractionated populations of blood mononuclear cells usually gives rise to αβ T-cell lines [14, 15], a finding that reflects the situation in vivo, where the vast majority of infected cells are CD4+ or CD8+ [16]. Infected cells express high levels of class I MHC and have markedly up-regulated expression of class II MHC [13].

### Features of Immunity

Experimental infection of susceptible cattle with *T. parva,* either by applying infected ticks or injecting infected tick homogenate, results in an acute fatal disease in the majority of animals. Treatment with a slow-release formulation of oxytetracycline at the time of infection delays the development of the parasite and allows animals to recover from infection [17]. Such animals are immune to subsequent challenge with the same isolate of the parasite [17, 18], and are able to withstand challenge with up to a 1,000-fold lethal dose of sporozoites [19]. Immunity has been shown to persist for at least 3.5 years in the absence of challege [20]. Much of the available information on the mechanisms of immunity to *T. parva* has been derived from studies utilizing this 'infection and treatment' model of immunization.

Following challenge of animals immunized by infection and treatment, parasitized lymphoblasts are transiently detected in the regional lymph node at the same time or only slightly later than they arise in unimmunized controls. This observation clearly indicates that the immunity engendered by infection and treatment does not prevent establishment of infection but operates by controlling infection at the level of the parasitized lymphoblast. Studies in which cattle have either been immunized or challenged with cultured autologous parasitized cells provide further evidence that neither the induction nor expression of immunity depends on exposure to sporozoites [21–23]. However, this does not preclude a role for sporozoite antigens in induction of protective responses (see later). Titration of cryopreserved sporozoite stabilates (homogenized infected ticks) in groups of cattle indicate that there is a narrow margin between the minimal infective dose and the minimum dose that will result in 100% mortality [24]. Thus, it is probable that the parasite inocula used to infect animals in infection and treatment regimes contain relatively small numbers of sporozoites that are unlikely to induce a strong immune response against this stage of the parasite. As discussed below, alternative immunization procedures utilizing sporozoites or sporozoite antigens have been shown to result in protection.

Studies with immune sera and monoclonal antibodies have failed to demonstrate expression of parasite-encoded antigens on the surface of parasitized lymphoblasts. Because of the apparent absence of such antigens and the intracellular location of the parasite throughout this stage of development, it has been inferred that the immunity induced by infection and treatment must be T-cell-mediated. This contention is supported by the demonstration of protection following adoptive transfer of lymphocytes from immune to naive twin calves [4]. Conversely, passive transfer of immune serum to susceptible animals failed to give any protection [25].

## Immune Responses to Sporozoites

Although available evidence suggests that protective immune mechanisms of cattle against *T. parva* are directed at the schizont-infected cell, there is little doubt that cattle respond to sporozoite antigens during challenge. Animals under heavy challenge in endemic areas develop sporozoite-specific serum antibodies that neutralize infectivity in vitro [26]. In addition, this activity can be shown to be effective against parasite stocks isolated from diverse geographical locations [27]. Similar neutralizing activity could be generated in cattle by hyperimmunization with lysates of sporozoites [28]. Although immunoprecipitation and Western blot analysis revealed that these sera recognize a number of parasite antigens [29], the major specificity appeared to be a 67-kD antigen, which was designated p67 [30]. The majority of monoclonal antibodies raised against sporozoites were specific for this determinant and most of these exhibited some degree of neutralizing activity. Immunolocalization studies with these reagents revealed that the antigen forms a loosely organized coat on the sporozoite surface [31].

The gene that encodes p67 has recently been cloned and characterized [32]. It contains two open reading frames that are separated by a 29-base intron and its predicted amino acid sequence comprises 709 residues. Although the protein contains seven N-linked glycosylation sites, there is currently no evidence that the expressed product is a glycoprotein. The gene has been expressed in recombinant form using a number of different systems including *Escherichia coli* [33], baculovirus [34] and vaccinia virus [McKeever, unpubl. data]. Although all of these systems have been evaluated in immunization trials, most information on the vaccine potential of p67 is derived from experiments using antigen produced in *E. coli*. In an experiment involving 9 cattle immunized on five occasions with saponin-formulated NS1-p67, a C-terminal fusion of the antigen with a portion of the NS1 influenza virus protein, 6 animals were protected against severe disease arising from a 70% lethal challenge with stabilated sporozoites [33]. A series of subsequent experiments involving over 86 cattle have consolidated this observation, establishing that immunization with recombinant p67 gives rise to protection in approximately 70% of vaccinates. Of those protected, a proportion show no signs of infection, while the remainder develop only mild parasitosis with negligible clinical signs. In line with observations of neutralizing activity in endemic sera, it has been established that p67-immunized cattle exhibit a similar degree of immunity against heterologous challenge [27]. A similar immunization regime based on a modified recombinant antigen formulated in a proprietary adjuvant is, at the time of writing, under evaluation in preliminary field trials [A.J. Musoke, pers. commun.].

The reasons behind the failure of a proportion of cattle to generate protective immunity to p67 have not been determined. All immunized animals generate strong specific antibody responses and no correlation has been established between protection and antibody titre, isotype, avidity or epitope specificity [35]. However, it is still possible that the variation in protection relates to antibody function. Elimination of pathogens after antibody binding requires a number of additional events, some of which are effected by polymorphic elements. For instance, it has been established that polymorphism in the FcRIIa receptor is associated with failure to clear bacterial respiratory infections in humans [36]. It is also conceivable that the protection is engendered by p67-specific T cells targeted at the recently infected cell. In this regard, ultrastructural studies have revealed that a portion of the sporozoite coat remains on the surface of the infected cell after invasion [30]. We have observed that bovine lymphocytes can process and present soluble antigen [McKeever, unpubl. data], so it is possible that p67-derived peptides are displayed on the parasitized cell in the early stages of infection, in association with class II MHC molecules. Conversely, activated lymphocytes, which have up-regulated expression of class II MHC, have been shown to be more susceptible to infection by sporozoites than their resting counterparts [37]. The observation of an approximately 30% failure rate in vaccination with p67 may be therefore related to MHC polymorphisms that either hinder appropriate responses or enhance infectivity of the parasite. Studies to examine the effects of cytokines generated from T-cell responses on the early development of the parasite in vitro have indicated an inhibitory role for several cytokines although in some instances the findings were contradictory. Thus, while Preston et al. [38] reported low levels of inhibition of establishment of infection by IL-1, IL-2, IFN-$\alpha$, IFN-$\gamma$ and

TNF-α, DeMartini and Baldwin [39] observed no inhibitory effect with IFN-γ and indeed demonstrated that many parasitized cell lines produce this cytokine. However, these authors did observe a modest inhibition of establishment of infection with TNF-α. More recently, Visser et al. [40] have reported that S-nitroso-N-acetyl-*D,L*-penicillamine, a nitric oxide releasing molecule, partially inhibits early development of the parasite in vitro. None of these mediators had any inhibitory effect on established parasitized cell lines. Further, more critical studies are required to determine whether or not cytokines have a role in controlling early development of the parasite. Although cattle immunized with native p67 generate specific proliferative T-cell responses, so far these have not been detected consistently in animals immunized with the recombinant product [33], whether protected or not, so that it has not been possible to determine whether vaccine failure is associated with this immune compartment.

To date, all p67 immunization trials have been based on challenge with stabilated sporozoites delivered by needle. A major difference between this and natural challenge is that the latter is delivered into a substantial inflammatory reaction provoked by the feeding tick. The significance of this remains to be determined, but, it has been shown that activated lymphocytes are considerably more susceptible to sporozoite invasion than their resting counterparts [37]. It is therefore possible that infection will establish more readily in p67-immunized cattle when derived from tick challenge although it could be argued that sporozoites will be more accessible to antibodies in the inflammatory exudate. In addition, while the 70% lethal challenge that has been employed in these trials was selected as being representative of that delivered by a tick in which only one salivary gland acinus is infected, it is known that substantially higher infection rates can occur in the field [41]. Animals are also usually subjected to multiple tick attachment under these conditions. Clarification of the significance of these issues await the results of preliminary field trials.

Should the p67-based vaccine prove efficacious in the field, a major consideration regarding its success will be the capacity of field challenge to boost immunity. Preliminary evidence suggests that p67-induced protection is not long-lived [A.J. Musoke, pers. commun.]. Although p67 antibodies are found in sera from cattle under heavy endemic challenge [26], sporozoite-specific responses are not prominent after primary exposure to the parasite [28]. Assuming that immunization with p67 results in the same spectrum of protection against field challenge as observed in laboratory trials, this issue has greatest relevance to those vaccinates in which infection fails to establish. Those animals that develop mild infections are known to generate parasite-specific CTL responses and resist subsequent challenge [33]. If p67-specific immunity is boosted by field challenge, neutralizing responses would be expected to persist in this population, provided a sufficient level of challenge is maintained. However, in situations where cattle are the principal reservoir of infection, it might be predicted that challenge would in fact wane as the source of infection for ticks progressively diminished. In the event that sporozoite challenge fails to boost p67-specific responses, animals that completely neutralize initial challenge will rapidly become susceptible. It is therefore likely that the most effective use of a p67-based vaccine will involve regular vaccination of the young calf population, along with newly introduced adults.

Significant opportunities for contact between buffalo and cattle persist in many areas where East Coast fever is endemic. Although conserved among cattle isolates, the p67 gene of buffalo-derived *T. parva* differs in the incorporation of a central insert and additional flanking polymorphisms [27]. Although there is still substantial homology between the two, a major question that remains unanswered regarding the sustainability of a p67-based vaccine strategy is that of whether the current recombinant, derived from the Muguga stock of *T. parva*, can give rise to a similar degree of protection against parasites of buffalo origin.

## Immune Responses to Parasitized Lymphocytes

Immunization of cattle by infection and treatment elicits a strong cytotoxic T lymphocyte (CTL) response which is detectable by direct assay of peripheral blood mononuclear cells (PBMC) for 2–3 days coinciding with remission of infection [5, 6]. A similar response is detected following challenge of immune animals [5, 7]. Memory CTL can also be demonstrated by stimulation of PBMC in vitro with autologous parasitized lymphoblasts either in bulk cultures or in limiting dilution assays [42, 43]. The CTL have been shown to reside within the CD8+ subset of T lymphocytes, are class I MHC-restricted and are specific for parasitized cells. The frequency of detectable CTL precursors (CTLp) in individual immune animals is relatively constant from about 5–6 weeks onwards, ranging from approximately 1:2,000 to 1:12,000 [44]. Following challenge with sporozoites, the frequency increases abruptly between 5 and 7 days reaching levels as high as 1:30 in efferent lymph from the lymph node draining the site of infection, and up to 1:600 in PBMC [45]. Clearance of parasites is followed by a return to prechallenge frequencies within 2–3 weeks.

The high frequency of CTLp detected in efferent lymph following challenge of immune animals has been exploited in experiments to examine the protective activity of CTL [45]. These experiments have utilized identical twin calves produced by embryo splitting. Efferent lymph lymphocytes collected 8–10 days after challenge of immune calves were depleted of CD4+ T cells, γδ T cells and B cells by complement-mediated lysis with specific antibodies and the surviving CD8-enriched cells transferred into the naive co-twins 1–3 days after inoculation with a lethal dose of sporozoites. Transfer of these cells into two calves resulted in marked attenuation of infection and recovery in contrast to control animals which developed high levels of parasitized cells and severe clinical disease. Although the transferred cells contained a significant residual population of cells that were negative for CD4 and CD8 and markers for B cells and γδ T cells, an additional calf that received cells from which the CD8+ T cells were also depleted, showed no evidence of protection. Hence the protective activity could be attributed to the CD8+ T cells. The results of these experiments coupled with the observed temporal association of CTL responses with resolution of primary and secondary infections with T. parva, indicate that CD8+ T cells play an important role in mediating immunity to the parasite. Whether they exert their effect solely by killing parasitized cells or by cytokine-mediated mechanisms has not been investigated in detail. As already discussed, there is some evidence that TNF-α and several other cytokines may inhibit early development of T. parva in lymphocytes [38–40]. However, none of the cytokines tested to date (IL-1, IL-2, IL-4, IL-6, IL-10, IFN-α, IFN-γ, TNF-α) inhibit the proliferation of established parasitized lines. In addition, RT-PCR analysis has revealed that T. parva-infected lymphoblasts themselves contain transcripts for a wide range of cytokines [46]. Since challenge of animals immunized by infection and treatment usually results in the appearance of parasitized cells in the regional lymph nodes at the same time or only slightly later than in susceptible control animals, it would appear that the immunity has little effect on early development of the parasite in vivo. The in vivo studies, therefore, suggest that these cytokines do not have a direct role as effector molecules, at least in animals immunized by infection and treatment. However, it is possible that they exert an indirect influence on parasite growth via their effects on other cell types such as macrophages.

Studies of the mechanisms of immunity to T. parva have concentrated mainly on the effector arm of the T-cell response. It is not yet known whether or not help from CD4+ T cells is required for induction of CD8+ T-cell responses. In this regard it is worth emphasizing that in the adoptive transfer studies referred to above, the transferred CD8+ cells were from an active response and may therefore have had little requirement for help. Studies of CD4+ T-cell-mediated responses to T. parva are complicated by the fact that parasitized cells stimulate proliferative responses in autologous PBMC from naive animals. Nevertheless, analyses of T-cell clones have clearly demonstrated that parasite-specific CD4+ T cells are generated following immunization [47–50]. CD4+ T cells respond specifically to parasitized cells and in some instances to glutaraldehyde-fixed parasitized cells and to extracts of parasitized cells added to antigen-presenting cells. Some clones have been shown to produce IFN-$\gamma$ indicating that they are Th1-like [50]. Given that parasitized lymphoblasts express high levels of both class I and class II MHC molecules, there is clearly the opportunity for specific CD4$^+$ cells to interact closely with CD8$^+$ T cells upon antigen recognition. The provision of CD4-mediated help could be potentially important in promoting a rapid CD8$^+$ T-cell response to ensure early control of infection. Available data also do not exclude a role for CD4$^+$ T cells as effectors. Although one study has reported parasite-specific CD4$^+$ T-cell clones with cytotoxic activity [51], CTL activity is not readily detected in CD4$^+$ T cells during primary and challenge infections or in primary cultures of PBMC from immune animals stimulated with parasitized cells.

## Parasite Strain Heterogeneity

Clear evidence of immunological heterogeneity in *T. parva* was first revealed in studies carried out to test the cross-protective properties of different isolates of the parasite in animals immunized by infection and treatment. Although immunization with a single isolate protected all animals against the homologous parasite, challenge with different isolates frequently resulted in disease in a proportion of the immunized animals [17, 18]. A similar outcome was observed when such animals were exposed to natural field challenge. However, heterogeneity appeared to be limited, because immunization with a cocktail of three isolates resulted in protection against experimental challenge with a range of different isolates [52]. Combinations of parasite isolates have also been used successfully to immunize against field challenge [53, 54]. A striking feature of the results obtained in these cross-immunization experiments is that failure of one parasite isolate to protect against another invariably occurred only in a proportion of the animals. Moreover, in many instances the effect was not reciprocal; whereas parasite A might fail to give complete protection against challenge with parasite B, parasite B would protect all animals against parasite A. These findings clearly indicated that protective immune responses can be restricted in specificity to some strains of the parasite and that this strain specificity can vary between animals.

A number of in vitro methods have been used to identify differences between isolates of *T. parva*. Genetic heterogeneity has been detected through restriction fragment length polymorphism (RFLP) analysis of repetitive parasite DNA sequences in Southern blots [55, 56]. Pulsed-field gel electrophoresis of purified parasite DNA digested with rare-cutter enzymes also reveals RFLP [57]. Heterogeneity at the protein level has been demonstrated using monoclonal antibodies that detect polymorphic determinants and through analysis of molecular weight differences in a major polymorphic schizont antigen [58–60]. That none of these differences shows an obvious correlation with the capacity of the different parasite populations to cross-protect is not surprising, given the genetic and antigenic complexity of the parasite.

## Parasite Strain Specificity of CTL Responses

The cytotoxic T-cell responses of immune cattle show restriction in specificity to some isolates of *T. parva* [7, 61, 62]. However, until recently, a clear relationship between the strain specificity of the CTL response and the ability of parasite populations to cross-protect had been difficult to establish. This was due in part to the fact that some of the parasite isolates used in experimental studies were themselves heterogeneous. DNA probes, monoclonal antibodies and CTL clones have all been shown to detect differences in cultured parasitized cell lines derived from the same isolate [59, 62]. The cell lines examined in these studies included cloned and uncloned lines, and it was clear from the findings that the uncloned lines had in each instance been selected by in vitro passage to contain predominantly one component of the starting population. Such cell lines are therefore not representative of the parent isolate. Because of potential heterogeneity in the parasite populations, all uncloned isolates of *T. parva* are referred to as stocks rather than strains.

The development of a method to obtain cloned populations of *T. parva* [63] opened the way for critical studies to investigate the immunological basis of parasite heterogeneity. The method involved twice cloning parasitized cell lines established by infection of lymphocytes in vitro with sporozoites at limiting dilution, followed by inoculation into the autologous animal for tick pick-up. The parasites in cell lines derived from these populations showed consistent profiles with parasite-specific DNA probes and monoclonal antibodies.

The relationship between parasite strain specificity of CTL responses and cross-protection has been investigated using two parasite populations, namely the Muguga stock and a cloned parasite derived from the Marikebuni stock (Marikebuni 3219). The former, although uncloned, has been used extensively in studies of CTL responses and has shown no evidence of heterogeneity in CTL epitopes within the stock. A proportion of animals immunized with the Muguga stock are susceptible to challenge with Marikebuni 3219 [44]. By contrast, heterogeneity in CTL epitopes in the Marikebuni stock can readily be detected with CTL clones [59, 62]. While immunization with the uncloned

Marikebuni stock protects all animals against challenge with Muguga, a proportion of animals immunized with Marikebuni 3219 are susceptible to challenge with Muguga [44].

A detailed analysis of the parasite strain specificity of the CTL response, utilizing limiting dilution cultures, was conducted in 22 cattle immunized by infection and treatment with the Muguga stock or Marikebuni 3219 [44]. All animals were subsequently challenged with a lethal dose of sporozoites of the reciprocal parasite population to determine the relationship between CTL specificity and immunity. With both parasites, some animals generated CTL that were specific for the parasite used for immunization whereas others mounted cross-reactive CTL responses. There was a close correlation between the specificity of the responses and susceptibility to challenge with the heterologous parasite: All animals with cross-reactive CTL were immune whereas those that had strain-specific CTL developed severe clinical reactions with abundant parasitized lymphoblasts in the lymph nodes. Unlike susceptible control animals, however, many of the latter animals recovered from the challenge infection, indicating that immunization had resulted in a low level of protection. Nevertheless, the results of this study provide further convincing evidence that CTL responses are important in protection. They also confirm that the strain specificity of the CTL response varies between animals immunized with the same parasite population.

The above findings might imply that some of the epitopes recognized by parasite-specific CTL are conserved in all parasite strains. However, studies in which CTL clones derived from animals immunized with the Muguga stock were tested on a wider range of target cell lines indicate that this is not the case. A total of 31 parasite-specific CTL clones comprising 6 sets of clones, each with a distinct MHC restriction specificity, were tested for cytotoxicity on different target cell lines derived from the Marikebuni stock [62, 64]. The parasites in these lines were shown to differ in genotype and/or in their reactivity with monoclonal antibodies. In all instances, the CTL clones killed some of the Marikebuni-infected cell lines but not others. Each set of clones with the same MHC restriction specificity displayed a similar pattern of strain specificity. By contrast, where clones with different MHC restriction specificities could be tested on the same target cells, they invariably exhibited different patterns of killing, indicating that the class I molecules were presenting different antigenic peptides. These findings provided evidence that, by selecting different epitopes, the class I molecules on parasitized cells could influence the strain specificity of the CTL responses. This notion has been reinforced by the results of limiting dilution analyses of the specificity of CTLp in immune animals of defined class I MHC phenotype. Molecular and functional studies of the bovine MHC have shown that cattle express two polymorphic class I genes, although serological typing for class I in most instances detects only the products of one locus [65, 66]. Analysis of the MHC restriction of CTL in a series of MHC-heterozygous cattle demonstrated that the response was restricted by the products of one of the MHC haplotypes in most animals [67]. Among the haplotypes represented there was a clear hierarchy in dominance, with certain haplotypes consistently acting as restriction elements in preference to others. In the case of one of the dominant haplotypes, for which the class I genes (A10 and KN104) have been defined, CTL induced by the Muguga stock were restricted entirely by the KN104 molecule in all animals examined, and in all but one of these animals they killed Muguga-infected targets but not Marikebuni-infected targets. These findings indicate that in many animals a single class I MHC molecule determines the epitopes that are recognized by CTL and thus can influence the specificity of the response. While, in the case of the Muguga parasite, there was an association of KN104 with Muguga-specific responses, this association was not absolute. Hence other factors such as the T-cell-receptor repertoire must also influence the fine specificity of the response.

## Immunodominance as a Determinant of Strain Specificity of CTL

Given the antigenic complexity of *Theileria* parasites and their intracytoplasmic site of replication, it might be expected that numerous peptides would be available for association with class I MHC molecules and recognition by CTL. However, as discussed above, the available evidence suggests that the CTL response in individual animals is focused on a limited number of epitopes. Additional findings indicate that an immunodominance phenomenon contributes to the restricted nature of the repertoire of CTL antigen specificities. In the course of comparing the specificity of CTL responses to the Muguga and Marikebuni 3219 parasites in identical twin calves, it was observed that in one set of twins carrying the A10 and KN104 specificities, the response was strain-specific in the Muguga-immunized animal and cross-reactive in the Marikebuni 3219-immunized animal, despite being entirely restricted by KN104 in both animals [67]. The in vivo relevance of this result was confirmed by the finding that the specificity of the responses was correlated with subsequent susceptibility to challenge with the reciprocal parasites. The result implied that the Muguga-immunized animal, although it mounted a strain-specific CTL response, was capable of responding to epitopes that are conserved between the two parasites. Further evidence to support this notion has been provided by an experiment in which the CTL response in two Muguga-immunized animals was compared before and after challenge with Marikebuni 3219 [67]. In both animals, immunization with Muguga produced a KN104-restricted Muguga-specific CTL response, whereas after challenge with Marikebuni 3219, which resulted in a severe clinical reaction followed by recovery, both animals developed a population of KN104-restricted CTL that recognized target cells infected with either parasite. These results indicated that individual animals generate a CTL response to only a restricted subset of the epitopes to which they are capable of responding in a given parasite. A similar immunodominance phenomenon has been observed in CTL responses to a number of human and murine viral infections. The most notable example is infection with human immunodeficiency virus in which a sequential shift of the CTL response from dominant to less dominant epitopes has been observed in some patients coinciding with the emergence of mutations in the most dominant epitopes [68, 69]. A parallel situation can be seen in the emergence of a KN104-restricted cross-reactive CTL response to *T. parva* following challenge with Marikebuni 3219 which presumably lacks the dominant strain-specific epitope(s) found in the Muguga parasite.

The molecular and cellular events that lead to immunodominance are not understood but are likely to involve variation in the concentrations of antigenic peptides bound to the presenting MHC molecules and the composition of the repertoire of T-cell receptors specific for the various peptide-MHC combinations. The former may be influenced by the relative abundance of the proteins containing antigenic peptides, the efficacy with which the peptides are processed and transported into the endoplasmic reticulum and their avidity of binding to class I MHC molecules. Restriction of the response to the most dominant epitopes presumably involves some form of competition at the level of T-cell recognition of infected cells.

The occurrence of immunodominance in CTL responses to *T. parva* has important implications for strategies to develop a vaccine against the parasite based on the use of antigens containing CTL epitopes. The strain-restricted nature of CTL responses and immunity following immunization with live parasites has been seen as a significant impediment to the development of such a vaccine. However, the effect of immunodominance is to exaggerate the parasite strain specificity of the response and hence to increase the likelihood that recovered animals will be susceptible to challenge with another strain of the parasite. The use in a vaccine of a delivery system that favours induction of CTL responses to different component antigens could overcome the problem of strain specificity. Although studies with CTL clones indicate that most if not all CTL epitopes show some polymorphism, available evidence suggests a mosaic distribution in which there is overlapping expression of epitopes among parasite strains, such that induction of CTL responses to a limited number of epitopes may be sufficient to provide protection in most animals against a wide range of strains [for further discussion, see 64]. Confirmation of this point awaits the identification and characterization of the parasite proteins containing CTL epitopes.

## Immune Responses to Primary Infection

The prevailing view of the pathogenesis of infection with *T. parva* in cattle is that the protective immune response is merely overwhelmed by the infection as a consequence of the inherent replicative capacity of parasitized cells. This notion is consistent with the finding that infected animals make an effective immune response and recover when parasite development is retarded by treatment with oxytetracycline at the time of infection. However, the reservoir host of *T. parva,* the African buffalo, does not develop disease [70] despite the fact that its cells are equally susceptible to infection and transformation by the parasite in vitro [71]. Studies of the cellular responses in cattle undergoing primary infection with *T. parva* also question this simple view of the pathogenesis of the disease.

In cattle infected with *T. parva* the lymph node draining the site of infection undergoes a dramatic 3- to 4-fold increase in size over a 1- to 2-day period around the time when parasitized cells are first detectable (usually 7–9 days after experimental infection) [72]. While increased recruitment of lymphocytes into the lymph node may contribute to this change, there is undoubtedly also a marked T-cell proliferative response in the node. Phenotypic analyses of lymph node cell aspirates and efferent lymph cells draining from the regional node have revealed up to 25% lymphoblasts in both populations at a time when less than 2% of the cells are parasitized [73]. The lymphoblasts are predominantly $CD8^+$ and contain a large subset of cells that are $CD8^+$ $CD2^-$ $CD3^+$ $\gamma\delta$ $TCR^-$, indicating that they are $\alpha\beta$ T cells [F. Houston and W.I. Morrison, unpubl. data]. Cells with this phenotype are rare in PBMC or lymph node cells from healthy cattle and they represent only a minor component of the lymphoblasts in the lymph nodes of immune animals after challenge with sporozoites. The clear distinction between the presence or absence of expression of CD2 on the $CD2^+$ $CD8^+$ and $CD2^-$ $CD8^+$ subpopulations in infected animals suggests that the $CD2^-$ $CD8^+$ cells are generated by expansion of a minor pre-existing population rather than by loss of expression of CD2. Analyses of their T-cell-receptor $V\beta$ gene usage have demonstrated that they are polyclonal in origin [F. Houston and W.I. Morrison, unpubl. data]. Preliminary studies of cytokine expression by RT-PCR indicate that they express IFN-$\gamma$ and IL-10. However, further analyses of the stimulatory requirements and function of these $CD2^-$ $CD8^+$ cells have been hampered by the inability to induce them to proliferate in vitro using a variety of specific and polyclonal stimuli.

In contrast to T-cell responses in immune cattle, parasite-specific CTL are not detected at any stage during primary infections with *T. parva*, either by direct assay of blood or lymph mononuclear cells or by limiting dilution assay of CTL precursors [5, 43]. In the latter assay, the majority of wells were overgrown by parasitized cells present in the responding populations, possibly precluding the detection of CTL precursors. To circumvent this problem, two animals were infected by inoculation with CD4+ T cells that had been purified by cell sorting and incubated in vitro with sporozoites for 48 h [74]. In separate experiments, this procedure had been shown to result in a lethal infection during which the parasite remained confined to CD4+ T cells. Limiting dilution assays with CD8+ T cells purified from these animals did not detect any specific CTLp up to day 10 of infection, i.e. several days after the onset of the in vivo T-cell response. That the primary response also lacks other effector functions is suggested by the fact that its onset coincides with a period of rapid multiplication of parasitized cells. Thus, the primary T-cell response to *T. parva* differs fundamentally from that observed following challenge of immune animals, both in the phenotype of the responding cells and the absence of obvious effector functions.

An important question raised by these findings is whether or not the T-cell response in naive animals contributes to the pathogenesis of the disease by potentiating the growth of parasitized cells. Evidence to support this idea comes from in vitro studies of the growth of parasitized cell lines. Recombinant IL-2 has been shown to enhance the growth of infected cells particularly at low cell densities [75, 76]; unsupplemented cells failed to grow when diluted beyond several hundred cells per microtitre well, whereas the use of medium containing IL-2 enabled them to be grown from a few cells per well. Similar, but less pronounced, growth-promoting activity has been observed with IL-1 and IL-10 [R.A. Collins and W.I. Morrison, unpubl. data]. Constitutive expression of the α chain of the IL-2 receptor (CD25) by cell lines was confirmed by detection of mRNA transcripts in Northern blots and by analysis of cell surface expression with specific antibodies [77]. In early studies, it was suggested that the parasitized cells themselves might be a source of IL-2 or other growth factors that could act in an autocrine or paracrine manner [75, 76]. Indeed, parasitized cell lines have been shown to contain mRNA transcripts for a number of cytokines, including IL-2; however, the profile of cytokine expression varied between cell lines, IL-10 being the only cytokine for which transcripts were consistently detected [46]. Growth-promoting activity has been detected in culture supernatants of some cell lines [75, 76]. Moreover, a role for stimulation via the IL-2 receptor in maintaining growth of some cell lines is indicated by the observations that antibody specific for CD25 partially inhibited proliferation of two cell lines [78], and that transfection of one of these cell lines with CD25 antisense RNA resulted in similar inhibition [79]. Studies of cells grown at low cell density also indicate that maintenance of growth is dependent on stimulation through cell-cell contact; these signals can be provided by the infected cells themselves or by uninfected leukocytes [78].

Whether the properties described for parasitized cell lines reflect those of parasitized cells in vivo or represent the end product of intensive selection imposed by in vitro passage remains to be determined. It is of note that during the early stages of infection in vivo parasitized cells are usually observed scattered singly rather than in clusters in the lymphoid tissues. Given the evidence that parasitized cells require external stimuli to proliferate at low cell concentrations, it seems likely that the primary T-cell response will contribute significantly to potentiation of the growth of parasitized cells. From an evolutionary point of view, the induction of an early host response that helps parasitized cells to multiply at low cell densities could be of considerable advantage to the parasite, provided it does not also subvert the responses that allow the host to control the infection. Since cattle are not the natural reservoir host of the parasite, their susceptibility to disease may reflect a lack of adaptation of the immune response such that it is heavily biased in favour of promoting parasite replication.

### Influence of Infected Cell Type on Pathogenesis

The capacity of *T. parva* to infect and transform purified populations of αβ T cells, γδ T cells and B cells in vitro at similar frequencies has already been discussed. However, the majority of parasitized cells in the tissues of infected cattle are CD4$^+$ or CD8$^+$ T cells, suggesting either that the cell types differ in their ability to replicate in vivo or that T cells are more likely to become infected in vivo. To distinguish between these possibilities, a series of experiments was carried out in which animals were inoculated with purified populations of autologous lymphocytes infected in vitro with *T. parva*. Previous studies had shown that 10$^5$ or more parasitized cells from freshly established cell lines produced severe disease when inoculated into the autologous animals, whereas similar inocula failed to infect allogeneic hosts [23]. However, animals that received 10$^5$ parasitized cells from cloned cell lines representing different cell phenotypes all developed relatively mild infections from which they recovered [15]. The reduced pathogenicity of the cloned cells was interpreted as being due to attenuation of the parasite or the ability of the host cells to replicate in vivo as a consequence of the more prolonged in vitro passage required to clone the cell lines. Therefore, a second approach was pursued that involved incubation of purified lymphocyte populations for 48 h in vitro with sporozoites prior to inoculation back into the autologous hosts [15]. Any sporozoites remaining in such cultures are no longer viable after 48 h, so infection of the host must therefore be initiated by the parasitized lymphocytes. As few as $3 \times 10^4$ autologous PBMC or purified CD4$^+$ or CD8$^+$ lymphocytes incubated with sporozoites induced severe, potentially lethal infections when injected into the autologous animals. By contrast, purified B cells treated in the same way produced mild self-limiting infections, even when 10 times more cells were used [15]. The prepatent period to detection of infection in the regional lymph node, which has been shown to be an indicator of the parasite dose received [23, 24], was not markedly different in animals that received B cells or T cells, indicating that the difference in outcome of infection is related to regulation of growth of the infected cells rather than merely reflecting the numbers of cells in which the parasite had established infection.

These findings clearly demonstrate that the cell type infected with *T. parva* influences the pathogenicity of the parasite. While the factors that determine the difference in pathogenic potential of parasitized B cells and T cells have not been investigated, some of the properties of parasitized cell lines have been compared. B-cell and T-cell lines have both been shown to express the IL-2 receptor and to be responsive to IL-2 [77]. Comparison of cytokine mRNA expression by a large number of parasitized cell lines of different phenotypes has failed to reveal any consistent differences between B-cell and T-cell lines, although individual lines showed different profiles [46]. Secretion of IFN-γ has been detected in both cell types [39]. We have also shown that B-cell and T-cell lines are both effective as stimulators and target cells in in vitro assays to induce and detect CTL, respectively, in PBMC from immune animals [W.I. Morrison and B.M. Goddeeris, unpubl. data]. However, given that parasitized T cells from established cell lines generally fail to reproduce severe infections when inoculated into the autologous animals [15], it is perhaps not surprising that studies of the properties of such cell lines have been uninformative in our understanding of the basis of the observed difference in growth of parasitized B cells and T cells in vitro.

There would appear to be two possible explanations for the difference in disease produced by B cells and T cells. First, infected B cells may be inherently limited in their capacity to sustain a high rate of replication in vivo; this might be related to a greater propensity of the parasites within B cells to undergo differentiation to merozoites, a process that in *T. annulata* is associated with a decrease in host cell proliferation [80]. Secondly, infected B cells and T cells may differ either in the types of immune responses they induce or in their susceptibility to host immune responses. Studies to resolve these issues should not only provide insight into the pathogenesis of East Coast fever but also yield clues as to how immune responses to the parasite might be manipulated to the benefit of the host.

## Concluding Remarks

Studies of the immune responses of cattle to *T. parva* indicate that control of infection can operate at two levels, namely by preventing establishment of infection with sporozoites and by elimination of parasitized lymphoblasts. The latter involves class I restricted CTL and is the principal mechanism of resistance in animals that have acquired immunity following recovery from a single infection. Immunity directed against the sporozoite is mediated by neutralizing antibodies and possibly also T-cell responses to cell-associated sporozoite antigens. In the field, such responses are only induced following repeated exposure to infected ticks. However, immunization of cattle with a recombinant sporozoite surface antigen has been shown to protect a proportion of animals against experimental sporozoite challenge. Field trials are under way to determine whether or not this method of immunization is effective against natural challenge. Identification of schizont antigens recognized by parasite-specific CTL, which could potentially be used for immunization, is the focus of current investigation.

Variation between animals in efficacy of the host immune response is a feature of the responses to both the sporozoite and intracellular stages of the parasite. In the case of antisporozoite responses the basis of this variation is unclear but manifests as differences in protection in animals that have antibodies of similar titre, isotype and specificity. CTL responses to parasitized lymphoblasts exhibit restricted parasite strain specificity that correlates closely with susceptibility to challenge with heterologous parasites. Variation between animals in the pattern of parasite strain specificity of the CTL response occurs and is determined in part by the class I MHC phenotype of the animal. An additional immunodominance effect, whereby animals respond only to a subset of the epitopes to which they are capable of responding, is an important factor in determining strain specificity of the CTL response.

In vitro studies of cell lines infected with *T. parva* indicate that parasitized cells express cytokine receptors and that their growth at low cell concentrations can be potentiated by cytokines and signals from cell-cell interactions. Cellular immune responses induced by the parasite, therefore, have the potential to control or enhance the growth of parasitized cells. That the latter occurs in responses to primary infections in cattle is suggested by the finding of a vigorous T-cell response that differs in phenotype from that in immune animals and apparently lacks antiparasite effector functions. The ability of the parasite to produce disease has also been shown to be influenced by the cell type that is infected, in that parasitized B cells, unlike T cells, give rise to mild self-limiting infections.

The information obtained from studies of immune responses to *T. parva* has been critical in the development of strategies to identify antigens for use in vaccination studies and in defining the types of antigen delivery systems that will be required for vaccination against different parasite stages. The findings also point to the potential of the parasite to induce T-cell responses that enhance disease pathogenesis, and highlight the need to gain a clearer understanding of the factors that determine the balance between responses that effect parasite clearance and those that potentiate parasite growth.

## References

1   Irvin AD, Morrison WI: Immunopathology, immunology and immunoprophylaxis of *Theileria* infections; in Soulsby EJL (ed): Immune Responses in Parasitic Infections: Immunology, Immunopathology and Immunoprophylaxis. Boca Raton, CRC Press, 1987, vol 3, pp 223–274.
2   Hulliger L, Wilde JKH, Brown CGD, Turner L: Mode of multiplication of *Theileria* in cultures of bovine lymphocytic cells. Nature 1983;203:728–730.
3   Irvin AD, Ocama JGR, Spooner PR: Cycle of bovine lymphoblastoid cells parasitised by *Theileria parva*. Res Vet Sci 1982;33:298–304.
4   Emery DL: Adoptive transfer of immunity to infection with *Theileria parva* (East Coast fever) between cattle twins. Res Vet Sci 1981;30:364–367.
5   Emery DL, Eugui EM, Nelson RT, Tenywa T: Cell-mediated immune responses to *Theileria parva* (East Coast fever) during immunisation and lethal infections in cattle. Immunology 1981;43:323–325.
6   Eugui EM, Emery DL: Genetically restricted cell-mediated cytotoxicity in cattle immune to *Theileria parva*. Nature 1981;290:251–254.
7   Morrison WI, Goddeeris BM, Teale AJ, Groocock CM, Kemp SJ, Stagg DA: Cytotoxic T-cells elicited in cattle challenged with *Theileria parva* (Muguga): Evidence for restriction by class I MHC determinants and parasite strain specificity. Parasite Immunol 1978;9:563–578.
8   Morrison WI, Taracha ELN, McKeever DJ: Contribution of T-cell responses to immunity and pathogenesis in infections with *Theileria parva*. Parasitol Today 1995;11:14–18.
9   Malmquist WA, Nyindo MBA, Brown CGD: East Coast fever: Cultivation in vitro of bovine spleen cell lines infected and tranformed by *Theileria parva*. Trop Anim Health Prod 1970;2:139–145.
10  Brown CGD, Stagg DA, Purnell RE, Kanhai GK, Payne RC: Infection and transformation of bovine lymphoid cells in vitro by infective particles of *Theileria parva*. Nature 1973;245:101–103.
11  Fawcett D, Musoke A, Voigt W: Interaction of sporozoites of *Theileria parva* with bovine lymphocytes in vitro. Tissue Cell 1984;16:873–884.
12  Shaw MK, Tilney LG, Musoke AJ: The entry of *Theileria parva* sporozoites into blood lymphocytes: Evidence for MHC class I involvement. J Cell Biol 1991;113:87–101.
13  Lalor PA, Morrison WI, Black SJ: Monoclonal antibodies to bovine leukocytes define heterogeneity of target cells for in vitro parasitosis by *Theileria parva*; in Morrison WI (ed): The Ruminant Immune System in Health and Disease. Cambridge, Cambridge University Press, 1986, pp 72–87.
14  Baldwin CL, Black SJ, Brown WC, Conrad PA, Goddeeris BM, Kinuthia SW, Lalor PA, MacHugh ND, Morrison WI, Morzaria SP, Naessens J, Newson J: Bovine T cells, B cells and null cells are transformed by the protozoan parasite *Theileria parva*. Infect Immun 1988;56:462–467.

15    Morrison WI, MacHugh ND, Lalor PA: Pathogenicity of *Theileria parva* is influenced by the host cell type infected by the parasite. Infect Immun 1996;64:557–562.

16    Emery DL, MacHugh ND, Morrison WI: *Theileria parva* (Muguga) infects bovine T lymphocytes in vivo and induces co-expression of BoT4 and BoT8. Parasite Immunol 1988;10:379–391.

17    Radley DE, Brown CGD, Burridge MJ, Cunningham MP, Kirimi IM, Purnell RE, Young AS: East Coast fever. 1. Chemoprophylactic immunization of cattle against *Theileria parva* (Muguga) and five theileria strains. Vet Pathol 1975;1:35–41.

18    Radley DE, Young AS, Brown CGD, Burridge MJ, Cunningham MP, Musisi FL, Purnell RE: East Coast fever. 2. Cross-immunity trials with a Kenya strain or *Theileria lawrencei*. Vet Parasitol 1975; 1:43–50.

19    Morzaria SP, Irvin AD, Voigt WO, Taracha ELN: Effect of timing and intensity of challenge following immunisation against East Coast fever. Vet Parasitol 1987;26:29–41.

20    Burridge MJ, Morzaria SP, Cunningham MP, Brown CGD: Duration of immunity to East Coast fever (*Theileria parva* infection of cattle). Parasitology 1972;64:511–515.

21    Pirie HM, Jarrett WFH, Crighton GW: Studies on vaccination against East Coast fever using macroschizonts. Exp Parasitol 1970;27:343–349.

22    Emery DL, Morrison WI, Buscher G, Nelson RT: Generation of cell-mediated cytotoxicity to *Theileria parva* (East Coast fever) after inoculation of cattle with parasitised lymphoblasts. J Immunol 1982;128:195–200.

23    Buscher G, Morrison WI, Nelson RT: Titration in cattle of infectivity and immunogenicity of autologous cell lines infected with *Theileria parva*. Vet Parasitol 1984;15:29–38.

24    Cunningham MP, Brown CGD, Burridge MJ, Musoke AJ, Purnell RE, Radley DE, Semphebwa L: East Coast fever: Titration in cattle of suspensions of *Theileria parva* derived from ticks. Br Vet J 1974;130:336–345.

25    Muhammed SI, Laeurman LH, Johnson LW: Effect of humoral antibodies on the course of *Theileria parva* infection (East Coast fever) of cattle. Am J Vet Res 1975;36:399–402.

26    Musoke AJ, Nantulya VM, Buscher G, Masake RA, Otim B: Bovine immune responses to *Theileria parva*: Neutralising antibodies to sporozoites. Immunology 1982;45:663–338.

27    Nene V, Musoke AJ, Gobright E, Morzaria SP: Conservation of the sporozoite p67 vaccine antigen in cattle-derived *Theileria parva* stocks with different cross-immunity profiles. Infect Immun 1996; 64:2056–2061.

28    Musoke AJ, Nantulya VM, Rurangirwa RF, Buscher G: Evidence for a common protective antigenic determinant on sporozoites of several *Theileria parva* strains. Immunology 1984;52:231–238.

29    Iams K, Hall R, Webster P, Musoke AJ: Identification of lambda gt11 clones encoding the major antigenic determinants expressed by *Theileria parva* sporozoites. Infect Immun 1990;58: 1828–1834.

30    Dobbelaere DA, Shapiro SZ, Webster P: Identification of a surface antigen on *Theileria parva* sporozoites by monoclonal antibody. Proc Natl Acad Sci USA 1985;82:1771–1775.

31    Webster P, Dobbelaere DAE, Fawcett DW: The entry of sporozoites of *Theileria parva* into bovine lymphocytes in vitro. Immunoelectron microscopic observations. Eur J Cell Biol 1985;36:157–162.

32    Nene V, Iams KP, Gobright E, Musoke AJ: Characterisation of the gene encoding a candidate vaccine antigen of *Theileria parva* sporozoites. Mol Biochem 1992;51:17–28.

33    Musoke A, Morzaria A, Nkonge C, Jones E, Nene V: A recombinant sporozoite surface antigen of *Theileria parva* induces protection in cattle. Proc Natl Acad Sci USA 1992;89:514–518.

34    Nene V, Inumaru S, McKeever DJ, Morzaria S, Shaw M, Musoke AJ: Characterisation of an insect cell-derived *Theileria parva* sporozoite vaccine antigen and immunogenicity in cattle. Infect Immun 1995;63:503–508.

35    Musoke AJ, Nene V, McKeever DJ: Epitope specificity of bovine immune responses to the major surface antigen of *Theileria parva* sporozoites; in Chanock RM, Brown F, Ginsberg HS, Norrby E (eds): Molecular Approaches to the Control of Infectious Diseases. Cold Spring Harbor, Cold Spring Harbor Laboratory Press, 1995, pp 57–61.

36    Sanders LA, Van De Winkel JG, Rijkers GT, Voorhorst-Ogink MM, De Haas M, Capel PJ, Zegers BJ: Fc gamma receptor IIa (CD32) heterogeneity in patients with recurrent bacterial respiratory tract infections. J Infect Dis 1994;170:854–861.

37    Shaw MK, Tilney LG, McKeever DJ: Tick salivary gland extract and interleukin-2 stimulation enhances susceptibility of lymphocytes to infection by *Theileria parva* sporozoites. Infect Immun 1993;61:1486–1495.

38    Preston PM, Brown CG, Richardson W: Cytokines inhibit the development of trophozoite-infected cells of *Theileria annulata* and *Theileria parva* but enhance the proliferation of macroschizont-infected cell lines. Parasite Immunol 1992;14:125–141.

39    DeMartini JC, Baldwin CL: Effects of gamma interferon, tumour necrosis factor alpha, and interleukin-2 on infection and proliferation of *Theileria parva*-infected bovine lymphoblasts and production of interferon by parasitised cells. Infect Immun 1991;59:4540–4546.

40    Visser AE, Abraham A, Bell-Sakyi LJ, Brown CGD, Preston PM: Nitric oxide inhibits establishment of macroschizont-infected cell lines and is produced by macrophages of calves undergoing bovine tropical theileriosis or East Coast fever. Parasite Immunol 1995;17:91–102.

41    Young AS, Leitch BL, Morzaria S, Irvin AD, Omwoyo PL, De Castro JJ: Development and survival of *Theileria parva* in *Rhipicephalus appendiculatus* exposed in the Trans-Mara, Kenya. Parasitology 1987;94:433–441.

42    Goddeeris BM, Morrison WI, Teale AJ: Generation of bovine cytotoxic cell lines specific for cells infected with the protozoan parasite *Theileria parva* and restricted by products of the major histocompatibility complex. Eur J Immunol 1986;16:1243–1249.

43    Taracha ELN, Goddeeris BM, Scott JR, Morrison WI: Standardization of a technique for analysing the frequency of parasite-specific cytotoxic T lymphocyte precursors in cattle immunised with *Theileria parva.* Parasite Immunol 1992;14:143–154.

44    Taracha ELN, Goddeeris BM, Morzaria SP, Morrison WI: Parasite strain specificity of precursor cytotoxic T cells in individual animals correlates with cross-protection in cattle challenged with *Theileria parva.* Infect Immun 1995;63:1258–1262.

45    McKeever DJ, Taracha ELN, Innes EL, MacHugh ND, Awino E, Goddeeris BM, Morrison WI: Adoptive transfer of immunity to *Theileria parva* in the CD8[+] fraction of responding efferent lymph. Proc Natl Acad Sci USA 1994;91:1959–1963.

46    McKeever DJ, Nyanjui J, Ballingall KT: In vitro infection with *Theileria parva* is associated with IL-10 expression in all bovine lymphocyte lineages. Parasite Immunol 1997;19:319–324.

47    Baldwin CL, Goddeeris BM, Morrison WI: Bovine helper T-cell clones specific for lymphocytes infected with *Theileria parva* (Muguga). Parasite Immunol 1987;9:499–513.

48    Brown WC, Sugimoto C, Grab DJ: *Theileria parva*: Bovine helper T cell clones specific for both infected lymphocytes and schizont membrane antigens. Exp Parasitol 1989;69:234–248.

49    Brown WC, Sugimoto C, Conrad PA, Grab DJ: Differential response of bovine T cell lines to membrane and soluble antigens of *Theileria parva* schizont-infected cells. Parasite Immunol 1989;11:567–583.

50    Brown WC, Lonsdale-Eccles, De Martini JC, Grab DJ: Recognition of soluble *Theileria parva* antigen by bovine helper T cell clones: Characterization and partial purification of the antigen. J Immunol 1990;144:271–277.

51    Baldwin CL, Iams KP, Brown WC, Grab DJ: *Theileria parva*: CD4[+] helper and cytotoxic T-cell clones react with a schizont derived antigen associated with the surface of *Theileria parva*-infected lymphocytes. Exp Parasitol 1992;75:19–30.

52    Radley DE, Brown CGD, Cunningham MP, Kimber CD, Musisi FL, Payne RC, Purnell RE, Stagg SM, Young AS: East Coast fever. 3. Chemoprophylactic immunization of cattle using oxytetracycline and a combination of *Theileria* strains. Vet Parasitol 1975;1:51–60.

53    Uilenberg G, Schreuder BEC, Silayo RS, Mpangala C: Studies on Theileriidae (Sporozoa) in Tanzania. IV. A field trial on immunisation against East Coast fever (*Theileria parva* infection of cattle). Tropenmed Parasitol 1976;27:329–336.

54    Morzaria SP, Irvin AD, Taracha E, Spooner PR, Voigt WP, Fujinaga T, Katende J: Immunisation against East Coast fever: The use of selected stocks of *Theileria parva* for immunisation of cattle exposed to field challenge. Vet Parasitol 1987;23:23–41.

55    Conrad PA, Iams K, Brown WC, Sohanpal B, Ole-Moiyoi OK: DNA probes detect genomic diversity in *Theileria parva* stocks. Mol Biochem Parsitol 1987;25:213–226.

56    Allsopp BA, Allsopp MTEP: *Theileria parva*: Genomic DNA studies reveal intra-specific sequence diversity. Mol Biochem Parasitol 1988;28:77–84.

57    Morzaria SP, Spooner PR, Bishop RP, Musoke AJ, Young JR: *Sfi I* and *Not I* polymorphisms in *Theileria* stocks detected by pulsed field gel electrophoresis. Mol Biochem Parasitol 1990;40: 203–212.

58    Minami T, Spooner PR, Irvin AD, Ocama JGR, Dobbelaere DAE, Fujinaga T: Characterisation of stocks of *Theileria parva* by monoclonal antibody profiles. Res Vet Sci 1983;35:334–340.

59    Toye PG, Goddeeris BM, Iams K, Musoke AJ, Morrison WI: Characterization of a polymorphic immunodominant molecule in sporozoites and schizonts of *Theileria parva.* Parasite Immunol 1991; 13:49–62.

60    Toye P, Gobright E, Nyanjui J, Nene V, Bishop R: Structure and sequence variation of the genes encoding the polymorphic, immunodominant molecule (PIM), an antigen of *Theileria parva* recognised by inhibitory monoclonal antibodies. Mol Biochem Parasitol 1995;73:165–177.

61    Goddeeris BM, Morrison WI, Teale AJ, Bensaid A, Baldwin CL: Bovine cytotoxic T-cell clones specific for cells infected with the protozoan parasite *Theileria parva*: Parasite strain specificity and class I major histocompatibility complex restriction. Proc Natl Acad Sci USA 1986;83:5238–5242.

62    Goddeeris BM, Morrison WI, Toye PG, Bishop R: Strain specificity of bovine *Theileria parva*-specific cytotoxic T cells is determined by the phenotype of the restricting class I MHC. Immunology 1990;69:38–44.

63    Morzaria SP, Dolan TT, Norval RAI, Bishop RP, Spooner PR: Generation and characterization of cloned *Theileria parva* parasites. Parasitology 1995;111:39–49.

64    Morrison WI: Influence of host and parasite genotypes on immunological control of *Theileria* parasites. Parasitology 1996;112:S53–S66.

65    Toye PG, MacHugh ND, Bensaid AM, Alberti S, Teale AJ, Morrison WI: Transfection into mouse L cells of genes encoding two serologically and functionally distinct bovine class I MHC molecules from a MHC-homozygous animal: Evidence for a second class I locus in cattle. Immunology 1990; 70:20–26.

66    Bensaid A, Kaushal A, Baldwin CL, Clevers H, Young JR, Kemp SJ, MacHugh ND, Toye PG, Teale AJ: Identification of expressed bovine class I MHC genes at two loci and demonstration of physical linkage. Immunogenetics 1991;33:247–254.

67    Taracha ELN, Goddeeris BM, Teale AJ, Kemp SJ, Morrison WI: Parasite strain specificity of bovine cytotoxic T cell responses to *Theileria parva* is determined primarily by immunodominance. J Immunol 1995;155:4854–4860.

68    Phillips RE, Rowland-Jones S, Nixon DF, Gotch FM, Edwards JP, Ogunlesi AO, Elvin JG, Rothbard JA, Bangham CRM, Rizza CR, McMichael AJ: Human immunodeficiency virus genetic variation that can escape cytotoxic T cell recognition. Nature 1991;354:453–459.

69    Nowak MA, May RM, Phillips RE, Rowland-Jones S, Lalloo DG, McAdam S, Klenerman P, Köppe B, Sigmund K, Bangham CRM, McMichael AJ: Antigenic oscillations and shifting immunodominance in HIV-1 infections. Nature 1995;375:606–611.

70    Grootenhuis JG, Leitch BL, Stagg DA, Dolan TT, Young AS: Experimental induction of *Theileria parva lawrencei* carrier state in an African buffalo (*Syncerus caffer*). Parasitology 1987;94: 425–431.

71    Baldwin CL, Malu MN, Kinuthia SW, Conrad PA, Grootenhuis JG: Comparative analysis of infection and transformation of lymphocytes from African buffalo and Boran cattle with *Theileria parva* subsp. *parva* and *T. parva* subsp. *lawrencei.* Infect Immun 1986;53:186–191.

72    Morrison WI, Buscher G, Murray M, Emery DL, Masake RA, Cook RH, Wells PW: *Theileria parva*: Kinetics of infection in the lymphoid system of cattle. Exp Parasitol 1981;52:248–260.

73    Emery DL: Kinetics of infection with *Theileria parva* (East Coast fever) in the central lymph of cattle. Vet Parasitol 1981;9:1–16.

74    Taracha ELN: Investigation of cytotoxic T-lymphocyte responses of cattle to *Theileria parva* by limiting dilution analyses; PhD thesis, Brunel University 1992.

75    Brown WC, Logan KS: Bovine T-cell clones infected with *Theileria parva* produce a factor with IL-2-like activity. Parasite Immunol 1986;8:189–192.

76    Dobbelaere DAE, Coquerelle TM, Roditi IJ, Eichhorn M, Williams RO: *Theileria parva* infection induces autocrine growth of bovine lymphocytes. Proc Natl Acad Sci USA 1988;85:4730–4734.

77  Dobbelaere DAE, Prospero TD, Roditi IJ, Kelke C, Baumann I, Eichhorn M, Williams RO, Ahmed JS, Baldwin CL, Clevers H, Morrison WI: Expression of Tac antigen component of bovine interleukin-2 receptor in different leukocyte populations infected with *Theileria parva* or *Theileria annulata.* Infect Immun 1990;8:3847–3855.

78  Dobbelaere DAE, Roditi IJ, Coquerelle TM, Kelke C, Eichhorn M, Williams RO: Lymphocytes infected with *Theileria parva* require both cell-cell contact and growth factor to proliferate. Eur J Immunol 1991;21:89–95.

79  Eichhorn M, Dobbelaere DAE: Partial inhibition of *Theileria parva* infected T cell proliferation by antisense IL-2R alpha-chain RNA expression. Res Immunol 1995;146:88–99.

80  Shiels BR, Kinnaird J, McKellar S, Dickson J, Ben Miled L, Melrose R, Tait A: Disruption of synchrony between parasite growth and host cell division is a determinant of differentiation to the merozoite in *Theileria annulata.* J Cell Sci 1992;101:99–107.

Prof. W.I. Morrison, Institute for Animal Health, Compton Laboratory,
Compton/nr.Newbury, Berks RG20 7NN (UK)
Tel. +44 1635 577261, fax +44 1635 577263, e-mail samantha.cook@bbsrc.ac.uk

Liew FY, Cox FEG (eds): Immunology of Intracellular Parasitism.
Chem Immunol. Basel, Karger, 1998, vol 70, pp 186–199

..........................

# Immunobiology of African Trypanosomiasis

*Jeremy M. Sternberg*

Department of Zoology, University of Aberdeen, UK

The African trypanosomes (*Trypanosoma brucei* sp.) are parasites of humans and domestic animals in sub-Saharan Africa, causing the disease trypanosomiasis or sleeping sickness [1]. Unlike the other parasites described in this volume these kinetoplastid protozoa are extracellular. As such, they have evolved remarkable immune-evasion mechanisms which shed light on fundamental differences between intracellular and extracellular modes of parasitism. This review will cover recent advances in the immunology of African trypanosomiasis. *T. brucei* is generally divided into three subspecies according to their infectivity to humans and the characteristics of the disease they cause. *T. b. rhodesiense* and *T. b. gambiense* cause sleeping sickness in man in East and West Africa respectively, while *T. b. brucei* is restricted to wild animal hosts due to lytic factors in human serum. Genetic evidence [2] suggests that *T. b. brucei* and *T. b. rhodesiense* are indistinguishable apart from the human infectivity trait which is itself unstable, and for the purposes of this review these subspecies will be referred to as *T. brucei*. Trypanosomiasis is a typical zoonosis, and the reservoir of infection in wild animals means that disease eradication is likely to be unattainable. It is estimated that there are 50 million people at risk from infection, with the reported 100,000 cases per annum likely to be a considerabe underestimate due to the lack of effective monitoring in many areas [3]. *T. brucei* infects laboratory rodents readily, and as a result the mouse model has been used for almost all immunological studies. Different inbred strains of mice exhibit a spectrum of resistance to *T. brucei* both in terms of survival time and parasitaemia. However, all eventually succumb to the parasite. Genetic analysis has shown resistance to be under polygenic control [4], but the nature of the factors involved is not known.

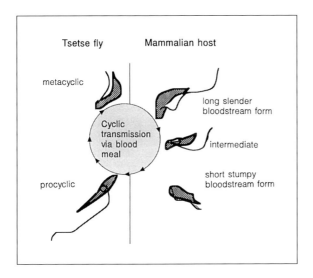

*Fig. 1.* Diagram illustrating the main stages of the life cycle of *T. brucei.*

## Life Cycle

The life cycle of *T. brucei* is shown in figure 1. Infection is initiated when the tsetse fly commences a blood meal. Mammalian-infective metacyclic trypanosomes, which have developed in the vector salivary gland, are inoculated subcutaneously along with tsetse saliva. In natural infections, these parasites replicate at the point of injection [5], causing an acute skin reaction (chancre). The chancre formation involves lymphocyte and mast cell recruitment and degranulation [6]. This part of the natural infection process is poorly understood at the immunological level, as it is completely bypassed in experimental mouse infections with both syringe passage and infected fly bites resulting in intraperitoneal inoculation. Over a period of 7–14 days the metacyclic parasites differentiate to the long slender (LS) bloodstream trypomastigotes which migrate via the local draining lymph nodes into the bloodstream, where proliferation by binary fission occurs. While the LS form multiplies exponentially, the African trypanosomes seem to have evolved a mechanism to prevent an uncontrolled parasitaemia which would rapidly overwhelm the host. The LS forms differentiate via an intermediate stage into $G_0$ arrested short stumpy (SS) trypomastigotes. This phenomenon aids the maintenance of chronic infection, a prerequisite for efficient transmission under conditions of low vector density. The cue for the LS to SS differentiation is as yet unidentified, although it has been suggested that it is mediated by a parasite-produced paracrine factor as the process also occurs in axenic culture [7]. It is the SS forms which are able to continue development after uptake by the vector in the blood meal, thus completing the life cycle. Although intracellular stages of the parasite have been reported in the past [8], it is now universally accepted that this parasite is extracellular both in the mammalian host and in the vector.

## Immunity and Antigenic Variation

The exquisite system of antigenic variation exhibited by *T. brucei* has for many years dominated consideration of the immunology of trypanosomiasis. Although first elucidated by serological methods, the biochemistry and molecular biology of antigenic variation are now well understood [9, 10]. The metacyclic and bloodstream form trypanosomes are uniformly coated with a glycoprotein, the variant surface glycoprotein (VSG). This is a GPI-anchored structure of 60 kD with conserved but buried C-terminal sequences, and a highly polymorphic N-terminus forming the exposed domain. Each parasite genotype contains a repertoire of up to 1,000 different VSG genes, distributed throughout the genome as 'basic copy' genes. At any one time, only a single VSG gene is actively transcribed at a telomeric expression site. Antigenic variation is driven by three main processes. Two of these are translocation events, namely duplicative transposition (gene conversion) and reciprocal recombination (nonduplicative transposition) which bring basic copy genes into an expression site. The third mechanism, telomeric in situ activation, involves rearrangements at a distant upstream promoter. Variant antigen switching occurs in a spontaneous nonprogrammed manner at a surprisingly high rate of $10^{-4}$–$10^{-5}$ per cell division [11]. Antigenic variation leads to the characteristic fluctuating parasitaemia of trypanosomiasis, as successive variant antigen types elicit an antibody response and are destroyed. The primary component of the antibody response to VSG is a T-cell-independent IgM response [12]. However, T-cell-dependent B-cell responses are also involved in eliciting VSG-specific IgG. It is possible that these two types of response are determined by the physicochemical properties of the VSG. The VSG coat on intact trypanosomes acts essentially as a T-independent antigen while nonvariant buried T-cell epitopes are presented to T cells only after phagocytosis of dying or opsonized trypanosmes [13]. As will be discussed below, this T-cell-mediated response plays a significant role in establishing the cytokine response profile in trypanosome infections. While antigenic variation is clearly an important immune-evasion strategy, there are circumstances where it is circumvented by other host-factors conferring resistance to the parasite. The best example of this is in the 'trypanotolerant' N'Dama breed of cattle which successfully control parasitaemias at a very low level [14]. This phenomenon has led to the study of another immunological facet of trypanosomiasis, immunosuppression, and the mechanisms underlying it.

### Immunosuppression during Trypanosomiasis

Immunosuppression is a well-characterized feature of trypanosomiasis, both in experimental rodent models [15, 16], domestic animals [17] and humans [18]. The effects of trypanosomiasis on the immune system have been extensively studied in experimental mice. At the macroscopic level, there are striking alterations in the architecture and cellularity of the lymphoid system. These include splenomegaly accompanied by a massive accumulation of B cells and null cells, and lymph node enlargement. During murine African trypanosomiasis there is a dramatic suppression of both B- and T-cell responses to specific antigens and mitogens in the spleen, lymph nodes and peripheral blood [19]. This suppression, which cannot be accounted for by the dilution in specific lymphocyte density which occurs in lymphoid tissues due to nonspecific proliferative responses, affects both primary and secondary responses to T-cell-dependent specific antigens as well as T-cell-independent responses. These effects, rather than dircetly mediated by the parasite, involve intermediate cells, and in particular suppressor macrophages [19–21]. Concurrent with this suppression of specific lymphocyte responsiveness, trypanosomiasis is also associated with a massive polyclonal B-cell activation in both experimental and natural hosts. This is manifest in elevated IgM levels, auto-antibody production, and elevated B-cell background proliferation [22]. While the mechanism responsible for nonspecific B-cell activation remains unknown, in recent years there has been considerable progress in our understanding of the mechanisms underlying immunosuppression during trypanosomiasis.

### Suppressor Macrophage Activity in Trypanosomiasis

Immunosuppression in trypanosome-infected animals, closely associated with the occurrence of suppressor macrophages [19], has been demonstrated in vivo in cell transfer experiments and in vitro using co-culture techniques. For example, as few as 40,000 peritoneal or splenic macrophages from trypanosome-infected donor mice were capable of causing a 50% suppression of recipient mitogen response after syngeneic cell transfer [20]. In co-culture experiments, macrophages from infected mice also suppressed the proliferative responses of lymphocytes from naive mice in vitro. Moreover, in splenocyte cultures from infected mice, normal proliferative responses could be restored by eliminating suppressor macrophages with the lysosomotropic agent *L*-leucine methyl ester and reconstitution with macrophages from uninfected mice [20].

Phenotypic analysis of macrophages in *T. brucei*-infected mice has indicated increased class II MHC expression [23], release of reactive oxygen intermediates [24], prostaglandin-$E_2$ ($PGE_2$) release [25, 26] and nitric oxide (NO) production [27]. These characteristics are typical of macrophage activation. An important function of activated macrophages in *T. brucei* infection is the destruction of opsonized and phagocytosed trypanosomes [28]. However, activated macrophages are also mediators of immunosuppresion.

Two activated macrophage products, $PGE_2$ [29] and NO [30], have been investigated as mediators of immunosuppression using specific inhibitors, indomethacin in the case of $PGE_2$ and $N^G$-methyl-*L*-arginine (*L*-NMMA) in the case of NO. Suppression was measured using in vitro antigen and mitogen-driven T-cell proliferation assays on lymphocytes from *T. brucei*-infected mice. Indomethacin, partially restored proliferative responses in both splenic [24] and lymph node [31] cell populations and elevated $PGE_2$ synthesis was observed in both spleen and lymph node cell cultures from infected mice. Analysis of lymph node cell culture supernatants from infected mice also showed a suppression of IL-2 production which was restored after the addition of indomethacin [31]. Thus, prostaglandins are one effector product of suppressor macrophages. To date there has been no test of this hypothesis in vivo in indomethacin-treated experimental mice, nor are there any data available on prostaglandins in bovine or human trypanosomiasis.

The use of NO synthase inhibitors such as *L*-NMMA and Nω-nitro-*L*-arginine methyl ester (*L*-NAME) also led to a partial abrogation of suppressor macrophage activity in splenocyte cultures from trypanosome-infected mice [27] and when used in combination with indomethacin there was a complete restoration of proliferative responses [25]. Therefore, NO is a second significant suppressive product of macrophages from trypanosome-infected mice. Indeed, NO production directly correlates with suppressor macrophage activity in macrophage adoptive transfer experiments [32]. The role of NO during murine *T. brucei* infection has been studied in vivo. When trypanosome-infected mice were treated with the NO synthase inhibitor-*L*-NMMA, not only was there a significant restoration of mitogen-driven T-cell proliferation in the spleen, but also a significant reduction in the first parasitaemic peak [33]. This provides direct evidence that NO is an infection-exacerbating factor during murine trypanosomiasis. It has also been proposed that NO released by bone-marrow macrophages may be a causal factor in the dyserythropoiesis associated with

*T. brucei* infection as in vivo *L*-NAME treatment of infected mice leads to a recovery from anaemia [34]. In human trypanosomiasis, while no studies of suppressor macrophages have been reported, there is evidence for NO synthesis during acute infection, based on one report of elevated serum nitrate concentration [35]. In this study, sera from trypanosomiasis patients in Mozambique showed highly significant increases in serum nitrate, an indirect marker for systemic NO synthase activity. Further studies of NO synthesis in macrophages from trypanosomiasis patients are now required and the African trypanosomes look set to provide an excellent system in which to test the controversial relevance of iNOS in human disease [36].

As a suppressive mediator in trypanosomiasis, NO does not significantly affect parasite proliferation. While *T. brucei* is effectively killed by either chemically generated or macrophage released NO in vitro [37, 38], the addition of physiological concentrations of red blood cells to such culture systems totally abolishes any inhibition of parasite growth [38]. This is a result of haemoglobin offering a high-affinity sink for NO in the form of met-haemoglobin. Thus *T. brucei* occupies an ideal niche in the bloodstream where it is protected from NO-mediated damage.

While the suppressor macrophage products described above are clearly damaging to the host, trypanosome infections also result in a significant release of TNF-$\alpha$, which was originally identified as the cachexia-inducing factor in chronic trypanosomiasis [39]. In contrast to NO and prostaglandins, TNF-$\alpha$ has a far more ambiguous role. In one study it was found that after priming with trypanosome lysates to induce TNF-$\alpha$ production, *T. brucei*-infected mice had lower parasitaemias than unprimed controls [40]. Concomitant treatment with neutralizing antibody to TNF-$\alpha$ completely restored the control level of parasitaemia and reduced the duration of survival [40]. Subsequent studies have shown that TNF-$\alpha$ is directly trypanolytic through a route which, while unrelated to the TNF-$\alpha$-mammalian TNF receptor interaction, remains unidentified [41].

### IFN-$\gamma$ in Trypanosomiasis

Given the potential significance of macrophage activation in trypanosomiasis, it is logical to turn to the nature of the macrophage-activating factor(s), at least one of which is likely to be IFN-$\gamma$, the synthesis of which is significantly up-regulated following infection with African trypanosomes in humans [42] and experimental rodents [43–45].

Recent studies have shown three independent potential sources of IFN-$\gamma$ during murine trypanosomiasis. First, Mansfield's group [46], studying T-cell

*Table 1.* Production of IFN-γ and NO ex vivo by spleen cells at day 6 of infection with *T. brucei* EATRO2340

|  | Naive | Infected | Infected + ASGM1 | Infected nu/nu |
|---|---|---|---|---|
| IFN-γ release | 3.0 ± 1.0 | 142 ± 6.0 | 64 ± 6.0 | 36 ± 1.0 |
| NO release | ND | 3.4 ± 0.01 | 0.80 ± 0.01 | 0.75 ± 0.15 |

Illustrative results from naive, infected, infected anti-ASGM1-treated and infected nude mice are presented. IFN-γ expressed as units/$5 \times 10^5$ cells/48 h. NO synthesis expressed as nmol nitrate/$5 \times 10^5$ cells/48 h.

responses to trypanosome antigens, identified VSG-specific CD4$^+$ cells in both the spleen and peritoneal cavity. These cells, while showing the inhibition of proliferative responses typical in trypanosome infection (see above) nevertheless secreted IFN-γ in response to VSG. Therefore, one element of IFN-γ production is a typical Th1 cell response to VSG peptides presented by class II MHC.

A second source of IFN-γ is a CD8$^+$ T-cell population which is directly activated by a trypanosomal factor, trypanosome-derived lymphocyte triggering factor (TLTF), which was originally identified by gel filtration resolution of crude *T. brucei* lysates and enrichment of an activity involved in promoting rat and human mononuclear cell IFN-γ production [47]. Subsequently, monoclonal antibodies to TLTF have allowed its purification as a 42–45 kD polypeptide [48]. TLTF triggers IFN-γ production in CD8$^+$ cells only and in an antigen nonspecific manner as evidenced by its activity in essentially pure T-cell populations [45]. There is a further source of IFN-γ in murine trypanosomiasis, as revealed in experiments on trypanosome infections in nu/nu mice lacking αβ T cells (table 1). Nude mice continue to produce reduced but significant IFN-γ and NO responses, and preliminary evidence suggests that this is likely to be from NK cells. In studies of NK-cell activity in *T. brucei* infection using YAC-cell target-specific cytolysis, there is a significant activation of splenic NK cells at days 2–4 of infection [unpubl. data]. Treatment of infected animals with anti-asialo-GM1 under conditions which completely neutralize this NK-cell activity in vivo leads to a significant reduction in serum IFN-γ as well as macrophage activation measured in terms of NO production (table 1). Interestingly, a contribution of NK-cell activity to pathogenesis in murine trypanosomiasis is also revealed by experiments showing prolonged survival time in beige mice infected with *T. brucei* [49]. In summary, at least three separate sources of IFN-γ drive macrophage activation and result in the deleterious effects on the host immune system described above.

In contrast to the inhibitory effect on host immune responses resulting from macrophage activation, IFN-γ has a stimulatory effect on the growth of the parasite. The proliferative response of the trypanosome to IFN-γ has been demonstrated in axenic culture [50] and is proposed to be a component of a bidirectional set of interactions in which the trypanosome released factor TLTF triggers CD8$^+$ T cells to release IFN-γ [45]. This model is supported by observations of T. brucei infection in specific gene-deleted mice. In T. brucei-infected IFN-γ –/– mice, parasitaemias were consistently lower, and survival time longer than in the wild type. In contrast with IFN-γ receptor –/– mice, parasitaemia rose more rapidly with a shorter survival time and this was ascribed to higher levels of unbound plasma IFN-γ [50]. This remarkable apparent specific interaction of a trypanosome with a host cytokine is not without precedent, as it has been established that T. brucei also interacts in a growth-regulatory manner with human epidermal growth factor via an erb-B-like specific membrane receptor [51, 52].

## Mechanisms of Macrophage Activation in Trypanosomiasis

In view of the acute macrophage activation occurring in murine and possibly human trypanosomiasis and its resultant pathological consequences, research efforts have been aimed at identifying the parasite factors involved. In early studies, Grosskinsky and Askonas [53] identified a soluble fraction from homogenized T. brucei which depressed antibody formation against sheep red blood cells in plaque assays. This activity was evident when the homogenate was co-incubated with peritoneal macrophages prior to addition to the responder cells. While crude fractionation of these homogenates indicated that the suppressive component was a lipid [54], this approach has yielded no further information.

Meanwhile, it was also proposed that the active factor involved in inducing immunosuppression was VSG which, when directly injected into mice, caused both polyclonal B-cell activation [55] and the inhibition of specific B-cell responses [56]. Again these experimental approaches appear to have proceeded no further and illustrate the difficulties involved in isolating biological activities in crude parasite products using indirect assays of effector activity.

Only in the last few years have there been renewed attempts to identify the active parasite components, largely as a result of the development of in vitro macrophage activation systems. These offer a direct measure of suppressor macrophage-inducing activity in simple bioassays. In one set of experiments,

*Table 2.* Induction of iNOS and prostaglandin synthesis in J-774 cells through the co-stimulatory activities of *T. brucei* lysate and IFN-γ.

| | Nitrite synthesis, $\mu M$ | Nitrite synthesis in presence of *L*-NMMA | PGE$_2$ synthesis pg/ml | PGE$_2$ synthesis the presence of indomethacin (10 μg/ml) |
|---|---|---|---|---|
| J-774 cells ($10^5$ cells) | 0.5 | 0.2 | 30 | 12 |
| J-774 + *T. brucei* lysate ($3 \times 10^7$ parasite equivalent) | 0.9 | 0.7 | 35 | 12 |
| J-774 + *T. brucei* lysate + IFN-γ (100 U/ml) | 22.2 | 0.8 | 1,000 | 30 |

the macrophage hybridoma cell line, 2C11-12P, was pulsed with opsonized parasites [57]. This stimulus caused the release of TNF-α, unidentified factors involved in suppression of T-cell proliferation and the stimulation of IFN-γ production in murine lymph node cells.

In another approach it has been shown that a trypanosome-secreted factor directly co-stimulates macrophage activation in the presence of IFN-γ. When axenically cultivated trypanosomes were added to primary murine peritoneal macrophage cultures, the bloodstream forms but not procyclic trypanosomes induced NO synthesis in the presence of IFN-γ as a co-stimulator [58]. This parasite-derived activity was named TMAF (trypanosomal macrophage-activating factor). As both live parasites and conditioned medium caused NO synthesis, it appears that the macrophage-activating factor is a soluble secretory component of the parasite. This was confirmed in experiments in which the live trypanosomes were separated from the responder macrophages in diffusion chambers. Similar experiments have been carried out using J-774 cells as responder cells and both NO and prostaglandin synthesis (table 2) were induced. The requirement for both IFN-γ and trypanosome factors as triggers for these responses is typical of the two-stimulus system of macrophage activation involved in the regulation of iNOS transcription in murine macrophages. While IFN-γ, acting through IFN regulatory factor gene-1, is the primary stimulus [59], other defined secondary stimuli include LPS [60], zymosan [61], and phagocytosis of the micro-organisms *S. aureus* and the protozoan *Leishmania major* [62].

Currently there is no information on the biochemical nature of TMAF. However it is of interest that TMAF activity is absent in procyclic *T. brucei* [58] again raising the question of whether VSG is involved in the process as discussed above. The VSG coat represents 10% of total parasite protein [3]

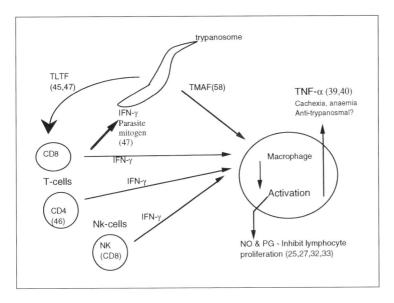

*Fig. 2.* Diagram representing the emerging network of T-cell, macrophage and trypanosome interactions. Numbers in parentheses refer to references.

and is released in a soluble form by live trypanosomes [64]. However, attempts to date to mimic any macrophage-activating factor with purified sVSG have met no success [Sternberg, unpubl. data].

## Discussion and Conclusions

It is becoming increasingly evident that the textbook model of *T. brucei* infection as a parasite which survives and proliferates within the mammalian host by means of antigenic variation is incomplete. In particular, it is clear that the trypanosome is involved in a web of interactions mediated by parasite factors and host cytokines. A summary of those mentioned in this review is presented in figure 2. The overall picture is that of a response dominated by macrophage activation and Th1 cytokines being manipulated via as yet uncharacterized parasite factors to enable the prolonged survival of the trypanosomes in the bloodstream. This presents an intriguing contrast to the Th1-mediated immune-effector mechanisms evident with intracellular trypanosomatids such as *Leishmania* [65]. The role of NO has provided some surprises and, rather than being host-protective, it is a significant contributor to immune-dysfunction. However the situation of NO being beneficial for the parasite is not unique to *T. brucei*. Recent work on the role of NO in the control of *Trypanosoma cruzi* infection in mice has also produced some unexpected results which suggest that low concentrations of NO promote parasite growth. The close association of iNOS activity with intracellular parasite nests revealed by immunohistochemistry provides a further example of NO acting as a double-edged sword in a protozoan infection [66]. The various parasite-released factors proposed to interact with macrophages are either poorly or not at all characterized, and this presents an urgent challenge. Also, it will be important to determine the relevance of the response to trypanosomiasis in the mouse model to that in human infection. Certainly the preliminary results from human trypanosomiasis patients showing elevated nitrate levels in infection sera [35] do indicate macrophage activation and *T. brucei* has been shown to cause both IFN-$\gamma$ production [45] and suppressed proliferation [67] in human PBMC in vitro.

## References

1   Seed JR, Hall JE: Trypanosomes causing disease in man in Africa; in Kreier JP, Baker JR (eds): Parasitic Protozoa. San Diego, Academic Press, 1992, vol II, pp 85–155.
2   Godfrey DG, Baker RD, Rickman LR, Mehlitz D: The distribution, relationships and identification of enzyme variants within the subgenus Trypanozoon. Adv Parasitol 1990;29:1–74.
3   World Health Organisation: World Health Report 1996. Fighting Disease, Fostering Development. Geneva, WHO, 1996.
4   De Gee ALW, Levine RF, Mansfield JM: Genetics of resistance to African trypanosomes. VI. Heredity of resistance and variable surface glycoprotein-specific immune responses. J Immunol 1984;140:283–288.
5   Luckins AG, Gray AR: An extravascular site of development of *Trypanosoma congolense*. Nature 1978;272:613–614.
6   Luckins AG, McIntyre N, Rae PF: Multiplication of *Trypanosoma evansi* at the site of infection in the skin of rabbits and cattle. Acta Trop 1991;50:19–27.
7   Hamm B, Schindler A, Mecke D, Duszenko M: Differentiation of *Trypanosoma brucei* bloodstream trypomastigotes from long slender to short stumpy-like forms in axenic culture. Mol Biochem Parasitol 1990;40:13–22.
8   Jenni L, Rudin W, Schell KF: Extravascular and vascular distribution of *Trypanosoma b. gambiense* in *Microtus montanus* after cyclical transmission; in Van Marck EAE (ed): From Parasitic Infections to Parasitic Disease. Basel, Karger, 1983, pp 95–102.
9   Pays E, Steinert M: Control of antigen gene expression in African trypanosomes. Annu Rev Genet 1988;22:107–126.
10  Borst P: Discontinuous transcription and antigenic variation in trypanosomes. Annu Rev Biochem 1986;55:701–732.
11  Turner CMR, Barry JD: High frequency of antigenic variation in *Trypanosoma brucei rhodesiense* infections. Parasitology 1989;99:67–75.
12  Campbell GH, Esser KM, Weinbaum FI: *Trypanosoma rhodesiense* infection in B-cell-deficient mice. Infect Immun 1977;18:434–438.
13  Mansfield J: T-cell responses to the trypanosome variant surface glycoprotein: A new paradigm? Parasitol Today 1994;10:267–270.
14  Morrison WI, Murray M, Akol GWO: Immune responses of cattle in African trypanosomiasis; in Tizard I (ed): Immunology and Pathogenesis of Trypanosomiasis. Boca Raton, CRC Press, 1985, pp 103–131.

15  Murray PK, Jennings FW, Murray M, Urquhart GM: The nature of immunosuppression in *Trypanosoma brucei* infections in mice. Immunology 1974;27:815–824.

16  Murray PK, Jennings FW, Murray M, Urquhart GM: The nature of immunosuppression in *Trypanosoma brucei* infections in mice. II. The role of the T and B lymphocytes. Immunology 1974;27: 825–840.

17  Ilemobade AA, Adsegboye DS, Onoviran O, Chima JC: Immunodepressive effects of trypanosomal infection in cattle immunized against contagious bovine pleuropneumonia. Parasite Immunol 1982; 4:273–282.

18  Greenwood BM, Whittle HC, Molyneux DH: Immunosuppression in Gambian trypanosomiasis. Trans R Soc Trop Med Hyg 1973;67:846.

19  Bancroft GJ, Askonas BA: Immunobiology of African trypanosomiasis in laboratory rodents; in Tizard I (ed): Immunology and Pathogenesis of Trypanosomiasis. Boca Raton, CRC Press, 1985, pp 76–101.

20  Borowy NK, Sternberg JM, Schreiber D, Nonnengasser C, Overath P: Suppressive macrophages occurring in murine *Trypanosoma brucei* infection inhibit T-cell responses in vivo and in vitro. Parasite Immunol 1990;12:233–246.

21  Flynn JN, Sileghem M: The role of the macrophage in induction of immunosuppression in *Trypanosoma congolense*-infected cattle. Immunology 1991;74:310–316.

22  Mayor-Withey KS, Clayton CE, Roelants GE, Askonas BA: Trypanosomiasis leads to extensive proliferation of B, T and null cells in spleen and bone marrow. Clin Exp Immunol 1978;34:359–363.

23  Grosskinsky CM, Ezekowitz RAB, Berton G, Gordon S, Askonas BA: Macrophage activation in murine African trypanosomiasis. Infect Immune 1983;39:1080–1086.

24  Vray B, De Baetselier P, Ouaissi A, Carlier, Y: *Trypanosoma cruzi* but not *Trypanosoma brucei* fails to induce a chemiluminescent signal in a macrophage hybridoma cell line. Infect Immun 1991;59: 3303–3308.

25  Schleifer KW, Mansfield JM: Suppressor macrophages in African trypanosomiasis inhibit T cell proliferative responses by nitric oxide and prostaglandins. J Immunol 1993;151:5492–5503.

26  Fierer J, Salmon JA, Askonas BA: African trypanosomiasis alters prostaglandin production by murine peritoneal macrophages. Clin Exp Immunol 1984;58:548–556.

27  Sternberg J, McGuigan F: Nitric oxide mediates suppression of T-cell responses in murine *Trypanosoma brucei* infection. Eur J Immunol 1992;22:2741–2744.

28  Van Velthuysen M-LF, Mayen AEM, Van Rooijen N, Fleuren GJ, De Heer E, Bruijn JA: T-cells and macrophages in *Trypanosoma brucei*-related glomerulopathy. Infect Immun 1994;62:3230–3235.

29  Phipps RP, Stein SH, Roper RL: A new view of prostaglandin E regulation of the immune response. Immunol Today 1991;12:349–352.

30  Mills CD: Molecular basis of suppressor macrophages. J Immunol 1991;146:2719–2723.

31  Sileghem M, Darji M, Remels L, Hamers R, De Baetselier P: Different mechanisms account for the suppression of interleukin-2 production and the suppression of interleukin-2 receptor expression in *Trypanosoma brucei*-infected mice. Eur J Immunol 1989;19:119–124.

32  Mabbott NA, Sutherland IA, Sternberg JM: Suppressor macrophages in *Trypanosoma brucei* infection: Nitric oxide is related to both suppressive activity and lifespan in vivo. Parasite Immunol 1995;17:143–150.

33  Sternberg JM, Mabbott NA, Sutherland IA, Liew FY: Inhibition of nitric oxide synthesis leads to reduced parasitemia in murine *Trypanosoma brucei* infection. Infect Immun 1994;62:2135–2137.

34  Mabbott NA, Sternberg JM: Bone-marrow nitric oxide production and the development of anemia in *Trypanosoma brucei*-infected mice. Infect Immun 1995;63:1563–1566.

35  Sternberg JM: Elevated serum nitrate in *Trypanosoma brucei rhodesiense* infections: Evidence for inducible nitric oxide synthesis in trypanosomiasis. Trans R Soc Trop Med Hyg 1996;90:395.

36  Albina JE: On the expression of inducible nitric oxide synthase by human macrophages: Why no NO? J Leukoc Biol 1995;58:643–649.

37  Vincendeau P, Daulouede S, Vegret B, Darde ML, Bouteille B, Lemesre JL: Nitric oxide-mediated cytostatic activity on *Trypanosoma brucei gambiense* and *T. b. brucei*. Exp Parasitol 1992;75:353–360.

38  Mabbott NA, Sutherland IA, Sternberg JM: *Trypanosoma brucei* is protected from the cytostatic effects of nitric oxide under in vivo conditions. Parasitol Res 1994;80:687–690.

39   Beutler B, Cerami A: The biology of cachectin/TNF: A primary mediator of the host response. Annu Rev Immunol 1989;7:625–655.

40   Magez S, Lucas R, Darji A, Songa EB, Hamers R, De Baetselier P: Murine tumour necrosis factor plays a protective role during the initial phase of the experimental infection with *Trypanosoma brucei brucei*. Parasite Immunol 1993;15:635–641.

41   Lucas R, Magez S, De Leys R: Mapping the lectin-like activity of tumour necrosis factor. Science 1994;263:814–817.

42   Bonfanti C, Caruso A, Bakhiet M, Olsson T, Turano A, Kristensson K: Increased levels of antibodies to IFN-γ in human and experimental African trypanosomiasis. Scand J Immunol 1995;41:49–52.

43   Bancroft GJ, Sutton AG, Morris AJ, Askonas BA: Production of interferons during experimental African trypanosomiasis. Clin Exp Immunol 1983;52:135–143.

44   Bakhiet M, Olsson T, Van Der Meide P, Kristensson K: Depletion of CD8⁺ T cells suppresses growth of *Trypanosoma brucei brucei* and interferon-gamma production in infected rats. Clin Exp Immunol 1990;81:195–199.

45   Olsson T, Bakhiet M, Hojeberg B, Ljungdahl A, Edlund C, Anderson G, Ekre H, Fung-Leung W, Mak T, Wigzell H, Fiszer U, Kristensson K: CD8 is critically involved in lymphocyte activation by a *T. brucei brucei*-released molecule. Cell 1993;72:715–727.

46   Schleifer KW, Filutowicz H, Schopf LR, Mansfield JM: Characterisation of T helper cell responses to the trypanosome variant surface glycoprotein. J Immunol 1993;150:2910–2919.

47   Olsson T, Bakhiet M, Edlund C, Höjeberg B, Van der Meide P, Kristensson K: Bidirectional activating signals between *Trypanosoma brucei* and CD8⁺ T cells: A trypanosome-released factor triggers interferon-γ production that stimulates parasite growth. Eur J Immunol 1991;21:2447–2454.

48   Bakhiet M, Olsson T, Edlund C, Hojeberg B, Holmberg K, Lorentzen J, Kristensson K: A *Trypanosoma brucei brucei*-derived factor that triggers CD8⁺ lymphocytes to interferon-γ secretion: Purification, characterisation and protective effects in vivo by treatment with a monoclonal antibody against the factor. Scand J Immunol 1993;37:165–178.

49   Jones JF, Hancock GE: Trypanosomiasis in mice with naturally occurring immunodeficiencies. Infect Immun 1983;42:848–851.

50   Bakhiet M, Olsson T, Mhlanga J, Buscher P, Lycke N, Van der Meide P, Kristensson K: Human and rodent interferon-gamma as a growth factor for *Trypanosoma brucei*. Eur J Immunol 1996;26: 1359–1364.

51   Sternberg JM, McGuigan F: *Trypanosoma brucei*: Mammalian epidermal growth factor promotes the growth of the African trypanosome bloodstream form. Exp Parasitol 1994;78:422–424.

52   Hide G, Gray A, Harrisson CM, Tait A: Identification of an epidermal growth factor receptor homologue in African trypanosomes. Mol Biochem Parasitol 1989;36:51–60.

53   Grosskinsky CM, Askonas BA: Macrophages as primary target cells and mediators of immune dysfunction in African trypanosomiasis. Infect Immun 1981;33:149–155.

54   Sacks DL, Bancroft G, Evans WH, Askonas BA: Incubation of trypanosome-derived mitogenic and immunosuppressive products with peritoneal macrophages allows recovery of biological activities from soluble parasite fractions. Infect Immun 1982;36:160–168.

55   Diffley P: Trypanosomal surface coat antigen causes polyclonal lymphocyte activation. J Immunol 1983;131:1983–1986.

56   Oka M, Yabu Y, Ito Y, Takayanagi T: Polyclonal B-cell simulative and immunosuppressive activities at different developmental stages of *Trypanosoma brucei gambiense*. Microbiol Immunol 1988;32: 1175–1177.

57   Darji A, Beschin A, Sileghem M, Heremans H, Brys L, DeBaetselier P: In vitro simulation of immunosuppression caused by *Trypanosoma brucei*: Active involvement of gamma interferon and tumor necrosis factor in the pathway of suppression. Infect Immun 1996;64:1937–1943.

58   Sternberg J, Mabbott N: Nitric oxide-mediated suppression of T-cell responses during *Trypanosoma brucei* infection: Soluble trypanosome products and interferon-γ are synergistic inducers of nitric oxide synthase. Eur J Immunol 1996;26:539–543.

59   Kamijo R, Harada H, Matsuyama T, Bosland M, Gerecitano J, Shapiro D, Le J, Koh SI, Kimura T, Green SJ, Mak TW, Taniguchi T, Vilcek J: Requirement for transcription factor IRF-1 in NO synthase induction in macrophages. Science 1994;263:1612–1615.

60    Isobe K-I, Nakashima I: Feedback suppression of staphylococcal enterotoxin-stimulated T-lympho-
      cyte proliferation by macrophages through inductive nitric oxide synthesis. Infect Immun 1992;60:
      4832–4837.
61    Cunha FQ, Moss DW, Leal LMCC, Moncada S, Liew FY: Induction of macrophage parasiticidal
      activity by *Staphylococcus aureus* and exotoxins through the nitric oxide synthesis pathway. Immuno-
      logy 1993;78:563–567.
62    Cunha FQ, Assreuy J, Moncada S, Liew FY: Phagocytosis and induction of nitric oxide synthase
      in murine macrophages. Immunology 1993;79:408–411.
63    Mansfield JM: Immunology and immunopathology of African trypanosomiasis; in Mansfield JM
      (ed): Parasitic Diseases. New York, Dekker, 1981, vol 1, pp 167–226.
64    Bulow R, Nonnengasser C, Overath P: Release of the variant specific glycoprotein during differenti-
      ation of bloodstream to procyclic forms of *Trypanosoma brucei*. Mol Biochem Parasitol 1989;32:
      85–92.
65    Milon G, Del Giudice G, Louis JA: Immunobiology of experimental cutaneous Leishmaniaisis.
      Parasitol Today 1995;11:244–247.
66    Rottenburg ME, Castanos-Velez E, DeMesquita R, Laguardia OG, Biberfeld P, Orn A: Intracellular
      colocalisation of *Trypanosoma cruzi* and inducible nitric synthase. Eur J Immunol 1996;26:3203–
      3213.
67    Kierszenbaum F, Muthukkumar S, Beltz LA, Sztein MB: Suppression by *Trypanosoma brucei
      rhodesiense* of the capacities of human T-lymphocytes to express interleukin-2 receptors and prolifer-
      ate after mitogenic stimulation. Infect Immun 1991;59:3518–3522.

Jeremy M. Sternberg, Department of Zoology, University of Aberdeen,
Aberdeen AB24 2TZ (UK)
Fax +44 1224 272396, e-mail j.sternberg@aberdeen.ac.uk

......................
# Author Index

# Subject Index